THE THREAT OF PANDEMIC INFLUENZA

Are We Ready?

Workshop Summary

prepared for
Forum on Microbial Threats
Board on Global Health

Stacey L. Knobler, Alison Mack, Adel Mahmoud, Stanley M. Lemon,
Editors

INSTITUTE OF MEDICINE
OF THE NATIONAL ACADEMIES

THE NATIONAL ACADEMIES PRESS
Washington, D.C.
www.nap.edu

THE NATIONAL ACADEMIES PRESS   500 Fifth Street, N.W.   Washington, DC 20001

NOTICE: The project that is the subject of this report was approved by the Governing Board of the National Research Council, whose members are drawn from the councils of the National Academy of Sciences, the National Academy of Engineering, and the Institute of Medicine. The members of the committee responsible for the report were chosen for their special competences and with regard for appropriate balance.

This project was supported by the U.S. Department of Health and Human Services' National Institutes of Health (Contract No. N01-OD-4-2139, TO#129), Centers for Disease Control and Prevention (200-2000-00629, TO#25), and Food and Drug Administration; U.S. Agency for International Development; U.S. Department of Defense (Contract No. DAMD-17-03-P-1331), U.S. Department of State; U.S. Department of Veterans Affairs (V101(93)P-2159); U.S. Department of Agriculture; American Society for Microbiology; Aventis Pasteur; Burroughs Wellcome Fund; Pfizer; GlaxoSmithKline; and The Merck Company Foundation. Any opinions, findings, conclusions, or recommendations expressed in this publication are those of the author(s) and do not necessarily reflect the view of the organizations or agencies that provided support for this project.

This report is based on the proceedings of a workshop that was sponsored by the Forum on Microbial Threats. It is prepared in the form of a workshop summary by and in the name of the editors, with the assistance of staff and consultants, as an individually authored document. Sections of the workshop summary not specifically attributed to an individual reflect the views of the editors and not those of the Forum on Microbial Threats. The content of those sections is based on the presentations and the discussions that took place during the workshop.

Library of Congress Cataloging-in-Publication Data

The threat of pandemic influenza : are we ready? : workshop summary / prepared for Forum on Microbial Threats, Board on Global Health ; Stacey L. Knobler ... [et al.], editors.
    p. ; cm.
Includes bibliographical references.
ISBN 0-309-09504-2 (pbk.) — ISBN 0-309-54685-0 (pdf)
    1. Influenza—Epidemiology. 2. Influenza—Government policy—United States.
[DNLM: 1. Influenza—prevention & control. 2. Communicable Disease Control—organization & administration. 3. Disease Outbreaks—prevention & control. 4. Influenza Vaccines. 5. Influenza, Avian—prevention & control.] I. Knobler, Stacey. II. Institute of Medicine (U.S.). Forum on Microbial Threats.
    RA644.I6T48 2005
    614.5′18—dc22
                                        2005000369

Additional copies of this report are available from the National Academies Press, 500 Fifth Street, N.W., Lockbox 285, Washington, DC 20055; (800) 624-6242 or (202) 334-3313 (in the Washington metropolitan area); Internet, http://www.nap.edu.

For more information about the Institute of Medicine, visit the IOM home page at: **www.iom.edu.**

The serpent has been a symbol of long life, healing, and knowledge among almost all cultures and religions since the beginning of recorded history. The serpent adopted as a logotype by the Institute of Medicine is a relief carving from ancient Greece, now held by the Staatliche Museen in Berlin.

COVER: A detailed section of a stained glass window 21 × 56″ depicting the natural history of influenza viruses and zoonotic exchange in the emergence of new strains was used to design the front cover. Based on the work done at St. Jude Children's Research Hospital supported by American Lebanese Syrian Associated Charities (ALSAC) and the National Institute of Allergy and Infectious Diseases (NIAID). Artist: Jenny Hammond, Highgreenleycleugh, Northumberland, England.

"Knowing is not enough; we must apply.
Willing is not enough; we must do."
—Goethe

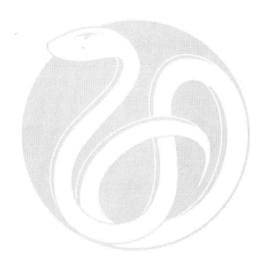

INSTITUTE OF MEDICINE
OF THE NATIONAL ACADEMIES

Adviser to the Nation to Improve Health

THE NATIONAL ACADEMIES
Advisers to the Nation on Science, Engineering, and Medicine

The **National Academy of Sciences** is a private, nonprofit, self-perpetuating society of distinguished scholars engaged in scientific and engineering research, dedicated to the furtherance of science and technology and to their use for the general welfare. Upon the authority of the charter granted to it by the Congress in 1863, the Academy has a mandate that requires it to advise the federal government on scientific and technical matters. Dr. Bruce M. Alberts is president of the National Academy of Sciences.

The **National Academy of Engineering** was established in 1964, under the charter of the National Academy of Sciences, as a parallel organization of outstanding engineers. It is autonomous in its administration and in the selection of its members, sharing with the National Academy of Sciences the responsibility for advising the federal government. The National Academy of Engineering also sponsors engineering programs aimed at meeting national needs, encourages education and research, and recognizes the superior achievements of engineers. Dr. Wm. A. Wulf is president of the National Academy of Engineering.

The **Institute of Medicine** was established in 1970 by the National Academy of Sciences to secure the services of eminent members of appropriate professions in the examination of policy matters pertaining to the health of the public. The Institute acts under the responsibility given to the National Academy of Sciences by its congressional charter to be an adviser to the federal government and, upon its own initiative, to identify issues of medical care, research, and education. Dr. Harvey V. Fineberg is president of the Institute of Medicine.

The **National Research Council** was organized by the National Academy of Sciences in 1916 to associate the broad community of science and technology with the Academy's purposes of furthering knowledge and advising the federal government. Functioning in accordance with general policies determined by the Academy, the Council has become the principal operating agency of both the National Academy of Sciences and the National Academy of Engineering in providing services to the government, the public, and the scientific and engineering communities. The Council is administered jointly by both Academies and the Institute of Medicine. Dr. Bruce M. Alberts and Dr. Wm. A. Wulf are chair and vice chair, respectively, of the National Research Council.

www.national-academies.org

vii

Reviewers

All presenters at the workshop have reviewed and approved their respective sections of this report for accuracy. In addition, this workshop summary has been reviewed in draft form by independent reviewers chosen for their diverse perspectives and technical expertise, in accordance with procedures approved by the National Research Council's Report Review Committee. The purpose of this independent review is to provide candid and critical comments that will assist the Institute of Medicine (IOM) in making the published workshop summary as sound as possible and to ensure that the workshop summary meets institutional standards. The review comments and draft manuscript remain confidential to protect the integrity of the deliberative process.

The Forum and the IOM thank the following individuals for their participation in the review process:

Neil Ferguson, Department of Infectious Disease Epidemiology, Imperial College, London
Frederick Hayden, Division of Infectious Diseases, University of Virginia
Clement S. Lewin, Chiron Vaccines
Arnold Monto, School of Public Health, University of Michigan, Ann Arbor
Peter Palese, Department of Microbiology, Mount Sinai School of Medicine
Eve Slater, Former Assistant Secretary for Health, U.S. Department of Health and Human Services

An additional technical review was provided by **John H. Barton,** George E. Osborne Professor of Law, Emeritus, Stanford Law School. The review of this report was overseen by **Elena O. Nightingale,** Scholar-in-Residence, IOM, who was responsible for making certain that an independent examination of this report was carried out in accordance with institutional procedures and that all review comments were carefully considered. Responsibility for the final content of this report rests entirely with the editors and individual authors.

Preface

The Forum on Microbial Threats (previously named the Forum on Emerging Infections) was created in 1996 in response to a request from the Centers for Disease Control and Prevention and the National Institutes of Health. The goal of the Forum is to provide structured opportunities for representatives from academia, industry, professional and interest groups, and government to examine and discuss scientific and policy issues that are of shared interest and that are specifically related to research and prevention, detection, and management of emerging infectious diseases. In accomplishing this task, the Forum provides the opportunity to foster the exchange of information and ideas, identify areas in need of greater attention, clarify policy issues by enhancing knowledge and identifying points of agreement, and inform decision makers about science and policy issues. The Forum seeks to illuminate issues rather than resolve them directly; hence, it does not provide advice or recommendations on any specific policy initiative pending before any agency or organization. Its strengths are the diversity of its membership and the contributions of individual members expressed throughout the activities of the Forum.

ABOUT THE WORKSHOP

Most infectious disease experts believe that a future influenza pandemic is inevitable. Yet despite the legacy of the 1918 "Spanish flu," which killed an estimated 20 million people,[1] and the additional deaths, social

---

[1] For more detailed estimates of the numbers of deaths caused by the 1918 influenza outbreak, see Barry's section in Chapter 1.

disruption, and economic losses that resulted from pandemics in 1957 and 1968, the general public appears relatively unconcerned about the next "killer flu," which is conservatively expected to cause between 2 and 8 million deaths. Considerably more attention has been focused on protecting the public from terrorist attacks than from the far more likely and pervasive threat of pandemic influenza. Meanwhile, the danger mounts as the world's capacity to produce vaccines shrinks and pandemic avian H5N1 influenza—which has infected many people and killed at least 32 to date—takes hold in southeast Asia.

Research has identified three essential prerequisites for the start of a pandemic: transmission of a novel viral subtype to humans; viral replication causing disease in humans; and efficient human-to-human transmission of the virus. Since 1997, the first two prerequisites have been met on four occasions; the most recent occurred early this year in Vietnam and Thailand. With H5N1 at or near endemic levels in poultry in many parts of Asia, the world stands at the verge of pandemic and is likely to remain there for years. A recent expert consultation convened by the World Health Organization concluded that "the unpredictability of influenza viruses and the speed with which transmissibility can improve mean that the time for preparedness planning is right now."

To address these urgent concerns, the Institute of Medicine's Forum on Microbial Threats hosted a public workshop on June 16 and 17, 2004. Through invited presentations and discussions among participants, the workshop informed the Forum, the public, and policy makers of the likelihood of an influenza pandemic and explored issues critical to the preparation and protection of the global community. Topics and questions considered during the workshop's presentations and discussions included the following:

- Learning from the past: pandemics and other threats to public health
- Global preparations against pandemic influenza
- Preparing the United States for pandemic influenza
- State and local preparation measures
- Strategies to prevent and control transmission in birds and other animals
- Biomedical approaches to preventing or controlling a pandemic
- Legal issues in pandemic prevention and control
- Improving preparedness: surveillance, prediction, and communication

ACKNOWLEDGMENTS

The Forum on Microbial Threats and the Institute of Medicine (IOM) wish to express their warmest appreciation to the individuals and organizations who gave valuable time to provide information and advice to the Forum through their participation in the workshop. A full list of presenters can be found in Appendix A.

The Forum is indebted to the IOM staff who contributed during the course of the workshop and the production of this workshop summary. On behalf of the Forum, we gratefully acknowledge the efforts led by Stacey Knobler, director of the Forum, Elizabeth Kitchens, research associate, Laura Sivitz, research associate, and Katherine Oberholtzer, research assistant, who dedicated much effort and time to developing this workshop's agenda, and for their thoughtful and insightful approach and skill in translating the workshop proceedings and discussion into this workshop summary. We would also like to thank the following IOM staff and consultants for their valuable contributions to this activity: Patrick Kelley, Alison Mack, Bronwyn Schrecker, Elena Nightingale, Eileen Choffnes, and Kate Giamis.

Finally, the Forum also thanks sponsors that supported this activity. Financial support for this project was provided by the U.S. Department of Health and Human Services' National Institutes of Health, Centers for Disease Control and Prevention, and Food and Drug Administration; U.S. Department of Defense; U.S. Department of State; U.S. Department of Veterans Affairs; U.S. Department of Agriculture; American Society for Microbiology; Aventis Pasteur; Burroughs Wellcome Fund; U.S. Agency for International Development; Pfizer; GlaxoSmithKline; and The Merck Company Foundation. The views presented in this workshop summary are those of the editors and workshop participants and are not necessarily those of the funding organizations.

Adel A.F. Mahmoud, *Chair*
Stanley M. Lemon, *Vice-Chair*
Forum on Microbial Threats

In Memoriam

John R. La Montagne
1943–2004

This publication from the Forum on Microbial Threats is dedicated to the memory and legacy of John R. La Montagne, Ph.D., Deputy Director of the National Institute of Allergy and Infectious Diseases (NIAID) of the National Institutes of Health, who unexpectedly died on November 2, 2004, en route to an international meeting on public health. As a founding member of the Forum and a continued supporter and participant in its activities, his contributions deeply enriched the national and international dialogue on emerging and reemerging infectious diseases research. In addition to his service to the Forum, John's outstanding grasp of the science, his global perspective, and his unwavering interest and support have been of critical importance to efforts of the Institute of Medicine focusing on the Children's Vaccine Initiative, AIDS research, and vaccines for malaria.

As a quiet but tireless champion, he helped to spearhead some of the most important recent global efforts to fight infectious diseases and to improve the health of children and adults everywhere. For nearly 30 years, John's thoughtful demeanor and even-handed approach led the way in tackling some of nature's greatest challenges to humankind. Relevant to this workshop summary, his work at NIAID began as the Influenza Program Officer, but it grew to include key leadership roles, including the directorship of the Division of Microbiology and Infectious Diseases. His influence has been incalculable on both national and international programs related to the development of vaccines for pertussis, rotavirus, AIDS, influenza, and malaria; new drugs for tuberculosis; and, more recently, biodefense research. In all of his work, John brought the human and public health dimensions to the efforts of laboratory research. He served the nation and the world immeasurably well, and we are better for it.

For the leadership, wise counsel, humor, and friendship that he shared with us and so many others, the Forum is deeply grateful. John will be greatly missed by all who knew him.

Contents

Summary and Assessment[1]

Most infectious disease experts believe that the world stands on the verge of an influenza pandemic (Chen et al., 2004; WHO, 2004a; Webby and Webster, 2003). Yet despite the legacy of the 1918 "Spanish flu," estimated to have killed at least 20 million people,[2] and the additional deaths, social disruption, and economic losses that resulted from pandemics in 1957 and 1968, the general public appears relatively unconcerned about the next "killer flu." Considerably more attention has been focused on protecting the public from terrorist attacks than from the far more likely and pervasive threat of pandemic influenza—an event conservatively expected to cause between 2 and 8 million deaths (WHO, 2004a).

Meanwhile, the danger mounts as the world's capacity to produce vaccines shrinks and H5N1 reaches endemic levels in poultry in many parts of Asia. A recent expert consultation convened by the World Health Organization (WHO) concluded that "the unpredictability of influenza viruses and the speed with which transmissibility can improve means that the time for preparedness planning is now" (WHO, 2004a).

To address these urgent concerns, the Institute of Medicine's (IOM) Forum on Microbial Threats convened the workshop *Pandemic Influenza:*

---

[1]The assessments contained in the summary are based on the presentations and discussion periods of the workshop. They reflect the assessments of individuals and the editors and cannot be construed as the deliberations, consensus, or recommendations of a formally constituted study committee of the Institute of Medicine.

[2]For a more detailed description of how estimates have been determined for the numbers of deaths caused by the 1918 influenza outbreak, see Barry's section in Chapter 1.

1

Assessing Capabilities for Prevention and Response on June 16 and 17, 2004. Participants discussed the history of influenza pandemics and the potentially valuable lessons it holds; the 2003–2004 H5N1 avian influenza outbreak in Asia and its implications for human health; ongoing pandemic influenza preparedness planning at global, regional, national, state, and local levels; strategies for preventing and controlling avian influenza and its transmission within bird and animal populations; and a broad range of medical, technical, social, economic and political opportunities for pandemic preparedness, as well as the many obstacles that stand in the way of this goal.

ORGANIZATION OF WORKSHOP SUMMARY

This workshop summary report is prepared for the Forum membership in the name of the editors as a collection of individually authored papers and commentary. Sections of the workshop summary not specifically attributed to an individual reflect the views of the editors and not those of the Forum on Microbial Threats, its sponsors, or the Institute of Medicine. The contents of the unattributed sections are based on the presentations and discussions that took place during the workshop.

The workshop summary is organized within chapters as a topic-by-topic description of the presentations and discussions. Its purpose is to present lessons from relevant experience, delineate a range of pivotal issues and their respective problems, and put forth some potential responses as described by the workshop participants.

Although this workshop summary provides an account of the individual presentations, it also reflects an important aspect of the Forum philosophy. The workshop functions as a dialogue among representatives from different sectors and presents their beliefs on which areas may merit further attention. However, the reader should be aware that the material presented here expresses the views and opinions of the individuals participating in the workshop and not the deliberations of a formally constituted IOM study committee. These proceedings summarize only what participants stated in the workshop and are not intended to be an exhaustive exploration of the subject matter or a representation of consensus evaluation.

SECURING THE FUTURE

Over the course of 2 days of wide-ranging, intense, and detailed discussion, several themes recurred and were elaborated upon from multiple perspectives. By the end of the proceedings, many of these ideas were surrounded by considerable clarity and a sense of urgency. These pervasive observations, described below, are grouped according to their ability to be accomplished in the near term or, following additional research or resolution, in the future. What can be said and was echoed throughout the discussions—if the question is: "Are we ready for a pandemic influenza?," the answer is "no."

Addressing Unmet Needs

Close Gaps in Global Surveillance[3]

Many countries lack infectious disease surveillance capabilities. Disturbingly, some of the most glaring gaps in surveillance occur in Asia, where H5N1 avian influenza has infected and killed scores of people since 1997. Developed countries' interests would be well served by funding improved influenza surveillance in such flu "hot spots." In addition to increasing surveillance capacity, replacing the current economic disincentives to early reporting of disease with incentives for surveillance, timely disease detection, and access to vaccines and antivirals will greatly increase the chance of catching and containing an emerging pandemic strain before or soon after it emerges.

U.S. data on severe illness and death from influenza are also inadequate. Improved data would more effectively inform priorities for prevention and treatment investments and strategies made at the local, state, regional, and national levels (e.g., immunization and preparedness planning). Importantly, improved real-time surveillance and disease reporting could provide an early warning for an emerging pandemic outbreak.

Integrate Animal and Public Health Communities[4]

Influenza surveillance, research, and pandemic response planning should reflect the zoonotic nature of the disease. Improved communication and the development of professional relationships among veterinary and medical researchers and agriculture and public health officials would encourage a greater appreciation in both communities for the implications of animal diseases in human populations, and for human practices that promote or prevent zoonoses. Current lack of integrated funding for influenza surveillance within the animal and human populations collectively now

---

[3]Buranathai (2004); Cox (2004); Gellin (2004); Gostin (2004a); Meltzer (2004); Stöhr (2004); Webster (2004a).

[4]Cardona (2004); Nguyen (2004); Sibartie (2004); Stöhr (2004); Swayne (2004); Webster (2004a).

works against such integration. Better coordination between public and private funders of research and disease surveillance will be necessary.

Explore Compensation for Preemptive Culling of Animals[5]

As is the case with surveillance, encouraging farmers (or even entire countries) to curtail or prevent a human pandemic by sacrificing their poultry or livestock is in the interests of global public health. A variety of options should be explored to support this outcome in a variety of settings, from individual farmers in low-resource settings to industrial poultry and livestock producers in wealthy countries.

Promote the Use of Rapid, Inexpensive Influenza Diagnostics[6]

Cheap, simple diagnostic tests would improve influenza surveillance in animals and humans. Polymerase chain reaction (PCR) testing is the best current option, but the international veterinary community has yet to adopt PCR. As a result, the first farm to be culled in the recent H7N7 outbreak in The Netherlands was delayed 4 days as officials waited for virus isolation results. Increased use and improved diagnostics for influenza will also promote more prudent and effective use of both vaccines and antiviral drugs.

Increase Demand for Annual Influenza Immunization and Antiviral Therapy and Prophylaxis[7]

Demand for influenza vaccine drives supply. After last year's severe flu season and this year's unanticipated vaccine shortages, the public may respond well to a pro-immunization campaign, perhaps one that introduces the hazards of pandemic influenza. It will be important to include in that message the distinction between the protective effect of an antiviral influenza vaccine and additional vaccination that would be necessary to respond to a pandemic strain. A similar argument can be made for increasing interpandemic demand for antiviral drugs, which to date have low demand. More interpandemic use of antivirals means the greater production and greater supply of them for use in an outbreak situation. Moreover, increasing physician experience with and public awareness of antiviral medications should support their effective use in responding to a pandemic.

---

[5]Buranathai (2004); Meltzer (2004); Soebandrio (2004); Webster (2004a).
[6]Koch (2004); Nguyen (2004); Swayne (2004); Webster (2004a); see Perdue in Chapter 5.
[7]Brown (2004); Fedson (2004a); Gellin (2004); Hosbach (2004); Nowak (2004).

Create International Stockpiles of Antiviral Drugs and Vaccines[8]

A dedicated supply of vaccines and antiviral drugs is necessary for a rapid response to the first cases of a potential pandemic influenza strain (e.g., through ring immunization and/or targeted antiviral prophylaxis). This plan would probably require a smaller investment, and possibly offers greater benefit in relation to cost, than the aforementioned strategy of compensating farmers for preemptive culling of poultry or livestock in areas affected by avian influenza. However, this strategy is unlikely to work unless an international agreement to create such stockpiles is in place when the next pandemic arrives; otherwise, stockpiles and production of vaccines and antiviral drugs are expected to be nationalized. Additionally, these antiviral stockpiles need to be placed in geographically high-volume points of care (e.g., outpatient clinics, emergency rooms, occupational health sites, student health facilities, nursing homes, pharmacies) for rapid access to therapy that does not rely on a visit to a physician for an effective pandemic response. If stockpiles of vaccines are to be developed and relied upon, it is clear that the range of factors contributing to the recent crises in seasonal influenza production and deployment will need to be overcome.

Establish Protocols for Research During a Pandemic[9]

When the next influenza pandemic emerges, it will be essential to gain a greater understanding of the clinical, epidemiological, and biological nature of influenza—but this will only be possible if research protocols and the laboratory networks to pursue them are established before a pandemic strikes. As Klaus Stöhr of WHO observed, "We have to invest more into planning research, into having protocols ready, and having networks of scientists in place and eager to contribute before the next pandemic virus emerges." For example, protocols to estimate vaccine efficacy could be implemented immediately upon the commencement of immunization in response to a pandemic, and could even be conducted during the annual flu season.

Goals for Research

Determine the Molecular Basis of Influenza Pathogenesis[10]

Much remains to be understood about the molecular basis of influenza pathogenesis, host immune response, immune protection, immune enhance-

---

[8]Brown (2004); Gellin (2004); Hosbach (2004); Longini (2004a); Stohr (2004).
[9]Grundy (2004); see Hayden in Chapter 3.
[10]Taubenberger (2004); Webster (2004a).

ment, virulence, and transmissibility. H5N1 variants provide an opportunity to study all of these phenomena. Breakthroughs in these areas of scientific understanding could rapidly lead to more effective and more easily produced countermeasures to an influenza pandemic.

Predict Pandemic Potential of Influenza Isolates[11]

As knowledge of the molecular pathology of influenza expands, it should become possible to predict the threat posed by a particular strain by analyzing key sequences in its genome. While there has been one probable case of human-to-human transmission (ProMED-mail, 2004e) to date, the fact that H5N1 has not yet accomplished infectious human-to-human transmission begs the question, "why not?" Risk assessment tools based on influenza viral genomics may one day provide an answer—and perhaps prevent the unnecessary culling of poultry or livestock following outbreaks of avian influenza.

Increase the Efficacy of Influenza Vaccines[12]

Limited supplies of vaccine could go further if their antigen content could be adjusted to provide the lowest effective dose to each recipient, and if they could be safely made more effective with an adjuvant. Several participants suggested the need for the United States and Europe to view this problem as a joint effort and work together to assure that the entire set of needs for improving influenza vaccines is addressed and shared.

An atmosphere of 11th-hour urgency surrounded many of the workshop presentations and participant discussions. The potential for catastrophe is immense, but that potential has been evident, and largely ignored, since 1918. The power of vaccines to prevent influenza is well proven, but the capacity to produce them—as recent events confirm—is limited so as to put them out of reach of the vast majority of the global population. If the initial cases of an emerging human influenza strain are detected, and if antiviral drugs were quickly administered to the close contacts of index cases, transmission could be stifled—but those are big "ifs" in a world where early reporting of influenza carries dire economic consequences and where nations are expected to nationalize stockpiles and production of antiviral drugs and vaccines in response to a threatened pandemic. What should be done to prevent the loss of millions of lives, and the evidence for doing it, is quite clear. What is missing—as evidenced by the clarion calls of

---

[11]Taubenberger (2004); Webster (2004a).
[12]Epstein (2004); Fedson (2004a); Gellin (2004).

workshop presenters—is the political will to support such efforts before the next pandemic renders them futile. However, developments during the writing of this report might suggest that the tide is changing. The World Health Organization has called for an unprecedented summit of national public health leaders, vaccine manufacturers, and leading researchers to expand the plans and possibilities for responding to a pandemic influenza threat— now a growing concern among many nations and leaders (see, http://www.who.int/en/) (Marchione, 2004).

THE STORY OF INFLUENZA: 1918 AND BEYOND

To expand on some of the key messages described above, the following text summarizes workshop presentations and discussions concerning preparedness for influenza outbreaks at every level of government and society and the prospects for preventing or mitigating the next pandemic.

Although historical evidence of probable encounters with virulent influenza date back to the 16th century, chronicles of the disease often begin with the 1918 pandemic (see Barry in Chapter 1). By that time, science was sufficiently sophisticated to characterize the most lethal infectious outbreak in recorded history, and even to anticipate that such an event would occur. As a result of its staggering mortality, the brunt of which was borne by young adults, the 1918 influenza pandemic remains a focus of scientific inquiry; the origin of the virus remains to be determined. Most recently, the "source" of its exceptional virulence has been discovered, and these findings suggest it is due to the hemagglutinin (HA) gene (Kobasa et al., 2004). Workshop participants discussed progress to date in addressing these critical issues. They also considered the consequences of deeply flawed public and official responses to the 1918 flu and their implications for the management of future pandemics and other public health crises.

Current estimates place the death toll from the approximately year-long 1918 pandemic at 50 to 100 million.[13] A "herald wave" of influenza in the spring of that year produced a relatively mild disease, as described in Western medical journals (Taubenberger, 2004). The second pandemic wave struck violently in early autumn, spreading and killing with astounding rapidity. The unusually severe symptoms of this so-called Spanish flu included cyanosis, internal and external hemorrhage, and intense pain (see Barry in Chapter 1). Limited reliable mortality statistics from the United States show that the highest number of flu deaths occurred in people aged 25 to 29 years and that more than twice as many people aged 20 to 34 died

---

[13]For a more detailed description of how estimates have been determined for the numbers of deaths caused by the 1918 influenza outbreak, see Barry's section in Chapter 1.

than did people older than 50 (see Barry in Chapter 1). Pregnant women had the highest case fatality (the number of deaths among people with clinically diagnosed illness) of any group in this country, a phenomenon that has been reported in other influenza outbreaks (see Barry in Chapter 1). Local estimates of case fatality varied widely across the globe and in some circumstances (e.g., among populations never before challenged by influenza and troops stationed in close quarters) reportedly exceeded 20 percent.

Patterns of Pandemic-Associated Mortality

Despite the devastation caused by the 1918 virus, it produced what was in many ways a typical influenza pandemic (see Taubenberger in Chapter 1) (Taubenberger, 2004). Most pandemics arrive in waves, albeit generally separated by years, rather than months. In the United States, with an aggregate case fatality of 2.5 percent, more than 97 percent of people with clinically reported influenza recovered from the disease; serological studies, conducted in the 1930s on people alive during the pandemic, suggest that less than 1 percent of people exposed to the virus died of flu. Prior exposure to pandemics in the mid-1850s and around 1890 apparently provided protection against the 1918 virus, resulting in relatively low mortality in people aged 35 and older. Thus the crucial uniqueness of the 1918 pandemic lay not in its virulence, but in the disproportionate number of deaths it caused among young adults, as reflected in its famously "W-shaped" pattern of mortality (Figure S-1).

Several workshop participants are studying this trend, described by presenter Jeffery Taubenberger as "the one issue that desperately needs to have a biological explanation before we can actually draw any lessons from 1918" (Taubenberger, 2004). Hypotheses under investigation include a genetic feature of the virus that targeted young adults; an intrinsic characteristic of their immune systems that produced a deadly response to viral infection; and—perhaps most likely—a deadly interaction between this virus and the young adult immune system.

Epidemiological analyses of the 1918 pandemic further highlight the dramatic shift in age-adjusted mortality as compared with subsequent years in which influenza was epidemic (Simonsen, 2004). Such studies also show that the profound impact of the 1918 flu on young adults was not limited to the second, autumnal wave of the disease, but could be detected in the initial herald wave and in influenza seasons for several years after the pandemic's peak. Similar age shifts in mortality also marked the two subsequent influenza pandemics in 1957 and 1968, which caused far fewer deaths than the 1918 flu.

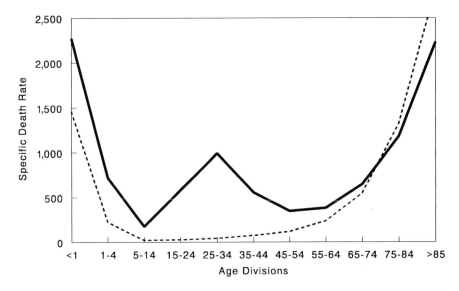

FIGURE S-1 Influenza and pneumonia mortality by age, United States. Influenza and pneumonia specific mortality by age, including an average of the inter-pandemic years 1911–1915 (dashed line) and the pandemic year 1918 (solid line). Specific death rate is per 100,000 of the population in each age division.
SOURCES: Grove and Hetzel (1968); Linder and Grove (1943); U.S. Department of Commerce (1976).

Clues to Lethality and Adaptation

It remains unclear why the 1918 influenza virus was so deadly to otherwise healthy young adults. Historical data suggest its virulence was due in part to its novelty to people under the age of 30, who were not exposed to similar viral antigens during the apparent pandemics of the mid- and late 19th century. Children between the ages of 5 and 10 years were diagnosed with flu at higher than average rates, yet had the lowest mortality rates of any age group; that outcome may reflect a weak T-cell response to the virus, which is known to spare this age group from mortality due to measles (Taubenberger, 2004). By contrast, young adults may have mounted an unusual—and deadly—immune response to the 1918 virus. This possibility is supported by death records from Kentucky which, when analyzed on a year-by-year basis, reveal a precipitous rise to a peak in flu deaths beginning at age 17 and ending with a more gradual drop beginning around age 30 (Taubenberger, 2004). Researchers have also found epidemiological evidence that in the United States, people infected with tuberculosis (TB)—a relatively common infection in 1918, particularly among young males—

were more likely than others to die of influenza (Noymer and Garenne, 2000). However, contradictory evidence from 120 autopsy reports of influenza victims showed that none had evidence of TB in the lungs, leading to the speculation that TB could have had a protective effect (Taubenberger, 2004). Genetic features of the 1918 virus have also been examined for clues to its deadliness, but none of the mutations identified have been shown to correlate with virulence (see Taubenberger in Chapter 1). Such genomic studies are, however, revealing the genetic basis of viral adaptation to human infection and transmission. For example, research on the 1918 hemagglutinin gene and its product suggest that a single amino acid change allowed the avian-like virus to bind to a human receptor (Kobasa et al., 2004); it was speculated that a similar change in the avian H5 gene—now circulating among birds infected with pandemic H5N1 influenza—would make it easier for the avian virus to infect humans.

Applying Lessons Learned from Past Pandemics

There is particular pressure to recognize and heed the lessons of past pandemics in the shadow of the worrisome 2003–2004 flu season. At the time of this report's release, 44 confirmed human cases of H5N1 avian influenza occurred in Thailand and Vietnam; 32 (72 percent) of these patients, mostly children and young adults, have died of the disease (ProMED-mail, 2004a; WHO, 2004d). Six of those confirmed deaths have occurred in Vietnam during a resurgence of the avian flu epidemic since July 2004, as this report was being prepared (ProMED-mail, 2004b,c). Concurrently, Thailand has confirmed four deaths since July 2004 (ProMED-mail, 2004d,v), with one case possibly having been transmitted from daughter to mother (ProMED-mail, 2004e).[14,15]

In addition, an early-onset, severe form of influenza A (H3N2) made headlines when it claimed the lives of many children in the United States in late 2003. As a result, stronger than usual demand for annual flu vaccine outstripped the vaccine supply, of which 10 to 20 percent typically goes unused (Hosbach, 2004). Because statistics on pediatric flu deaths had not been collected previously, it is unknown if the 2003–2004 season witnessed a significant change in mortality patterns. However, in response to these deaths, the Centers for Disease Control and Prevention's (CDC's) Advisory

---

[14]Editor's note: During the production process, further evidence suggests the daughter transmitted H5N1 to her mother and this report also suggests she transmitted H5N1 to her aunt (Ungchusak et al., 2005).

[15]Editor's note: It should be noted that during the production process of this report there were 12 additional deaths in Vietnam during January 2005 and the first case and death in Cambodia, bringing the total number of deaths to 45 (ProMED-mail, 2005).

Committee on Immunization Practices now recommends that beginning in 2004–2005, children aged 6 to 23 months (and their close contacts) receive the annual flu vaccine (Harper et al., 2004).

During the writing of this report, another vaccine shortage was making headlines. On October 5, 2004, British authorities suspended Chiron Corporation's license for vaccine production due to contamination problems during the manufacturing process (ProMED-mail, 2004f). Currently one of only two suppliers of the influenza vaccine to the United States, Chiron was expected to provide approximately half of the supply of vaccines to the United States this flu season. As a result, the U.S. Department of Health and Human Services is urging healthy adults to forego the shot this year in an effort to conserve the remaining doses for the youngest, oldest, and sickest Americans, who are the most vulnerable to influenza (CDC, 2004b). However, problems with distribution of vaccine supply to providers well placed to serve the at-risk populations and the unwillingness of many healthy adults to sacrifice on behalf of these at-risk individuals continue to complicate this public health strategy. Difficulty finding the vaccines, long lines, and frustration have caused many to even cross the border into Canada to be immunized (Americans cross border for flu shots, 2004).

Both of these shortages reveal the historic lack of adequate attention and preparedness to the threat of influenza and the complications presented by the vaccine development and production process. This continued crisis demonstrates how fragile the method of vaccine production is and has brought to light our lack of investments for alternative forms of vaccine production. Most importantly, these shortages raise questions about our ability to respond to an influenza crisis or pandemic if we cannot provide routine influenza vaccine in a typical influenza season. The outrage expressed and extreme measures taken recently by some individuals do not suggest that the population is adequately prepared to respond rationally to a future crisis.

A series of recent avian influenza epidemics, discussed in detail below, can be seen to foreshadow pandemic human influenza in an age of globalization. In several cases, the virus has spread rapidly across entire countries, necessitating the destruction and disposal of millions of domestic birds. None of these viruses has proven readily transmissible among humans, but several workshop participants recognized that this development—a recipe for pandemic influenza—may be only a few mutations away (Figure S-4). It was also noted that although there is no historical precedent for an influenza pandemic spawned by highly pathogenic avian influenza virus in poultry, flu "does something different every time" (Taubenberger, 2004). To more reliably predict the threat posed by emerging avian influenza strains, the complex, and largely unknown, spectrum of genetic variability among these viruses must be better understood.

On the other hand, as pointed out by presenter Lone Simonsen, there may be predictive value in features shared by the three 20th-century influenza pandemics (see Simonsen in Chapter 1). Mortality data from the three pandemics provide important insights into how the pandemic evolves over time, and shows that younger age groups (ages 64 and younger) are at the highest risk for severe outcomes. Similar observations in future influenza surveillance may suggest an emerging pandemic. Several workshop participants noted a need for further historical epidemiological research, particularly toward extending our understanding of the two probable 19th-century pandemics for use in preparing for future outbreaks.

Public Communication: A Cautionary Tale

The 1918 influenza pandemic also has much to teach, by negative example, about public communication in times of crisis (see Barry in Chapter 1). Because the pandemic struck when the world was caught up in its first global war, public officials and the media were particularly reluctant to diminish public morale by announcing the arrival of a plague. Indeed, the pandemic's nickname, "Spanish flu," is unlikely to reflect the origin of the pandemic, but rather the fact that it was first announced in the relatively uncensored press of Spain, a noncombatant nation.

In the United States (and probably in other Western countries as well), public officials and the media played down—and in some cases, lied about—the pandemic's approach, its severity, and its probable course. The public responded to this breach of trust with inaction: uncharacteristically, throughout the United States, calls for public assistance and sacrifice for the sake of the common good went unheeded. As the credibility of public authorities crumbled, so did social order. There is no more powerful demonstration of the need for clear and truthful communications in a public health emergency (the subject of additional discussion below) than the social chaos visited on the United States during the 1918 influenza pandemic.

TODAY'S PANDEMIC THREAT: H5N1 INFLUENZA

The past decade has seen increasingly frequent and severe outbreaks of highly pathogenic avian influenza (Webby and Webster, 2003) (see Li et al., in Chapter 2, p. 116). The current, ongoing epidemic of H5N1 avian influenza in Asia is unprecedented in its scale, in its geographical distribution, and in the economic losses it has caused (WHO, 2004b). But the prospect for the future is far more worrisome: recent evidence suggests that H5N1 has accumulated mutations that have made it increasingly infectious and deadly in mammals (Chen et al., 2004).

The first documented direct infection of humans by H5N1 occurred in 1997, by a virus that originated among Chinese geese and found its way into Hong Kong poultry markets (Webster, 2004b). There it re-sorted with other viral subtypes in both quail and duck to produce a strain that killed 6 of 18 people it was known to have infected. By acting quickly to cull every domestic bird in the country—about 1.5 million animals—Hong Kong thwarted the continued progress of this deadly strain, which has not since been detected. The parental H5N1 strain continued to evolve in geese and recombine with other avian influenza viruses, however, yielding more novel viruses that infected additional bird species and, eventually, humans. In late 2002, coincident with the arrival of migratory birds, an emergent H5N1 variant began to kill resident waterfowl in two Hong Kong parks (Guan et al., 2004). In February 2003, H5N1 virus was isolated from a 33-year-old man and his 9-year-old son in Hong Kong. They had become ill with a pneumonia-like disease upon returning from a trip to Fujian Province in China to celebrate the lunar New Year; the man's 8-year-old daughter had died of a similar illness while abroad, and the man died as well.

Reports from the 2003–2004 Asian Epidemic

This reemergence of a species-jumping, highly pathogenic H5N1 strain foreshadowed the next year's epidemic. In late 2003, H5N1 began to appear in domestic poultry and spread rapidly across Asia; by mid-February, outbreaks had been confirmed in South Korea, Vietnam, Japan, Thailand, Cambodia, China, Laos, and Indonesia (CDC, 2004a). The highly integrated poultry industry that connects farms and markets throughout China, Vietnam, Thailand, and Indonesia provided ample opportunity for widespread viral transmission, but several species of birds that migrate long distances across the epidemic area may also have spread the virus (Li et al., 2004; Webster, 2004b). As a result, tens of millions of birds died of influenza and hundreds of millions were culled to protect humans after 34 confirmed human cases of H5N1 influenza in Thailand and Vietnam resulted in 23 deaths. Among the first 10 human cases, which occurred in Vietnam in December 2003 and January 2004, none had a pre-existing medical condition, and all but one were known to have been in direct contact with poultry within 3 days before their symptoms appeared (Tran et al., 2004). Eight of these 10 patients died (Figure S-2).

Recent evidence also indicates that H5N1 has infected pigs in Vietnam (but are not yet established in the population) (Webster, 2004a), a white tiger and a clouded leopard (both in captivity) in Thailand, and domestic cats; all of the felines had eaten raw chicken (ProMED-mail, 2004g; Lovgren, 2004). During the preparation of this report, further confirmation of H5N1 infection has been shown in tigers (Keawcharoen et al., 2004;

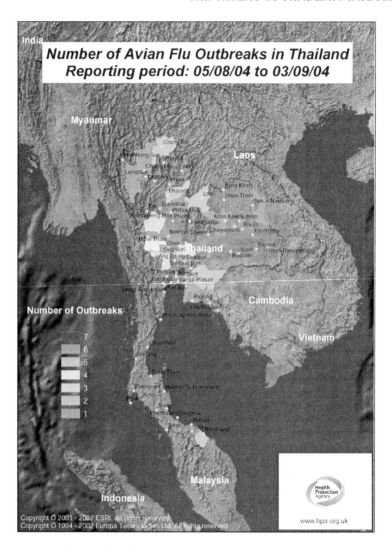

FIGURE S-2 The map displays the most recent reporting of avian influenza outbreaks in Thailand as published by the Office International des Epizooties (OIE, 2004). The mapping has been produced on a provincial basis, requiring "Bangkok Province" (as named in the data source: OIE, 2004) to be mapped to Krung Thep Province. Access to improved geographical data, e.g., sub province, would enable the mapping to be more precise, making full use of the level of detail published by OIE. Produced by: Microbial Risk Assessment Team, HPA Porton Down. In collaboration with colleagues at ProMED-mail, Oracle Corporation, and Environmental Systems Institute, Inc. (UK) Health Protection Agency are developing a mapping front end to the ProMED website.
SOURCE: Health Protection Agency (2004).

ProMED-mail, 2004h) and domestic cats (Kuiken et al., 2004) through the ingestion of raw chicken. The Thailand Zoo tiger outbreak killed more than 140 tigers, causing health officials to make the decision to cull all the sick tigers in an effort to stop the zoo from becoming a reservoir for H5N1 influenza (ProMED-mail, 2004i; ProMED-mail, 2004w). A study of domestic cats showed H5N1 virus infection by ingestion of infected poultry and also by contact with other infected cats (Kuiken et al., 2004).

Throughout Asia, affected countries responded to the avian flu epidemic with time-tested strategies: surveillance to detect the outbreak and monitor the progress of control efforts; culling potentially infected birds; disinfection of affected facilities, including the safe disposal of dead and culled birds; and educating poultry farmers and the general public about the threat posed by H5N1 avian influenza. Yet each country's circumstances and their handling of the epidemic were unique, as illustrated by workshop presentations by agricultural and public health officials from Indonesia, Vietnam, and Thailand. The diversity of these responses, and their resulting outcomes, offer important lessons for the control of future avian flu outbreaks—a key protection against a human pandemic.

Indonesia

Although Indonesia was one of the first Asian countries to experience cases of H5N1, which was identified in Central Java in August 2003, a comprehensive control strategy was not initiated until November (Soebandrio, 2004). By that time, the disease had spread throughout Java and had also been detected on the islands of Bali, Sumatra, and Borneo. This late start, along with the fact that the epidemic had spread widely and affected many small farms, made disease control a daunting challenge. Nevertheless, a strong effort was made to cull all domestic birds on all farms and facilities where H5N1 was detected. Surveillance for human infection was also conducted among more than 1,000 people (80 percent of whom had direct contact with poultry; the others as controls) in affected provinces; no positive cases were found by Reverse Transcriptase (RT)-PCR.

Unlike most other affected countries, Indonesia also instituted mass vaccination of healthy domestic birds against H5N1, followed by routine vaccination (China has a similar policy; other Asian countries are considering it [ProMED-mail, 2004j]) (Soebandrio, 2004). This is a risky strategy, because vaccinated birds can develop asymptomatic infections that allow virus to spread, mutate, and recombine (ProMED-mail, 2004j). Intensive surveillance is required to detect these "silent epidemics" in time to curtail them. In Mexico, for example, mass vaccination of chickens against epidemic H5N2 influenza in 1995 has had to continue in order to control a persistent and evolving virus (Lee et al., 2004). The prospects, advantages, and limitations of vaccination as a means to control avian influenza (and prevent the infection of other animals, including humans) are further discussed below. Indonesia's decision to vaccinate poultry against H5N1 was, however, strongly influenced by the fact that illegal vaccine of questionable quality, some of which may have harbored live influenza virus, was already being used throughout the country (ProMED-mail, 2004k; Soebandrio, 2004). To accompany its offer of a free, safer alternative to illegal vaccine, the Indonesian government launched a multimedia public awareness campaign on avian influenza (Soebandrio, 2004).

Vietnam

In Vietnam, the avian influenza outbreak was recognized comparatively quickly, but several factors hindered effective action to control influenza (see Nguyen in Chapter 2; Nguyen, 2004). These included an initial lack of engagement of the highest levels of government in the institution and enforcement of control measures; a delay in imposing a ban on the movement and consumption of poultry; and disagreement within the country's scientific community as to how to gauge the threat influenza posed to human health. However, once the grave danger of H5N1 was recognized, the Vietnamese government took action to bring the outbreak rapidly under control through culling in infected premises and a ban on the movement and consumption of poultry. Vietnam's political structure and media were instrumental in educating the public and gaining popular support for infectious control efforts. CDC also played a key role in quelling the epidemic by providing the Vietnamese government with training and materials for the rapid diagnosis of H5N1.

Vietnam was, however, widely criticized for announcing that H5N1 was controlled on March 30, only 15 days after its last human victim died (ProMED-mail, 2004l,m). Successful eradication of avian influenza is generally believed to take at least 2 to 3 years. Nevertheless it is easy to understand why a country where the poultry industry is important not only to economic stability, but as an affordable source of protein for a growing population would be powerfully motivated to pronounce the end of this devastating epidemic (Nguyen, 2004). Nor is it surprising that expert predictions of a resurgence of influenza in Vietnam were realized, with devastating consequences, as described below (ProMED-mail, 2004l).

Thailand

Two features of Thailand's response to the avian flu epidemic merit particular attention: the degree to which the country was prepared to address the outbreak, and its willingness to compensate farmers for their losses. When surveillance for highly pathogenic H5N1 first detected the virus in

Thailand in January 2004, officials adapted the country's established emergency response plan, which specifies chains of command and communications, to address the threat (see Buranathai in Chapter 2; Buranathai, 2004).

Approximately 75,000 cloacal samples from poultry in every village in the country were tested for the virus within a 2-week period, followed by culling and disinfection of the 160 premises found to be infected. In addition, all poultry within 5 kilometers of each of the infected farms were preemptively culled, and the movement of all poultry within a 50 to 60 kilometer radius was controlled. A second round of active surveillance and culling was performed from mid-February through early March, when the epidemic was deemed to be under control. The country then reverted to passive agricultural surveillance while maintaining active clinical surveillance for human cases. Thailand is currently investigating the possibility of using vaccination against future avian flu outbreaks. The country has the necessary manufacturing capacity, but at present prohibits livestock vaccination due to the aforementioned risks.

Thailand's generous emergency compensation policy, also in place prior to the recent epidemic, became even more generous in response to farmers' losses (Buranathai, 2004). Rather than the standard 75 percent of market price, farmers whose infected flocks were culled received their full market value. This strategy backfired, however, when struggling farmers infected their flocks so as to recoup losses sustained as a result of decreased demand for poultry products. While many workshop participants identified compensation for farmers' losses as a key strategy in the control of avian influenza, this example highlights the difficulty of designing a compensation policy that truly supports the goal of infection control.

The Puzzling Present and Worrisome Future of Avian Flu

In addition to the Asian epidemic, unprecedented numbers of outbreaks of diverse subtypes of avian influenza arose during the 2003–2004 flu season in locations including British Columbia and three separate regions of the United States (Figure S-3) (Webster, 2004a). In several of these instances, a few nonfatal cases of human infection were also identified (ProMED-mail, 2004n). Meanwhile, the Asian H5N1 epidemic continued to smolder. In July 2004 it reignited, resulting in multiple outbreaks in Vietnam and Thailand and a single outbreak in China; hundreds of thousands of birds were culled in both Vietnam and Thailand in an attempt to contain the epidemic (ProMED-mail, 2004o). Since July, Vietnam has confirmed that six more people have died from H5N1 influenza (ProMED-mail, 2004b,c), and Thailand has confirmed four more deaths (ProMED-mail, 2004d,v), with one case possibly having been transmitted from human to human (ProMED-mail, 2004e).

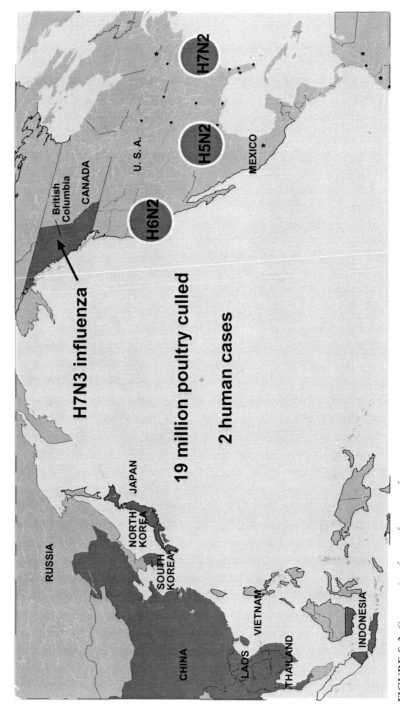

FIGURE S-3 Converging forces for a perfect storm.

The possibility that H5N1 is gaining momentum is especially troubling in light of recent evidence that the virus has become increasingly pathogenic toward mammals (Chen et al., 2004). Between 1999 and 2002, researchers periodically isolated samples of the virus from asymptomatically infected southern Chinese ducks (a natural reservoir for the H5N1 and other avian influenzas) and tested each isolate for its ability to infect a mouse model. Recently, a new study reported that domestic ducks infected with H5N1 shed more virus for longer periods and the majority do so asymptomatically. This suggests that ducks might now be acting as a "silent" reservoir for the virus and may play an increased role in transmitting H5N1 to both poultry and humans (WHO, 2004c). The results reveal a progressive increase in virulence (based on the virus's ability to replicate in mice) and lethality over time. Viewed in light of the proliferation of H5N1 influenza in Asia and the numerous concurrent outbreaks of other avian flu subtypes, these findings led one of the investigators, workshop presenter Robert Webster, to the ominous conclusion that "flu has got something going at the moment that we don't fully understand."

THE PLANNED RESPONSE TO PANDEMIC THREAT

The odds of detecting, controlling, and even preventing the spread of an influenza virus with pandemic potential have improved dramatically since 1918, when the disease was recognized by symptoms alone; it was not until 1933 that a virus was determined to cause influenza (Noymer and Garenne, 2000). In 1957 and 1968, although surveillance of new viral subtypes was theoretically possible, pandemic viruses were not identified until after outbreaks had occurred in Asia (WHO, 1999). Today, international programs permit the characterization of thousands of viral isolates each year and support worldwide surveillance and communications networks. These efforts are informed by expanding scientific understanding of viral molecular biology and evolution, and bolstered by simultaneous preparations against the threat of bioterrorism.

Yet major challenges to pandemic preparedness remain to be overcome. The world's growing—and increasingly urbanized—population and the speed and volume of international travel create abundant opportunities for widespread viral transmission. A recent example illustrating these vulnerabilities was reported when two eagles were smuggled into Belgium from Thailand. Customs officials at Brussels airport found and seized the birds, which were then discovered to be infected with H5N1 and immediately culled at the quarantine holding zone. For precautionary measures, the other birds being held in the quarantine zone were also destroyed and all the people in direct contact with the eagles were monitored and tested for H5N1 infection. To date, no one has tested positive for the virus (ProMED-mail, 2004p).

Some countries will respond to a pandemic with abundant resources and expertise, but many others remain essentially defenseless. Even populations wealthy enough to obtain vaccine are unlikely to get enough to prevent significant morbidity and mortality from pandemic influenza, unless more rapid vaccine production methods or novel prophylactic vaccines can be introduced before the next pandemic strikes (see also upcoming section on vaccines).

Global Preparations

WHO plays a central role among the many international and nongovernmental organizations that contribute to global preparations against pandemic influenza. Its 1999 *Influenza Pandemic Plan* provides a model of flexible contingency planning and outlines "the separate but complementary roles and responsibilities for WHO and for national authorities when an influenza pandemic appears possible or actually occurs" (WHO, 1999). The basic precepts of that plan were tested and proved effective during the global response to severe acute respiratory syndrome in 2003, which WHO coordinated (IOM, 2004). Many countries have based their pandemic influenza plans on the 1999 WHO document, which provides guidance on the issues to be addressed and actions to be undertaken by each nation in the event of a threatened or actual pandemic (Stöhr, 2004).

The WHO influenza pandemic plan has two main objectives:

• To assess the risk posed by new viruses, primarily the responsibility of WHO; and
• To manage risk when a virus appears capable of causing widespread and serious disease, an authority that rests largely with national governments (see below) (WHO, 1999).

Recognizing that new influenza strains may infect and even kill humans without causing a pandemic—as was the case with swine flu in the United States in 1976 and avian influenza in Hong Kong in 1997—the plan presents a range of responses ("preparedness levels") appropriate to each prepandemic and pandemic phase. WHO's specific contributions to influenza pandemic preparedness and response are summarized in Box S-1. Parts of the 1999 document have been revised to reflect knowledge gained from the recent lethal transmission of H5N1 avian influenza to humans and the recommendations and conclusions of a consultation convened by WHO in March 2004 in response to these cases (WHO, 2004a).

In addition to the activities listed in Box S-1, which can largely be characterized as reactive to a threatened pandemic, WHO has begun to pursue strategies to avert an influenza pandemic—a goal long considered to

---

BOX S-1
International Pandemic Planning and Response:
The Role of the World Health Organization (WHO)

Specific contributions by WHO to influenza pandemic preparedness and response include:

• Providing model national pandemic plans and self-assessment tools to guide countries in planning for pandemic influenza
• Conducting, coordinating, and supporting surveillance to detect and report emerging influenza strains
• Promoting free and rapid sharing of surveillance information
• Reporting outbreaks
• Providing medical support (diagnosis, treatment, personal protective equipment) to affected countries
• Supporting the prompt implementation of non-medical interventions at the international level
• Advocating for equity in vaccine and antiviral drug distribution on behalf of developing countries; potentially managing an international antiviral stockpile
• Coordinating research to characterize possible pandemic strains
• Promoting the importance of risk communication to public health authorities, health care providers, and the public
• Developing a prototype strain vaccine and providing standardizing reagents to pharmaceutical companies for vaccine development
• Assessing the effectiveness of various non-medical interventions

SOURCE: Stöhr (2004).

---

be impossible (Stöhr, 2004). To stop, or even slow, a pandemic would require an internationally coordinated, "all-out" response in the early stages of human-to-human transmission (WHO, 2004a). Such an effort would necessitate balancing agricultural and public health interests—which frequently conflict with regard to infection control measures for zoonoses—and a coordinated approach by animal and human health authorities to influenza surveillance and reporting (Stöhr, 2004).

National Preparations

While global preparations against pandemic influenza focus on detecting and defining risk, national governments must determine how to manage the threat posed by an actual or potential pandemic. National governments must be prepared to respond to a developing—and largely unpredictable—pandemic, and in "an atmosphere of considerable scientific uncertainty and fragile public confidence," as described in the report of the recent WHO consultation (WHO, 2004a). In order to face these challenges, several countries have adopted WHO's model of contingency planning; Canada's plan, for example, stresses the documentation of response activities and outcomes so that timely adjustments can be made (Health Canada, 2004). Complete, partial, and draft pandemic influenza plans from several countries can be accessed through the WHO website (http://www.who.int/csr/disease/influenza/nationalpandemic/en/print.html).

In the United States, managing the risk of a pandemic influenza entails not only addressing key national issues through the Department of Health and Human Services (DHHS) and the Department of Homeland Security, but also the harmonization and coordination of state, local, and private-sector plans (GAO, 2000; Slater, 2004). The first U.S. pandemic preparedness plan was organized in 1978, following the emergence of H1N1 swine flu in 1976. The federal government's experience in responding to this threat revealed the importance of developing agreements with private- and public-sector players to assure the timely purchase, distribution, and administration of vaccines and drugs in advance of future infectious outbreaks (GAO, 2000; Millar, 1977). In a sense, the latest version of the U.S. pandemic plan has been under construction since the release of its predecessor nearly 25 years ago, but looming threats of avian influenza and bioterrorism, along with recent sobering estimates of the potential impact of pandemic influenza on the United States (Table S-1) have raised the plan's profile considerably (Gellin, 2004).

The DHHS National Vaccine Program Office is specifically responsible for the U.S. pandemic preparedness plan. Director Bruce Gellin described the contents of the latest version of this plan, which at the time of the meeting was nearing release in draft form. During the development of this report, it was posted on the Internet for a 60-day comment period, beginning on August 26, 2004 (see Chapter 3 for Executive Summary of the plan) (DHHS, 2004a). Beyond revisions to the draft plan based on comments received during this time, DHHS expects future updates based on advancements in the understanding of influenza biology and of the effectiveness of various control measures.

TABLE S-1 U.S. Impact Estimates for the Next Influenza Pandemic

	Number of People	Percentage
Deaths	89,000-207,000	.03-.07
Hospitalizations	314,000-733,000	.1-.3
Outpatient care	18,000,000-42,000,000	6-15
Total infected	43,000,000-100,000,000	15-35

Absent vaccination, health-related economic impacts = $71 to $166 billion

The three main objectives of the U.S. pandemic plan parallel those of other national pandemic preparedness plans, and of the WHO plan: to decrease the burden of disease, minimize social disruption, and reduce the economic impact associated with a pandemic (CDC, 2004c). It addresses surveillance; development and licensure of a vaccine against the strain; production of sufficient vaccine for the U.S. population and provision for its delivery; targeted distribution strategies for limited supplies of vaccine and antiviral medications; coordination with international, state, and local authorities; maintenance of medical care and other community services; and communication with community leaders, medical care providers, the public, and the media (Gellin, 2004). The plan includes the following elements (Gellin, 2004):

• A core plan, which describes the protocol for national coordination and decision-making, reviews key preparedness issues, and outlines response at national, state, and local levels.
• Two guides to aid planning by (1) state and local health departments and (2) public and private health care systems.
• Twelve annexes providing detailed and technical information on preparedness and response issues.

Additional efforts by the federal government to prepare for pandemic influenza at the national level include a $100 million DHHS initiative in 2003 to build U.S. vaccine production. Several agencies within DHHS—including the Office of the Secretary, the Food and Drug Administration (FDA), CDC, and the National Institute of Allergy and Infectious Diseases (NIAID)—are in the process of working with vaccine manufacturers to facilitate production of pilot vaccine lots for both H5N1 and H9N2 strains as well as contracting for the manufacturing of 2 million doses of an H5N1 vaccine. This H5N1 vaccine production will provide a critical pilot test of the pandemic vaccine system; it will also be used for clinical trials to evaluate dose and immunogenicity and can provide initial vaccine for early use in the event of an emerging pandemic. Other efforts include the introduction into the U.S. Senate of the Flu Protection Act of 2004, which aims to increase safeguards against both annual influenza and epidemic/pandemic preparation. Two Senate bills introduced in 2003 also address key influenza preparedness issues: boosting vaccine production[16] and promoting immunization against several diseases, including influenza.[17]

---

[16]Amendment to the Public Health Service Act to ensure an adequate supply of vaccines. S. 371, 108th Congress, 2nd Session (2003).
[17]Improved Vaccine Affordability and Availability Act. S.754, 108th Congress, 1st Session (2003).

State and Local Preparations

The most direct, most primary response to pandemic influenza will come from state and local authorities, public health officials, and providers of medical and other public services. Unlike a typical, localized public health emergency or natural disaster, a pandemic disease cannot be managed from outside the affected community; each community must face the possibility of responding to influenza with minimal external resources or support—or none at all (Gensheimer et al., 2003; Health Canada, 2004; Perrotta, 2004). If a pandemic is confirmed, governors will make most state-level decisions on infection control and case management; however, state health officials are generally responsible for overseeing pandemic preparations and resolving potential conflicts between state and federal governments on issues such as strategies for mass vaccination and disease containment (ASTHO, 2002). Logistical models for local response to pandemic influenza include the widely used Incident Command System, which has been adapted in some areas specifically to respond to infectious disease outbreaks, including pandemic influenza (ASTHO, 2002).

State and local health departments rely heavily on guidance from the federal government in formulating pandemic influenza plans (see Gensheimer in Chapter 3). According to a recent survey conducted by the Council of State and Territorial Epidemiologists (CSTE), 29 states have complete drafts or final plans to address pandemic influenza, and 14 have earlier drafts of a plan (Personal communication, Kristine Morris). In addition to the federal pandemic plan, resources available for state and local planning include CDC's guide for state and local officials and its online modeling tool, FluAid (CDC, 2000), which uses state-specific statistics to approximate the impact of a pandemic on an area (ASTHO, 2002). Tabletop exercises are being developed to help state and local officials rehearse and refine strategies for coping with a pandemic (DHHS, 2004a), much as simulations of bioterrorist attacks have been used to assess federal, state, and local preparedness (ASTHO, 2002; Vastag, 2002).

Several states, including Texas, Wisconsin, and California, are preparing for the next influenza pandemic as a complement or adjunct to preparations against bioterrorism (Perrotta, 2004; Shult, 2004; State of California, 2003). Wisconsin, for example, is establishing a common infrastructure for coping with bioterrorism and infectious disease outbreaks—and managing two or more such events simultaneously. Such efforts are made possible by federal funding for bioterrorism preparedness. Since September 11, 2001, DHHS has provided more than $3.7 billion to improve state public health emergency preparedness for bioterrorism, infectious disease outbreaks, and public health emergencies (DHHS, 2004b). These funds enable states and communities to conduct influenza-related activities including surveillance, planning, drills, and tabletop exercises.

Hospitals are a key focus of state and local influenza preparedness because a pandemic is likely to result in increased demand for health care services, staff shortages, and limited access to critical equipment and supplies (above predicted shortfalls in vaccines and antiviral medications) (DHHS, 2004b). Hospital surge capacities are extremely limited; for example, medical care capacity in a major urban center (Los Angeles County) recently proved insufficient even to address severe seasonal influenza (Glaser et al., 2002). In addition, of course, hospitals and hospital workers themselves become the sieves for infection spread as sick health care workers are required to report to work due to staff shortages, and spread their illness to immunocompromised patients, particularly the elderly, who visit emergency rooms and occupy beds on the wards.

Workshop participants expressed concern that much work remains to be done to establish pandemic planning at state and local levels. The presenters particularly noted a gap in planning and coordination between public health agencies and hospital administrators. Moreover, while most people who contract influenza will not require hospital care, many will need other support services such as home health care, delivery of prescription drugs, and meals (DHHS, 2004b). These needs, along with those for other essential community services (e.g., police, fire, utility, sanitary services) should be addressed in local pandemic planning and in infection control.

State and Local Surveillance

In addition to serving on the "front lines" of the response to pandemic influenza, state and local public health officials and health care providers are also largely responsible for implementing influenza surveillance in the United States. Surveillance programs and capacity vary considerably from state to state. The program in Texas, described by state epidemiologist Dennis Perrotta as "better than most," was modeled on a program run by Baylor University Medical School that tracks year-round respiratory illness in the Houston area (Perrotta, 2004). In the statewide program, participating physicians and hospitals collect swabs from people presenting with febrile illness during flu season. The swabs are analyzed by the state public health laboratory, which uses these results to create a statewide "picture" of respiratory viruses.

In Wisconsin, influenza surveillance is conducted through a network of public and private laboratories that track all emerging diseases and provide isolates to CDC for further testing (Shult, 2004). Small private laboratories and clinicians that conduct rapid diagnostic tests for flu also send their samples to the state laboratory for confirmation. Additional samples and patient information are obtained by clinicians who serve populations where new influenza strains are likeliest to emerge: preschool and school-age children in rural areas where swine and poultry are raised. The data are shared and compared with surveillance of animal respiratory diseases by the University of Wisconsin's veterinary diagnostic laboratory.

TOWARD PREPAREDNESS: OPPORTUNITIES AND OBSTACLES

Addressing Avian Influenza

Considerations of the pandemic threat posed by H5N1 avian influenza in Asia were augmented and enriched by further discussion of the global phenomenon of avian influenza, its impact on the poultry industry, and possible strategies for preventing and controlling its spread among birds and mammals, including humans. Participants noted the importance of surveillance to the effective control of influenza, as well as the limitations of predominant models of surveillance that focus on a single species or industry. In recognition of the need for a broader understanding of influenza behavior, the Office International des Épizooties (OIE), an international and intergovernmental organization that promotes worldwide solidarity in animal disease control, is developing influenza surveillance guidelines that encompass birds, domestic mammals, wildlife, and humans (see Sibartie in Chapter 4; Sibartie, 2004). Weeks after the workshop, the OIE, the Food and Agriculture Organization (FAO), and WHO announced plans to launch a jointly sponsored regional veterinary influenza network intended to strengthen surveillance and speed the diagnosis and reporting of emergent strains (ProMED-mail, 2004q).

Obstacles to Early Reporting

In the absence of a comprehensive surveillance network in place, the rapid reporting of early cases is essential to controlling an emergent infectious disease. All OIE member countries are therefore required to report certain diseases—including avian influenza—within 24 hours of their detection in animals. After an outbreak of H7N7 avian influenza in ducks in 2003, The Netherlands established its own early warning system for the disease. Unfortunately, the system's utility is limited by the fact that avian influenza has been relatively rare in The Netherlands, and is thus unlikely to be recognized by veterinarians (Koch, 2004).

Given existing obstacles to surveillance and early reporting, it is not surprising that in many instances, infection control for avian influenza has entailed mass culling of poultry. However, according to Dewan Sebartie of the OIE, that organization "recognizes that culling is no longer a viable option for certain countries for social, economic, technical, ethical and ecological reasons." Small farmers, for example, are unlikely to comply with culling policies because their flocks provide a lifeline of daily income; they cannot help but focus on their immediate and pressing need to sell their birds (Soebandrio, 2004). On a larger scale, the economic consequences of early reporting—to a country or region if many animals must be culled, or to a corporation raising millions of infected, and therefore potentially unprofitable, animals—present a massive barrier to disease control. One country, for example, experienced outbreaks of H5N1 over more than 6 months before admitting the situation to the OIE (Sibartie, 2004). In California, poultry producers kept their knowledge of a recent H6N2 avian influenza outbreak to themselves due to their fear of public rejection of poultry products; meanwhile, the disease spread across the western United States and has since become endemic (Box S-2).

The need to remove economic disincentives to the timely discovery and control of emergent avian influenza strains is clearly established. Providing compensation for culled animals could, at least in theory, remove a major disincentive to reporting for farmers in developing countries (however, see earlier discussion of Thailand's problematic compensation program). Several participants urged the creation of a fund by developed countries to compensate for culling of infected flocks in developing countries, as well as for the quarantine and isolation of humans should transmission occur (Meltzer, 2004). In developed countries, government-run mandated insurance policies, similar to policies currently in use to encourage reporting of Salmonella in eggs and poultry in the United States, could compensate the losses of poultry producers who report suspected or confirmed cases of avian influenza (Meltzer, 2004). Another option proposed by the OIE is to allow demonstrably biosecure regions of a country where avian influenza has been reported—or even biosecure farms within an affected area—to continue to export poultry products, because avian influenza is not a foodborne disease (Sibartie, 2004). This could, however, also be a disincentive for farms to certify the presence of avian influenza in their flocks and possibly their workers. It was also suggested that, given increased public interest in avian influenza, poultry from producers who can certify their chickens to be "influenza free" and their workers to be "influenza safe" through protection programs may be more desirable to consumers (Cardona, 2004).

Immunization of Poultry

Avian influenza vaccines increasingly are being viewed as a means of reducing the necessity for massive poultry culls, particularly in Asia. Together with culling, immunization can speed the eradication of avian influenza and, by decreasing the amount of virus shed by infected animals,

---

BOX S-2
H6N2 Avian Influenza in the Triangle of Doom

In February 2000, a low pathogenic H6N2 virus was detected for the first time in commercial egg layers in southern California, an area with a population of approximately 15 million chickens. At that time fewer than 10 farms were found to be infected with this low-pathogenic virus in an area with about 60 large farms ranging in size from about 30,000 to 1.2 million birds. The infection was asymptomatic—egg production and mortality were not affected—thus little was done to eradicate the virus. The state performed some vaccination of layer farms, but because it was not accompanied by depopulation or stamping-out, the measure proved futile.

Over the next 2 years, the virus persisted on some farms where it found a continual stream of naïve hosts. Sporadic infections occurred in additional farms in the area, bringing the total number of affected (H6N2 antibody positive) farms to 15. Three different genotypes of H6N2 virus were found to be circulating; in January 2002, one form emerged to cause clinical disease in San Diego County, where an infected flock suffered a 50 percent decrease in egg production and a 10-fold increase in mortality. The farmer had his birds tested, but during a 2-week period before the diagnosis was made, chicken manure was removed from the farm, young hens were brought in, and eggs continued to be taken to be processed. The virus immediately spread to approximately 10 farms and the outbreak continued to expand over the next 2 months.

A major expansion of the outbreak subsequently occurred in Turlock, a town in northern California where layer hens from several states were slaughtered and processed. Infected layer hens from southern California were sent to the Turlock plant, into the heart of a densely populated poultry region. Shortly thereafter, three egg-laying flocks in the Turlock region were found to be positive for avian influenza detected through passive surveillance; a drop in egg production prompted the producers to have the birds tested.

One week later a broiler flock was found to be positive for avian influenza at slaughter. Once the virus got into broilers, it spread very rapidly among turkeys and layers as well. This acceleration resulted from the unfortunate coincidence

---

reduce human exposure as well (ProMED-mail, 2004r; Sibartie, 2004). However, as several conference participants stressed, vaccination must be accompanied by strong surveillance to prevent the spread of asymptomatic infection among vaccinated birds. This can be accomplished either through the use of unvaccinated sentinel birds or of recombinant vaccines that elicit a distinct "marker" antibody (ProMED-mail, 2004s). Should a "silent epidemic" of influenza manage to erupt under these conditions, it could serve as an incubator for the evolution of a more deadly viral strain. This apparently occurred in Mexico after chickens were vaccinated against highly pathogenic H5N2 influenza in 1995; today, antigenically distinct variants of the vaccine strain are spreading among the country's poultry flocks (Lee et al., 2004).

that broilers are sent to slaughter at an optimal age for viral shedding, as well as from the large numbers of broilers that traveled to that facility. Millions of birds shedding viruses traveling in trucks to Turlock easily spread the infection to farms along the route. That is when the Turlock region, which is bound by three major highways, became known as the Triangle of Doom: a bird couldn't enter the area without becoming infected with H6N2. An estimated 35 million birds in California became infected with this H6N2 virus during a 4-month period beginning in March 2002.

Perhaps more astonishing than the extent and speed of this outbreak was the fact that no one outside the region heard much about it. The virus was not a feared H5 or H7 subtype, but the Triangle of Doom was also kept quiet by corporate decision-makers who feared that consumer demand would plummet if the public knew they were buying infected meat and eggs, safe though they may be to eat. Thus, other than the initial diagnosis of the broiler flock, all other diagnoses were made by corporate veterinarians, and the results were not released—not to the state or to other potentially affected states, not to the Office International des Épizooties, not even to neighboring farmers, who might have better protected their flocks from infection had they known about it. H6N2 has since become endemic in California, following its spread to farms that raise birds for the state's live fowl markets.

Eventually, the poultry producers in the Triangle of Doom developed a biosecurity plan to curtail the spread of the virus, and thereby restore egg and poultry production. The plan does not penalize farms that test positive for influenza, and it provides for the safe movement of eggs and broilers to market from infected facilities. These sorts of protections need to be offered to the industries that raise much of the poultry (and swine) in the United States in order to achieve complete surveillance and their cooperation in addressing avian influenza. Similar dense poultry and swine populations exist throughout the country. Any one of them could be the site of the next outbreak of an emergent influenza virus.

SOURCE: Cardona (2004).

Since the height of the Asian avian influenza in February 2004, the FAO has recommended vaccination against influenza "where appropriate and practical," but the practice remains prohibited in several Asian nations (ProMED-mail, 2004r). Japan and Korea, the only Asian countries that successfully controlled and eradicated H5N1 following the recent epidemic, did so through culling alone. Thailand is currently considering the possibility of immunization following a resurgence of H5N1 in July 2004, although as a major poultry exporter, it will surely take into consideration the European Union's ban on poultry imports from countries where chickens have been vaccinated against avian influenza. Vaccination against avian influenza is not widely practiced in the United States due to its high cost relative to profit margins for most of the poultry industry (see Swayne and Sibartie in Chapter 4; Swayne, 2004).

Preventing Interspecies Transmission

The intersecting and sometimes conflicting interests of commerce and public health were also evident in discussions on preventing transmission of avian influenza from wild to domestic birds, and from poultry to domestic animals and humans (for transmission pathways between species, see Figure S-4). Because wild waterfowl can carry the influenza A virus without developing signs of infection, influenza cannot realistically be considered an

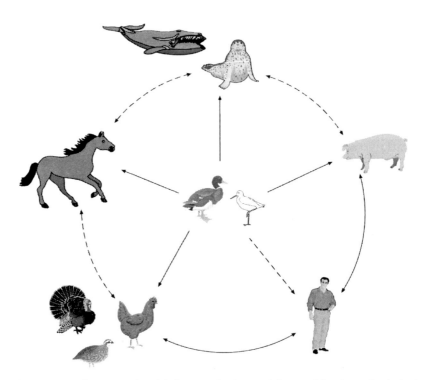

FIGURE S-4 The reservoir of influenza A viruses. The working hypothesis is that wild aquatic birds are the primordial reservoir of all influenza viruses for avian and mammalian species. Transmission of influenza has been demonstrated between pigs and humans and between chickens and humans but not between wild birds and humans (dotted lines). There is extensive evidence for transmission of influenza viruses between wild ducks and other species (solid lines). The five different host groups are based on phylogenetic analysis of the nucleoprotein genes of a large number of different influenza viruses.

eradicable disease (Webster, 1998). During the development of this report, it was reported that H5N1 avian influenza had been discovered in migratory birds in the Novosibirskaya region of Russia (ProMED-mail, 2004t). Preliminary data indicate that the virus was brought from south east Asia by migratory birds, such as ducks and geese (ProMED-mail, 2004t). Workshop discussants concurred that the best chance of averting a pandemic lies in stopping the further spread of epidemics in poultry populations, thereby reducing human exposure to the virus and limiting its opportunities for reassortment (Trampuz et al., 2004; Barclay and Zambon, 2004).

Live poultry markets provide near-optimal conditions for amplifying and perpetuating viruses due to the continuous movement of many bird species through the market (Webster, 2004b). These risks are multiplied when livestock and poultry are kept in close proximity and in crowded conditions, as is often the case in "wet markets" and in livestock (especially swine) and poultry feeding operations (Liu et al., 2003). Because neither practice is likely to end soon, participants agreed, the immediate focus of preventive efforts should be on making farms and markets safer through measures and regulations that reduce the possibility of contact between domestic and wild animals and between domestic mammals and poultry, as well as through efforts to protect workers from infection (see Swayne and Sibartie in Chapter 4).

Surveillance

Influenza surveillance at all levels—from global to local—has a common, practical goal: to detect events indicating unusually large or severe outbreaks of influenza as early as possible, and to determine the intensity and impact of influenza on populations. The first step toward this goal is to determine normal conditions, so that an unusual event can be recognized for what it is. Thus influenza surveillance must be stable, ongoing, and representative of populations on the basis of geography, demography, and severity of disease. The vital data that emerge determine vaccine strain selection and public health resource allocation and drive influenza prevention and control policy and planning for pandemic preparedness.

Surveillance findings also contribute to epidemiological research, most often as a springboard for more detailed investigation. In the case of influenza, surveillance has clarified essential questions regarding the clinical epidemiology of pandemics and the biological causes of epidemiological phenomena. Pursuing answers to these questions will require investment in planning research, designing protocols, and establishing networks of scientists ready to engage in these studies in advance of the next pandemic (Stöhr, 2004).

Global Surveillance

WHO has spearheaded global influenza surveillance efforts since 1948 and now coordinates a network of 110 national influenza centers in more than 80 countries (Cox, 2004; Stöhr, 2004). These laboratories isolate and characterize influenza viruses and collect epidemiological information; they also submit certain viruses for characterization to one of four WHO international collaborating centers in Atlanta, London, Melbourne, and Tokyo. These facilities analyze and compare thousands of viral strains each year in order to determine the antigen content of the three annual influenza vaccines, then prepare and distribute the candidate vaccine strain to manufacturers. While this network is strong in Western countries and was characterized as "sufficient" in Eastern Europe and the Middle East, it is riddled with strategic gaps in Africa as well as in Asia—an area of particular concern due to H5N1 (Stöhr, 2004). Laos and Cambodia, for example, lack national influenza centers and did not conduct routine influenza surveillance during the recent H5N1 epidemic; thus the extent of infection in human populations in those countries is unknown (Cox, 2004). Even in countries participating in WHO surveillance, the surveillance of the H5N1 epidemic was hindered by limited access to virus isolates (in part because laboratories in developing countries could not afford to ship isolates to international collaboration centers) and poor communication between veterinary and public health officials.

As a result of this experience, DHHS recently launched a $5.5 million initiative to create and enhance infrastructure for influenza surveillance in Asia (Cox, 2004). While this investment is likely to lead to immediate improvements in virologic surveillance in this important region, participants noted that it will be equally necessary—but much more difficult—to obtain epidemiological evidence of disease impact. The United States was described as a possible model for collecting both types of information on a national scale. Here, a network of 2,000 sentinel physicians monitor more than 8 million patient visits per year and submit reports and specimens to CDC; additional reports are provided by state and territorial epidemiologists and public health authorities in 122 U.S. cities.

Integration and Collaboration

It was frequently noted that influenza surveillance efforts at all governmental levels would benefit immensely from better integration between the animal and human health communities. While acknowledging that formal collaboration between the OIE and WHO has been limited to date, a forthcoming meeting promised to discuss information and strain sharing and the harmonization of surveillance methods between the two international organizations and their collaborators (Sibartie, 2004). The previously mentioned plan for a regional veterinary influenza network, jointly sponsored by the OIE, WHO, and the FAO, was announced weeks after the workshop (ProMED-mail, 2004u). The recent DHHS initiative will also support study of the animal–human interface in influenza, particularly as it enables predictions of human risk from animal influenza viruses (Cox, 2004).

Workshop participants also emphasized the need to strengthen international influenza surveillance through the sharing of:

- Timely information,
- Viral isolates,
- Reagents,
- Funding, and
- Expertise.

The global threat posed by influenza necessitates international collaboration that balances the health and economic needs of developing countries—essential participants in influenza surveillance—with the medical, scientific, and financial resources of developed countries.

Vaccines

Widely accepted as the most effective intervention against influenza in humans, vaccines significantly reduce morbidity and mortality during annual (interpandemic) flu seasons (Fedson, 2004a; Hosbach, 2004; Nichol, 2003). Considerable obstacles hinder the production of a vaccine against a pandemic strain of influenza, however. Planning and production of interpandemic flu vaccine require nearly a year to complete; experts estimate that if a pandemic were to strike today, 6 to 8 months would elapse from the identification of the viral strain to the initial release of vaccine if it were produced by standard methods (GAO, 2000). Moreover, given existing manufacturing capacity, vaccine availability would fall far short of projected demand, especially in countries without vaccine manufacturing facilities (Fedson, 2004b). Workshop participants considered the critical role of vaccine manufacturers in addressing a pandemic; methods and logistics for the development and production of a pandemic vaccine; and the challenges of equitably distributing it given the likelihood that demand will far outstrip supply (see Fedson in Chapter 3).

Supply and Demand

Above all, several workshop participants stressed the importance of building capacity to manufacture pandemic vaccine by accelerating demand for interpandemic influenza vaccines (Fedson, 2004a; Gellin, 2004; Hosbach, 2004; Nowak, 2004). Although annual influenza immunization rates have increased sharply over the past decade, from 135 to 292 million doses of flu vaccine worldwide (Fedson, 2004b), demand remains too weak for manufacturers to make investment in preparations for a rapid ramp-up of pandemic vaccine production. Currently only 75 to 85 million Americans (about one-quarter of the population) are immunized annually against influenza, and only 38 percent of health care workers receive influenza vaccination (see Hosbach in Chapter 3).

Because last year's early and virulent flu season, and particularly news of several child fatalities, ratcheted up vaccine demand in the United States, participants suggested that the country may be ripe for a pro-immunization campaign. In addition, the flu immunization season—now largely limited to October and November—could be extended into January, when peak rates of infection generally occur. This might have been possible in the United States during the 2003–2004 flu season if more vaccine doses had been preordered; instead, as rarely occurs, demand for vaccine exceeded supply. Because influenza vaccine cannot be stockpiled (due to antigenic shift and drift), it was also suggested that the federal government share the risk of investing in producing vaccine reserves, in preparation for either a severe annual flu season or in response to a threatened pandemic. This arrangement would help ensure that influenza vaccine supplies will meet a sharply increased demand (Hosbach, 2004) (see Figure S-5).

The subject of liability protection was also noted as crucial to the production of a pandemic vaccine. Manufacturers are loath to repeat the experience of the 1976 swine flu, when they produced 150 million doses of vaccine for a threatened pandemic that never occurred; only 45 million doses were used, and the immunization campaign was suspended after the vaccine was linked with Guillain-Barré syndrome (ASTHO, 2002). Participants also observed there is some likelihood that a pandemic vaccine could be offered as an Investigational New Drug as befits an emergency situation, demanding advance consideration of the complexities of administering an unlicensed vaccine in this context (Hosbach, 2004).

The effort to produce a pandemic vaccine promises to send shock waves beyond the drug manufacturing sector. Demand for syringes, vials, and other vaccine-related materials are likely to skyrocket, as will demand for the attention and resources of the FDA's Center for Biologics Evaluation and Research (CBER). That agency will need to significantly increase its own capacity in order to speed the testing of candidate vaccines. Efficient delivery of the vaccine must also be considered; currently, 85 percent of influenza vaccine in the United States is sold, distributed, and administered by private health care providers. Although participants recognized that this system is not perfect, they advised that in the midst of a pandemic

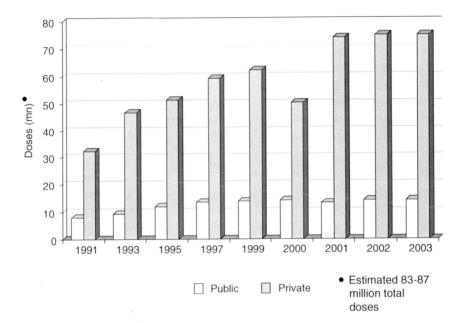

FIGURE S-5 The influenza vaccine market is increasingly a private purchase system. Public versus private demand.

it would be better to build on and improve current distribution networks rather than attempt to replace them. Pandemic vaccine production is expected to displace production of all other vaccines for 1 to 2 years; thus pediatric and other routinely used vaccines would require stockpiling to ensure their uninterrupted availability.

H5N1 "Pandemic-Like" Vaccines

In response to the threat posed by H5N1 in Asia, both the European Union (under the auspices of the European Medicines Evaluation Agency) and the United States (under the auspices of NIAID) have embarked on efforts to produce, and test in clinical trials, a vaccine against the viruses that infected and killed humans. However, divergent approaches are being taken to the initial development of these vaccines on either side of the Atlantic: While the U.S. researchers have given highest priority to assuring that the vaccine is safe and capable of protecting individual recipients against severe disease, the Europeans seek to balance safety with an antigen-sparing dosage level intended to maximize pandemic vaccine supply (see Fedson in Chapter 3).

Some workshop participants raised concerns that in the event of an imminent pandemic, the NIAID approach would provide enough vaccine to supply only a fraction of the U.S. population (Fedson, 2004a). Earlier European trials with other monovalent pandemic-like vaccines had successfully added adjuvant to gain immunogenicity at low doses, it was observed, and it was suggested that such a formulation would assure the largest possible vaccine supply. Americans and Europeans were also urged to develop a common process for funding the clinical trials needed to develop candidate pandemic vaccines. One workshop participant proposed that the candidate H5N1 vaccine, after validation for immunogenicity and reactogenicity, should be deployed as soon as possible in the at-risk populations of south east Asia and data should be collected and analyzed on its effectiveness.

The program officer for the National Institutes of Health (NIH) clinical trials for the H5N1 vaccine responded to these concerns by stating that NIAID, which is part of NIH, will initially focus on the safety and dose-related antigenicity of vaccines produced by currently licensed manufacturing processes. Although influenza vaccines formulated with adjuvants have not consistently enhanced immune responses in previous studies and have in some cases shown increased reactogenicity, NIAID expects to conduct direct comparisons of pandemic-like vaccines with and without adjuvants in the future.

Technical Innovations

Without the use of reverse genetics—the cloning of inactivated hemagglutinin and neuraminidase genes and their expression in a recombinant virus in cell culture—the seed strain for the H5N1 vaccine currently in clinical trials might never have been produced. Avian influenza viruses often grow poorly—and some kill—the embryonated eggs in which commercial viral seed stocks are grown (see Fedson in Chapter 3). During a pandemic, the use of reverse genetics would be expected to speed vaccine production significantly as compared with conventional egg-based methods. MedImmune Incorporated, the major patent holder for reverse genetic technology, permitted WHO to employ the method, free of charge, to prepare H5N1 seed strains and provide them to vaccine manufacturers in the United States and Europe (see MedImmune in Chapter 3; Coelingh, 2004). If a company eventually produces pandemic vaccine for profit, however, MedImmune and possibly other parties must be paid a royalty on its patented technology. Although this arrangement does not in theory restrict research on the use of reverse genetics in vaccine production, it was suggested that the necessity to license the technology discourages its use by pharmaceutical companies, few of whom make vaccines due to their already low profit margins. Moreover, MedImmune is not the sole patent holder in reverse genetic technology (Fedson, 2004b). In Europe, which produces more than 70 percent of the world's vaccine supply, reverse genetic vaccines also encounter significant regulatory hurdles due to their designation as genetically modified organisms (GMOs). In response to these challenges, European vaccine manufacturers have called for publicly funded international trials of all pilot lots of potential pandemic vaccines made by its companies that produce vaccine before the next pandemic occurs.

Workshop participants also discussed the possible replacement of egg-based viral propagation with mammalian cell culture methods that may lead to more rapid vaccine production. While cell culture may eventually prove viable, and sufficiently cost effective for vaccine manufacturers, participants recognized that egg-based production is the only proven and rigorously tested method of large-scale vaccine manufacture and is likely to remain so for several years to come. Fortunately, promising new methods for boosting antigen yields in egg-based vaccine systems, coupled with adjuvants and delivery devices to enhance vaccine supply and performance, could increase vaccine availability in the near term (Hosbach, 2004; Stöhr, 2004). Participants also learned of recent progress in a baculovirus-derived antigen production system for a recombinant, trivalent influenza vaccine that is expected to enter Phase III trials within months (Jones et al., 2003). In 1997, this method produced 1,700 doses of a vaccine against "Hong Kong" avian influenza in a total of 8 weeks.

Coping with Limited Vaccine Supplies

While encouraged by the variety of ways in which influenza vaccine may be made increasingly available, participants also emphasized the need to make just and optimal use of limited vaccine stocks in an imminent pandemic—and the challenges that could prevent this from happening. Chief among these hurdles is the fact that 95 percent of the world's vaccine is produced by countries accounting for only 12 percent of its population (see Fedson in Chapter 3). Thus in the widely expected event that vaccine-producing countries nationalize vaccine production in response to pandemic influenza, nearly 90 percent of the world's population would be denied timely access to vaccine. Participants therefore urged the negotiation of international agreements to ensure equitable vaccine distribution in advance of a pandemic. WHO also stresses the importance of developing and evaluating non-medical interventions for use in populations without access to a pandemic vaccine (Stöhr, 2004). At the national level, as discussed previously (with regard to pandemic planning) and subsequently (with regard to mathematical and economic models of pandemic impact), the probability of vaccine shortages necessitates the prioritization of recipients. Such a scenario is currently unfolding with the U.S. vaccine shortages for the

2004–2005 influenza season. The United States is attempting to prioritize the vaccine by urging healthy adults to forego the shot this year so that the remaining doses can go to the youngest, oldest, and sickest Americans, who are the most vulnerable to influenza. The two difficulties with this prioritization method are that the prioritization is voluntary and not enforced, allowing anyone to receive it, and it has been difficult for the health care industry to effectively distribute the limited supplies to individuals and facilities that need it most in different regions of the country.

Antiviral Drugs

Vaccines provide the best protection against influenza, but due to their limitations, as detailed in the previous section, they are not likely to protect the vast majority of people, particularly in the early phases of a pandemic. This breach could be filled by antiviral drugs, which have been shown to be effective in influenza treatment and prophylaxis (Longini et al., 2004; Monto, 2003); evidence indicates that antivirals also inhibit bacterial superinfection, a significant cause of influenza-related mortality in the elderly and other high-risk individuals (Petola and McCullers, 2004; Kaiser et al., 2000, 2003). Unlike vaccines, antivirals currently can be stockpiled in advance of a pandemic. Ensuring adequate supplies of antivirals and methods for effective mass distribution to higher-risk populations would be critical to any containment of a pandemic that could be achieved by antiviral prophylaxis (especially in lieu of adequate vaccine supply).

Of the two classes of antiviral agents, M2 inhibitors (amantidine and rimantidine) and neuraminidase inhibitors (zanamivir and oseltamivir), only the latter appear to be effective against current H5N1 avian influenza, considered to be the likeliest source of the next pandemic. Unfortunately, similar obstacles to those hindering vaccine use stand in the way of fighting flu with neuraminidase inhibitors. Only two manufacturers produce these compounds, and their existing surge capacity is unlikely to meet pandemic demand. One means to increase the availability of neuraminidase inhibitors is similar to that proposed for vaccines: to make greater use of the product in treating and preventing influenza in interpandemic seasons, with the expectation that capacity for its production will rise with demand; currently only 1.5 million oseltamivir treatments are produced per year.

Timely access to antiviral drugs is also a concern, because they would need to be administered early in a pandemic to provide effective prophylaxis against influenza. Thus in addition to setting priorities for the distribution of limited supplies of antiviral drugs, including how much of an emphasis to place on prophylaxis versus therapeutic use, pandemic preparations should provide for the rapid and efficient distribution of prophylactic doses. The draft U.S. pandemic plan assigns priority for antiviral prophylaxis to health care workers and other public service providers who are likely to be exposed to the virus and to workers who cull infected animals (Gellin, 2004). A plea was also made to award high priority to employees of pharmaceutical companies who are engaged in producing pandemic vaccine (Hosbach, 2004).

Stockpiles

Unlike vaccines, antiviral drugs can be stockpiled in anticipation of a pandemic. The strategic U.S. national stockpile has made an initial purchase of oseltamivir, and the federal government is studying various stockpiling options and distribution strategies for the future (Gellin, 2004). Oseltamivir may be stockpiled either as "active pharmaceutical ingredient" (API) or after formulation into pills or capsules; each model offers advantages and disadvantages (Brown, 2004). Reserves of oseltamivir, an oral suspension that can be used for either adults or children, are relatively inexpensive and have a shelf life of at least 5 years; however, the drug is relatively difficult to distribute and would require regulatory review because it is currently approved for sale only in capsule form. Oseltamivir capsules, sold under the name Tamiflu™, take longer to produce than the API and are not approved for use in people who weigh less than 88 pounds. Because much about the U.S. plan for pandemic use of antiviral drugs (and oseltamivir in particular) remains to be determined, manufacturers cannot predict the extent to which they can recoup the costs of increasing production capacity. Moreover, unlike vaccine manufacturers, antiviral drug producers recognize that stockpiling their product means that this expanded capacity may be used only once.

Participants also considered the possibility of creating an international stockpile (either as a single entity controlled by WHO, or a virtual stockpile contributed by participating countries from their national stockpiles) that could be made available to slow or contain a potential pandemic—or any emerging zoonosis—at an early stage. The effectiveness of such targeted antiviral prophylaxis has been suggested by studies of influenza transmission within families, and has also been explored through mathematical models of infectious disease transmission (see subsequent discussion on emerging technical tools). Several participants emphasized that negotiations to build such a stockpile should be undertaken immediately, given the likelihood that the production of antiviral drugs, as with vaccines, will be nationalized in the event of a pandemic. The need for such a stockpile was also demonstrated by the recent experience of WHO, which attempted to introduce antiviral prophylaxis early in the recent Asian H5N1 outbreak. The organization's order for neuraminidase inhibitors was not delivered for

2 weeks, and it was limited to 6,000 doses—too little and too late to avert a pandemic, if one had been imminent (Stöhr, 2004).

Inappropriate Use

Workshop participants were alerted to the danger posed by the inappropriate use of antiviral medications during a pandemic, as apparently occurred during the recent Asian H5N1 epidemic (Brown, 2004). Patients who take the drug for only 2 or 3 days gain significant relief from flu symptoms, but continue to shed virus (Treanor et al., 2000)—and virus that is potentially resistant to oseltamivir—if they do not complete the prescribed 5-day course. This is an especially worrisome trend and should be an area of future investigation given the scarcity of antiviral medications in the drug development pipeline that potentially could be substituted for oseltamivir should resistance to the drug develop during or before a pandemic.

Antiviral Resistance Surveillance

As antivirals are increasingly used for treatment of the Asian H5N1 epidemic, surveillance in both humans and animals (i.e., poultry, swine) for emergence of a drug-resistant strain is essential. Concerns are loss of drug efficacy, spread of resistant variants, and possible increased virulence or transmissibility of resistant variants. Recent reports have raised concerns that the frequency of antiviral resistance might be higher than previously observed when Tamiflu™ is used for treatment of influenza in infants and young children (Kiso et al., 2004). Further data on the frequency of resistance emergence, its relationship to dosing regimens and its consequences are needed for anti-influenza agents (NISN, 2004). It was suggested during discussion that a need exists for continued surveillance of antiviral susceptibility patterns in community isolates and for resistance transmission in high-risk epidemiological settings.

The Role of the Private Medical System

Although the American health care system is overwhelmingly privatized, little attention has been paid to private medicine's potential role in preparing for pandemic influenza. Thus the workshop presentation and discussion led by Gordon Grundy—a regional medical director for Aetna, one of the country's largest managed care insurance corporations—introduced a novel perspective and several new ideas to discussions of pandemic planning (see Chapter 3). Workshop participants considered how partnerships could be fostered between government and managed care organizations to better prepare the United States to cope with an influenza pandemic, the resources each partner could bring to the table, and some key issues that must be addressed by private health care organizations to prepare themselves for pandemic influenza.

Approximately two thirds of the U.S. population is insured by the more than 1,300 private health care plans that operate in this country (Grundy, 2004). A key mission of such plans is to control the expense of members' medical care; this is accomplished in part through "gatekeeping" measures that include requirements for referrals and restrictions on formularies. Although these policies are generally effective in holding down health care costs, health plan administrators realize these policies would hinder the medical response to a public health crisis such as pandemic influenza. Aetna and other insurers have therefore waived certain cost-containment measures in response to emergencies including the September 11, 2001, terrorist attacks, the 2003 blackout of the northeastern United States, and various natural disasters, and they could be expected to do so in the event of an influenza pandemic.

But the private health system has done little toward planning—or even considering—a coordinated response to pandemic influenza (Grundy, 2004). Likewise, few federal, state, or local officials have attempted to engage representatives of the private medical system in the pandemic planning process. In considering how such a partnership for pandemic planning might be initiated, participants advised that it represent a broad spectrum of health plans, perhaps under the aegis of an industry trade association. One such group, the Council for Affordable Quality Health Care, has taken on other public health initiatives, including a partnership with CDC to encourage appropriate antibiotic use.

Potential Contributions to Preparedness

Private health care organizations could contribute to pandemic preparedness in several ways. Their broad outreach capabilities could be used to educate their members about the risks posed by influenza, and they could provide incentives to encourage annual immunization, particularly for individuals at high risk for complications. Health plans could also offer financial incentives to physicians for providing services that prevent or mitigate the impact of pandemic influenza. The vast patient databases maintained by health plans could be used to contact and alert vulnerable members to an impending pandemic and instruct them in protective measures. Health plans could also help identify and establish facilities for mass immunizations in nontraditional sites (e.g., shopping malls). These same medical record database systems could also be utilized to provide surveillance data on emerging outbreaks of influenza to the public health system as a part of an early warning system to engage an effective response.

Managed care providers also have much to offer to the pandemic planning process (Grundy, 2004). Their detailed knowledge of the capacity and limitations of most community health care could be brought to bear on local or regional planning to accommodate a pandemic surge. Health plans could also recommend strategies to reduce this burden based on their expertise in providing cost-effective alternatives to intensive care and in optimizing the use of other health care resources. In return, health plans can best support the government's response to pandemic influenza if plan managers receive clear statements, directives, and recommendations as to their industry's role and responsibilities in that response. For example, health plan managers will need to know the priority targets for immunization and the rationale governing these choices, whether it is reducing overall morbidity and mortality, minimizing lost productivity, or safeguarding health care workers. Both partners also need to understand the financial consequences to private medicine of responding to (or simply weathering) pandemic influenza, and particularly how health care providers will be compensated for the services they provide during a pandemic.

In addition to encouraging participation by the private medical system in pandemic planning at all levels of government, workshop participants also urged private care providers—particularly hospitals and hospital systems—to make their own preparations for pandemic influenza. Issues that might be addressed by such plans include what to do when hospital resources are exhausted (send patients away? make arrangements for home health care for as many patients as possible?) and strategies for maintaining services when significant numbers of hospital workers and health care providers contract influenza. "To my knowledge, health plans do not have a comparable pandemic plan . . . to what is being discussed in the public sector," Dr. Grundy observed. "We do have contingency plans [for delivering critical messages to members], but I can tell you, we need a [pandemic] plan in my shop."

Emerging Technical Tools

Targeting Broadly Conserved Viral Features

Strain-specific immunization offers the best protection against influenza, but as previously discussed, is unlikely to be widely available in time to have a significant impact on the course of an imminent pandemic. It has long been recognized that people who have had influenza tend to have less severe symptoms upon subsequent infections with immunologically distinct viruses. This phenomenon, known as heterosubtypic immunity (Het-I), was first characterized in animal studies that began in the 1960s. Het-I is a non-sterilizing immunity—that is, it reduces symptoms but does not eliminate viral replication—induced by one influenza A subtype that protects against another (see Epstein in Chapter 5; Epstein, 2004). It can be induced in mouse models with live, wild-type viruses or inactivated viruses given mucosally, but has not been studied for the live attenuated viruses sometimes used in influenza vaccines. Although Het-I has not been demonstrated to occur in humans, accounts of the 1957 pandemic suggest that it occurred and that additional historical epidemiological investigation would reveal further evidence of its existence.

Researchers thus reasoned that if Het-I could be induced in humans through mass or routine immunization, there is the possibility that they would gain broad cross-protection against all influenza A subtypes, which should at least reduce mortality in a pandemic until a matched vaccine became widely available (Epstein, 2004). Vaccines could be made in advance and administered to prime immunity, and they could be used "off the shelf" in the event of a pandemic to reduce symptoms until a matched vaccine became widely available. Several proteins that are relatively conserved among all subtypes have proved promising targets for such a strategy, and have been shown to induce immunity that greatly reduced morbidity and mortality in mouse influenza models (Epstein, 2004; Epstein et al., 2002). These antigens were delivered in the form of DNA vaccines, which offer several advantages: They can be preserved at ambient temperatures, removing the need for a cold chain; because they are produced in bacterial cell culture, not in eggs or mammalian cell cultures, they might eventually be cheaper or faster to produce; and they permit investigation of the roles of individual viral proteins in immunity. However, it must be stated that although a DNA vaccine strategy may be effective in addressing pandemic influenza, it is years away from clinical use because no DNA vaccine has been shown to provide effective immune protection from disease (any disease) nor has one been registered with the FDA for future approval.

Another weapon that could be aimed at broadly conserved features among influenza A strains is RNA interference (RNAi) technology, which consists of short, complementary RNA sequences that inhibit protein expression. In this case, the target proteins are necessary for influenza A replication, of which several are relatively conserved among known viral subtypes. Prior studies on this technology have examined viral systems in vitro and in vivo, but few disease models have been explored. Recently, researchers from the CBER and CDC demonstrated that RNAi could protect against lethal virus challenge by H5N1, H1N1, and H7N7 in mice (Tompkins et al., 2004). A second group from the Massachusetts Institute of Technology produced similar results in mice against H1N1 using an intranasal plasmid delivery system that could be adapted for clinical use (Ge et al., 2004).

Although these initial results appear promising, workshop participants raised important challenges that must be resolved before taking this targeted approach to the clinic. Foremost among them is the need to examine the potential risk that immunization against conserved viral features could under some circumstances result in immunopathology (e.g., immune enhancement) rather than protection (Epstein, 2004). The cost of these measures—particularly RNAi, which would be classified as a drug therapy—is also prohibitively expensive as currently delivered.

Transgenic Suppression of Influenza Virus Replication in Chickens

Given that the next influenza pandemic is widely expected to be avian in origin and to emerge from domestic poultry (though perhaps detouring through pigs or another mammalian species on the way), it would seem desirable to inhibit the replication of influenza viruses in chickens, greatly reducing the danger of transmission to humans or other livestock. Recent developments in transgenic technologies and inhibitory strategies make possible the engineering of disease-resistant livestock, including influenza A-resistant chickens; meanwhile, research on the influenza virus has revealed promising strategies for inhibiting influenza replication (see Tiley and Sang in Chapter 5). In addition to RNAi, described above, influenza A replication potentially could be suppressed through the introduction of Mx genes—which block the expression of incoming viral genomes in several mammal and bird species, but not in chickens—and through the presence of RNA decoys, short sequences that mimic the binding sites of RNA proteins and thereby act as competitive inhibitors for transcription. By combining these strategies, researchers hope to achieve complete blockage of influenza replications and prevent the development of resistant viral strains; if they fall short of this goal, dangerous "silent epidemics" of sub-clinical infection could occur (see the earlier discussion of this phenomenon in relation to avian influenza vaccines).

Until recently, the lack of a delivery system suitable for engineering the chicken genome posed a major roadblock to developing influenza virus-resistant poultry. Thanks to the advent of lentiviral vectors, which can be prepared to very high concentrations and can successfully infect and integrate into the chromosomes of virtually any cell type, the first attempts to produce influenza-resistant transgenic birds are currently underway. If these efforts prove successful, researchers must then face the far more daunting challenge of demonstrating the system's long-term efficacy, and perhaps more importantly, its lack of detrimental effects on chickens, humans who consume poultry products, and the environment. While acknowledging that many people hold negative attitudes toward genetically modified organisms, presenter Laurence Tiley (see Chapter 5) observed that "even the direst GMO scare-mongering scenario" pales in comparison to that of another 1918.

Mathematical Models of Pandemic Containment

Mathematical modeling of pandemic scenarios added another dimension to a recurring topic of discussion: how to manage likely shortages of vaccines and antiviral medications (see Medema et al. in Chapter 5). Although models are not evidence of effectiveness, it was suggested by several presenters that they could be helpful decision-making tools during the crisis of a pandemic outbreak. One presentation described the use of a stochastic model that simulates daily contacts by a cross-section of Americans to examine the effects of epidemic influenza under various regimens of antiviral prophylaxis and/or vaccination (Longini, 2004; Longini et al., 2004; Monto, 2003). A strategy known as targeted antiviral prophylaxis (TAP), in which antiviral medications are given to people believed to be in close contact with index cases, was found to temporarily contain influenza transmission when 80 percent of all identifiable contacts were treated prophylactically for 4 weeks; similar results were obtained in simulations when 50 percent of the population in the model was immunized (Longini et al., 2004). The epidemic was extinguished when the TAP treatment was extended to 8 weeks, much as it was when 80 percent of the children in the model population were vaccinated. Vaccinating children, as opposed to adults, was found to increase the effectiveness of vaccination in this model (Longini et al., 2004).

Beyond the Biomedical Response

A comprehensive response to pandemic influenza should address far more than the disease itself. As several of the previously discussed pandemic plans have anticipated, a pandemic will introduce a plethora of legal and ethical dilemmas and political and economic consequences. It will also take place in a social context in which public perception of and reaction to an emergency strongly influences its impact. In light of these profound influences, workshop participants considered a variety of social perspectives on the coming pandemic: economic, legal, and ethical implications of various response options; opportunities for collaboration between public and private sectors; and public communication strategies to address both interpandemic and pandemic influenza.

"Insuring" the Pandemic Response

Pandemic preparations can be viewed as an insurance policy: an investment, accumulated over time, in anticipation of an eventual crisis (see Chapter 6) (Meltzer, 2004). The annual rate of investment in pandemic preparedness, the "premium" on the insurance policy, depends on the potential impact of pandemic influenza and its probability of occurrence in any given year. Using a relatively simple, conservative model, presenter Martin Meltzer and colleagues determined the total costs of a moderate (15 percent attack rate) and severe (35 percent attack rate) influenza pandemic, then calculated annual "premiums" to be paid on preparations against these losses based on the cost of vaccination (Meltzer et al., 1999).

The cost of vaccination, however, depends on the population segment that first receives the projected limited quantities of pandemic vaccine. Given the expected pattern of higher mortality in the elderly, it would be most cost effective to vaccinate high-risk people of working age, but more deaths would be prevented if the high-risk elderly are given priority (Meltzer et al., 1999). Only one of these outcomes can be maximized, so decision-makers must make the difficult choice among them. This requirement highlights the need for a system by which such a choice could be made, as well as a means to gain public understanding and support for the decision-making process (and thereby, for its outcome). Having chosen a goal, public health officials must be vigilant for changes in patterns of pandemic mortality, and be ready to adapt interventions to support the desired outcome.

To make optimal use of funds set aside for pandemic preparedness, decision-makers were advised to invest in activities that both ensure a strong pandemic response and enhance the response to annual influenza (Meltzer, 2004). These include improvements in surveillance (including support for surveillance in low-resource countries where a pandemic strain is likely to emerge), increasing vaccination rate among high-risk individuals (and perhaps providing a financial incentive to do so), and conducting planning and preparedness exercises to strengthen the response to a broad range of possible public health emergencies.

The Legal and Ethical Context

Legal authority should be brought to bear on nearly every facet of pandemic preparedness, from measures designed to reduce the risk of animal-to-human transmission of disease; to surveillance and detection procedures; to medical interventions to prevent or control the spread of infection; to the imposition of voluntary or mandatory quarantine and/or isolation measures; to travel limitations, trade restrictions, and border closures (see Gostin in Chapter 6) (Gostin, 2004b). Each of these interventions, while potentially beneficial to society, also imposes a burden on at least some of its members in the form of economic disadvantage, loss of political power, or sacrifice of human rights. Moreover, if these measures are to be effective, they should be imposed early in the course of a pandemic, before it can be scientifically ascertained whether they are actually warranted. Thus, it was argued, decision makers must undertake transparent and ethical deliberations in order to safeguard against the possibility of an unjustified and burdensome response to an apparent pandemic threat.

But public health law at many levels is not sufficiently robust to meet this daunting challenge. At the international level, efforts to ensure strong surveillance and response to infectious disease outbreaks are hampered by the outdated International Health Regulations, which are currently undergoing revision (Gostin, 2004a). Strong national infrastructures for public health law also need to be developed to support the delivery of essential services, assign public health powers, and safeguard human rights; unfortunately, no such foundation currently exists, because most public health statutes have been enacted in response to a specific (and therefore limited) threat or crisis. In response to this need, model public health laws are currently being developed for the United States (Center for Law and the Public's Health, 2001), and WHO is studying the development of a national public health law toolkit for worldwide distribution (Gostin, 2004b).

In addition to this legal framework, workshop participants were also urged to evaluate the ethics of public health interventions against pandemic influenza. Compelling ethical considerations include the need for transparency, the importance of anticipating and addressing stigmatization, the pursuit of human rights and social justice, and the fair distribution of scarce resources.

Coordinating Public and Private Sectors

The example of the Department of Veterans Affairs (VA) was used to illustrate a variety of opportunities for public–private partnership in addressing pandemic influenza, including the guaranteed advanced purchase of vaccine, the establishment of coordinated risk communications, the delivery of prophylaxis and treatment in home-based and other non-medical settings, and the removal of disincentives to sheltering in place for ill and exposed workers. Health policy within the VA system focuses on the use of information systems and outcomes measurement in clinical decision-making. This paradigm also supports the collection of standardized data that, if replicated in hospitals nationwide, could be used to build a national health information database—a possibility that has come one step closer to reality with the recent launch of a 10-year federal initiative to develop electronic medical records for most Americans (DHHS, 2004c).

Increasing Immunization Uptake

The previously described confluence of events that led to exceptionally high demand for immunization during the 2003–2004 flu season can be likened to a worst case scenario in order to increase uptake: let the disease come early, at the beginning of immunization season; let it be severe, strik-ing otherwise healthy people—even lethally, so that it makes headlines and causes medical experts to issue warnings of dire consequences. Unfortu-nately, a large component of this success depended on the timing and severity of the disease and so may not result in continued high immuniza-tion rates; however, this experience could also be seen as a dress rehearsal for communication during an influenza pandemic, with its attendant short-ages of vaccine and dire media reports.

Clear communication will be essential to obtaining adherence to mass vaccination campaigns during a pandemic, but it faces several challenges, particularly among people who consistently refuse annual flu shots. Mixed messages will be hard to avoid, particularly given the fact that only a minority (less than 40 percent) of health care workers are immunized each year. On the one hand, people with high priority to receive vaccine will need to be encouraged (and perhaps made afraid enough) to get it; others will need to be encouraged to wait calmly for their opportunity to receive vaccine while using non-medical measures to reduce their exposure to infec-tion. Unless public messages are tailored to gain the attention of specific segments of our racially and culturally diverse society, they are likely to be ignored.

The most effective way that public officials can avoid a damaging credibility problem in a pandemic, participants advised, is by sharing the dilemmas of pandemic control with the public in a productive and effective way—that is, by doing more than simply furnishing facts and figures. More research is needed to learn how to do this well; in the meantime, public health officials are advised to invest in targeted (as opposed to nuanced) and widely dispersed communications in order to sway as many "undecideds" as possible to the cause of influenza prevention and control (see Nowak in Chapter 6).

Public Communication Strategies

The history of public response to a variety of natural disasters demon-strates that people are capable of effective collective action in these circum-stances, and conversely, that failure to involve the general public in crisis response can increase the likelihood of social disruption (Glass and Schoch-Spana, 2002). Although it is widely believed that public support for a pandemic response can only be won through good communication, it is important to recognize that "good communication" is perceived differently by the communicator, who wants public cooperation and understanding in a time of crisis, and members of the public, who want inclusion, consider-ation, respect, expert guidance, and proof that officials have justly considered the public (see Schoch-Spana in Chapter 6). Risk communication,[18] a key component of the WHO pandemic plan and several national plans, attempts to bridge this gap by providing individuals and communities with information that allows them to make the best possible decisions about their well-being.

Systemic challenges make it difficult to get such messages out, however. Due to the multiplicity of contemporary media outlets, the significant decline in newspaper readership, and the lack of a public broadcast system (in the United States) public health messages should be broadly directed and more effectively coordinated among agencies and official channels that often compete for resources and notoriety. Although a more coordinated effort at the federal level is paramount, it was suggested that important information could be disseminated effectively through trusted sources in communities, such as physicians, neighborhood leaders, schools, or places of worship. It was also noted that official attitudes that equate overwhelming public requests for information with "panic" obscure an important opportunity for communication. Rather than view these demands as a distraction, communicators were advised to address the public's increased need for information as part of an emergency response (Schoch-Spana, 2000). Both the quality and quantity of information available to the public should address the fears as well as the facts about disease spread, and are key to promoting public security as well as more effective public health. Chapter 6 (see Schoch-Spana) describes the development of analytical tools for decision-makers to help them forge collaborations with the public during health crises.

REFERENCES

Americans cross border for flu shots. 2004. CNN. [Online]. Available: http://www.cnn.com/2004/HEALTH/conditions/10/20/fluvaccine.canada.ap/ [accessed November 10, 2004].

ASTHO (Association of State and Territorial Health Officials). 2002. *Nature's Terrorist Attack: Pandemic Influenza; Preparedness Planning for State Health Officials.* Washington, DC: ASTHO.

Barclay WS, Zambon M. 2004. Pandemic risks from bird flu. *BMJ* 328(7434):238–239.

Brown P. 2004 (June 16). *Ensuring an Adequate Stockpile of Antivirals.* Presentation at the Institute of Medicine Workshop on Pandemic Influenza: Assessing Capabilities for Prevention and Response. Washington, DC: Institute of Medicine Forum on Microbial Threats.

---

[18]Defined by CDC as the attempt by science or public health professionals to provide information that allows individuals, stakeholders, or an entire community to make the best possible decisions about their well-being, under nearly impossible time constraints, and to communicate those decisions, while accepting the imperfect nature of their choices (source: http://www.cdc.gov/communication/emergency/ercoverview.htm).

Buranathai C. 2004 (June 17). *Avian Influenza Outbreak in Thailand 2004.* Presentation at the Institute of Medicine Workshop on Pandemic Influenza: Assessing Capabilities for Prevention and Response. Washington, DC: Institute of Medicine Forum on Microbial Threats.

Cardona C. 2004 (June 17). Panel Discussion at the Institute of Medicine Workshop on Pandemic Influenza: Assessing Capabilities for Prevention and Response. Washington, DC: Institute of Medicine Forum on Microbial Threats.

CDC (Centers for Disease Control and Prevention). 2000. *FluAid Home.* [Online]. Available: http://www2.cdc.gov/od/fluaid/ [accessed November 10, 2004].

CDC. 2004a. Outbreaks of avian influenza A (H5N1) in Asia and interim recommendations for evaluation and reporting of suspected cases—United States. *MMWR* 53(05):97–100.

CDC. 2004b. *Interim Influenza Vaccination Recommendations—2004–05 Influenza Season.* [Online]. Available: http://www.cdc.gov/flu/protect/whoshouldget.htm [accessed November 10, 2004].

CDC. 2004c. *Pandemic Influenza Planning.* [Online]. Available: http://www.cdc.gov/programs/immun5.htm [accessed November 10, 2004].

Center for Law and the Public's Health. 2001. *Model State Emergency Health Powers Act and the Turning Point Model State Public Health Act.* [Online]. Available: http://www.publichealthlaw.net [accessed November 10, 2004].

Chen H, Deng G, Li Z, Tian G, Li Y, Jiao P, Zhang I, Liu Z, Webster RG, Yu K. 2004. The evolution of H5N1 influenza viruses in ducks in southern China. *Proc Natl Acad Sci USA* 101(28):10452–10457.

Coelingh K. 2004 (June 17). Panel Discussion at the Institute of Medicine Workshop on Pandemic Influenza: Assessing Capabilities for Prevention and Response. Washington, DC: Institute of Medicine Forum on Microbial Threats.

Cox N. 2004 (June 17). *Enhancing Influenza Surveillance: From the Global to Local Perspective.* Presentation at the Institute of Medicine Workshop on Pandemic Influenza: Assessing Capabilities for Prevention and Response. Washington, DC: Institute of Medicine Forum on Microbial Threats.

DHHS (Department of Health and Human Services). 2004a. *Pandemic Influenza Preparedness and Response Plan.* [Online]. Available: http://www.hhs.gov/nvpo/pandemicplan [accessed November 10, 2004].

DHHS. 2004b. *HHS Awards $849 Million to Improve Public Health Preparedness.* [Online]. Available: http://www.hhs.gov/news/press/2004pres/20040617.html [accessed November 10, 2004].

DHHS. 2004c. The decade of health information technology: Delivering consumer-centric and information-rich health care. *HHS Fact Sheet—HIT Report At-A-Glance.* [Online]. Available: http://www.hhs.gov/news/press/2004pres/20040721.html [accessed November 10, 2004].

Epstein SL. 2004 (June 16). *Strategies for Control of Influenza by Targeting Broadly Conserved Viral Features.* Presentation at the Institute of Medicine Workshop on Pandemic Influenza: Assessing Capabilities for Prevention and Response. Washington, DC: Institute of Medicine Forum on Microbial Threats.

Epstein SL, Tumpey TM, Misplon JA, Lo CY, Cooper LA, Subbarao K, Renshaw M, Sambhara S, Katz JM. 2002. DNA vaccine expressing conserved influenza virus proteins protective against H5N1 challenge infection in mice. *EID* 8(8):796–801.

Fedson DS. 2004a (June 16). Panel Discussion at the Institute of Medicine Workshop on Pandemic Influenza: Assessing Capabilities for Prevention and Response. Washington, DC: Institute of Medicine Forum on Microbial Threats.

Fedson DS. 2004b. Vaccination for pandemic influenza: A six point agenda for interpandemic years. *Pediatr Infect Dis J* 23:S74–S77.

GAO (General Accounting Office). 2000. *Influenza Pandemic: Plan Needed for Federal and State Response.* [Online]. Available: http://www.gao.gov/new.items/d014.pdf [accessed December 20, 2004].

Ge Q, Filip L, Bai A, Nguyen T, Eisen HN, Chen J. 2004. Inhibition of influenza virus production in virus-infected mice by RNA interference. *Proc Natl Acad Sci USA* 101(23):8676–8681.

Gellin B. 2004 (June 16). *U.S. Government Pandemic Influenza Preparedness Plan.* Presentation at the Institute of Medicine Workshop on Pandemic Influenza: Assessing Capabilities for Prevention and Response. Washington, DC: Institute of Medicine Forum on Microbial Threats.

Gensheimer KF, Meltzer MI, Postema AS, Strikas RA. 2003. Influenza pandemic preparedness. *EID* 9(12):1645–1648.

Glaser CA, Gilliam S, Thompson WW, Dassey DE, Waterman SH, Saruwatari M, Shapiro S, Fukuda K. 2002. Medical care capacity for influenza outbreaks, Los Angeles. *EID* 8(6):569–574.

Glass TA, Schoch-Spana M. 2002. Bioterrorism and people: How to vaccinate a city against panic. *Clinical Infectious Diseases* 34:217–223.

Gostin LO. 2004a. International infectious disease law: Revision of the World Health Organization's International Health Regulations. *JAMA* 291(21):2623–2627.

Gostin LO. 2004b (June 17). *Preparing the Legal System for Pandemic Influenza.* Presentation at the Institute of Medicine Workshop on Pandemic Influenza: Assessing Capabilities for Prevention and Response. Washington, DC: Institute of Medicine Forum on Microbial Threats.

Grove RD, Hetzel AM. 1968. *Vital Statistics Rates in the United States: 1940–1960.* Washington, DC: Government Printing Office.

Grundy G. 2004 (June 16). *Partnering with the Private Medical System.* Presentation at the Institute of Medicine Workshop on Pandemic Influenza: Assessing Capabilities for Prevention and Response. Washington, DC: Institute of Medicine Forum on Microbial Threats.

Guan Y, Poon LL, Cheung CY, Ellis TM, Lim W, Lipatov AS, Chan KH, Sturm-Ramirez KM, Cheung CL, Leung YH, Yuen KY, Webster RG, Peiris JS. 2004. H5N1 influenza: A protean pandemic threat. *Proc Natl Acad Sci USA* 101(21):8156–8161.

Harper SA, Fukuda K, Uyeki TM, Cox NJ, Bridges CB; Centers for Disease Control and Prevention Advisory Committee on Immunization Practices. 2004. Prevention and control of influenza: Recommendations of the Advisory Committee on Immunization Practices. *MMWR Recommendations and Reports* 53(RR-6):1–40.

Health Canada. 2004. *Canadian Pandemic Influenza Plan.* [Online]. Available: http://www.hc-sc.gc.ca/pphb-dgspsp/cpip-pclcpi/ [accessed December 20, 2004].

Health Protection Agency. 2004. *Number of Avian Flu Outbreaks in Thailand Reporting Period: 05/08/04 to 03/09/04.* [Online]. Available: http://www.hpa.org.uk/infections/topics_az/avianinfluenza/pdfs/Thailand_outbreak_map0904.pdf [accessed November 18, 2004].

Hosbach P. 2004 (June 16). *Vaccine Development and Production Issues.* Presentation at the Institute of Medicine Workshop on Pandemic Influenza: Assessing Capabilities for Prevention and Response. Washington, DC: Institute of Medicine Forum on Microbial Threats.

IOM (Institute of Medicine). 2004. *Learning from SARS.* Washington, DC: The National Academies Press.

Jones T, Allard F, Cyr SL, Tran SP, Plante M, Gauthier J, Bellerose N, Lowell GH, Burt DS. 2003. A nasal proteosome influenza vaccine containing baculovirus-delivered hemagglutinin induces protective mucosal and systemic immunity. *Vaccine* 21(25–26):3706–3712.

Kaiser L, Keene ON, Hammond JM, Elliott M, Hayden FG. 2000. Impact of zanamivir on antibiotic use for respiratory events following acute influenza in adolescents and adults. *Arch Intern Med* 160(21):3234–3240.

Kaiser L, Wat C, Mills T, Mahoney P, Ward P, Hayden F. 2003. Impact of oseltamivir treatment on influenza-related lower respiratory tract complications and hospitalizations. *Arch Intern Med* 163(14):1667–1672.

Keawcharoen J, Oraveerakul K, Kuiken T, Fouchier RAM, Amonsin A, Payungporn S, Noppornpanth S, Wattanodorn S, Theamboonlers A, Tantilertcharoen R, Pattanarangsan R, Arya N, Ratanakorn P, Osterhaus A, Poovorawan Y. 2004 (December). Avian influenza H5N1 in tigers and leopards. *Emerging Infectious Diseases*. [Online]. Available: http://www.cdc.gov/ncidod/EID/vol10no12/04-0759.htm [accessed December 10, 2004].

Kiso M, Mitamura K, Sakai-Tagawa Y, Shiraishi K, Kawakami C, Kimura K, Hayden FG, Sugaya N, Kawaoka Y. 2004. Resistant influenza A viruses in children treated with oseltamivir: Descriptive study. *Lancet* 364(9436):759–765.

Kobasa D, Takada A, Shinya K, Hatta M, Halfmann P, Theriault S, Suzuki H, Nishimura H, Mitamura K, Sugaya N, Usui T, Murata T, Maeda Y, Watanabe S, Suresh M, Suzuki T, Suzuki Y, Feldmann H, Kawaoka Y. 2004. Enhanced virulence of influenza A viruses with the haemagglutinin of the 1918 pandemic virus. *Nature* 431(7009):703–707.

Koch G. 2004 (June 17). *Some Lessons Learned from the Dutch Avian Influenza Outbreak 2003*. Presentation at the Institute of Medicine Workshop on Pandemic Influenza: Assessing Capabilities for Prevention and Response. Washington, DC: Institute of Medicine Forum on Microbial Threats.

Kuiken T, Rimmelzwaan G, van Riel D, van Amerongen G, Baars M, Fouchier R, Osterhaus A. 2004. Avian H5N1 influenza in cats. *Science* 306:241.

Lee CW, Senne DA, Suarez DL. 2004. Effect of vaccine use in the evolution of Mexican lineage H5N2 avian influenza virus. *J Virol* 78(15):8372–8381.

Li KS, Guan Y, Wang J, Smith GJ, Xu KM, Duan L, Rahardjo AP, Puthavathana P, Buranathai C, Nguyen TD, Estoepangestie AT, Chaisingh A, Auewarakul P, Long HT, Hanh NT, Webby RJ, Poon LL, Chen H, Shortridge KF, Yuen KY, Webster RG, Peiris JS. 2004. Genesis of a highly pathogenic and potentially pandemic H5N1 influenza virus in eastern Asia. *Nature* 430(6996):209–213.

Linder FE, Grove RD. 1943. *Vital Statistics Rates in the United States: 1900–1940*. Washington, DC: Government Printing Office.

Liu M, Guan Y, Peiris M, He S, Webby RJ, Perez D, Webster RG. 2003. The quest of influenza A viruses for new hosts. *Avian Diseases* 47:849–856.

Longini IM. 2004 (June 16). *Mathematical Modeling: Containing Pandemic Influenza with Vaccines and Antivirals*. Presentation at the Institute of Medicine Workshop on Pandemic Influenza: Assessing Capabilities for Prevention and Response. Washington, DC: Institute of Medicine Forum on Microbial Threats.

Longini IM Jr, Halloran ME, Nizam A, Yang Y. 2004. Containing pandemic influenza with antiviral agents. *Am J Epidemiol* 159:623–633.

Lovgren S. 2004. Cats can catch and spread bird flu, study says. *Stefan Lovgren for National Geographic News*. [Online]. Available: http://news.nationalgeographic.com/news/2004/09/0902_040902_birdflu.html#main [accessed November 10, 2004].

Marchione M. 2004. *Pandemic Risk Spurs Flu Vaccine Planning*. [Online]. Available: http://www.washingtonpost.com/wp-dyn/articles/A13922-2004Oct31.html [accessed November 10, 2004].

Meltzer M. 2004 (June 16). *"Insuring" a Better Response*. Presentation at the Institute of Medicine Workshop on Pandemic Influenza: Assessing Capabilities for Prevention and Response. Washington, DC: Institute of Medicine Forum on Microbial Threats.

Meltzer MI, Cox NJ, Fukuda K. 1999. The economic impact of pandemic influenza in the United States: Priorities for intervention. *Emerging Infectious Diseases* 5(5):659–671.

Millar JD. 1977 (June 27). The Swine Flu Program: An unprecedented venture in preventive medicine. Report to the Congress by the Comptroller General of the United States. HRD-77-115. Washington, DC: Department of Health, Education, and Welfare.

Monto AS. 2003. The role of antivirals in the control of influenza. *Vaccine* 21(16):1796–1800.

Nguyen TD. 2004 (June 17). *Retrospection into Avian Influenza Outbreak in Vietnam during 2003-04*. Presentation at the Institute of Medicine Workshop on Pandemic Influenza: Assessing Capabilities for Prevention and Response. Washington, DC: Institute of Medicine Forum on Microbial Threats.

Nichol KL. 2003. The efficacy, effectiveness, and cost-effectiveness of inactivated influenza vaccines. *Vaccine* 2003:1769–1775.

NISN (Neuraminidase Inhibitor Susceptibility Network). 2004 (August 13). Neuraminidase Inhibitor Susceptibility Network statement. *Weekly Epidemiological Record* 79:306–308. [Online]. Available: http://www.who.int/wer/2004/en/wer7933/en/ [accessed November 10, 2004].

Nowak G. 2004 (June 17). *Increasing Awareness and Uptake of Influenza Immunization*. Presentation at the Institute of Medicine Workshop on Pandemic Influenza: Assessing Capabilities for Prevention and Response. Washington, DC: Institute of Medicine Forum on Microbial Threats.

Noymer A, Garenne M. 2000. The 1918 influenza epidemic's effects on sex differentials in mortality in the United States. *Population and Development Review* 26(3):565–581.

OIE (Office International des Epizooties). 2004. *Disease Information*. 17(36). [Online]. Available: http://www.oie.int/eng/info/hebdo/a_current.htm#Sec0 [accessed December 21, 2004].

Perrotta D. 2004 (June 16). Panel Discussion at the Institute of Medicine Workshop on Pandemic Influenza: Assessing Capabilities for Prevention and Response. Washington, DC: Institute of Medicine Forum on Microbial Threats.

Petola VT, McCullers JA. 2004. Respiratory viruses predisposing to bacterial infections: Role of neuraminidase. *Pediatr Infect Dis J* 23:S87–S97.

ProMED-mail. 2004a. PRO/AH/EDR> Avian influenza, human—East Asia (52): update. Published date: October 4, 2004. Archive number: 20041004.2738. Available at http://www.promedmail.org.

ProMED-mail. 2004b (August 31). PRO/AD/EDR> Avian influenza, human—East Asia (38). Published date: August 31, 2004. Archive number: 20040813.2249. Available at http://www.promedmail.org. Source: WHO Outbreak News, 13 August 2004 [edited]: http://www.who.int/csr/don/2004_08_13/en/print.html. "Human cases of avian influenza: situation in Viet Nam."

ProMED-mail. 2004c (September 29). PRO/AH/EDR> Avian influenza, human—East Asia (49): Viet Nam. Archive number: 20040929.2692. Available at http://www.promedmail.org.

ProMED-mail. 2004d. PRO/AH/EDR> Avian influenza—Eastern Asia (98): Viet Nam, Thailand. Published date: July 27, 2004. Archive number: 20040727.2058. Available at http://www.promedmail.org.

ProMED-mail. 2004e. PRO/AH/EDR> Avian influenza, human—East Asia (46): Thailand, susp. Published date: September 25, 2004. Archive number: 20040925.2647. Available at http://www.promedmail.org.

ProMED-mail. 2004f. PRO/AH/EDR> Influenza vaccine 2004/2005—N. hemisphere (02): supply. Published date: October 5, 2004. Archive number: 20041005.2742. Available at http: //www.promedmail.org.

ProMED-mail. 2004g. Avian influenza—eastern Asia (78): Thailand, cats. Published date: June 17, 2004. Archive number: 20040617.1614. Available at http://www.promedmail.org. Source: The Messybeast Cat Resource Archive: 16 June 2004 [edited]: http://www.messybeast.com/zoonoses.htm. "Asian Bird Flu." Byline: Sarah Hartwell.

ProMED-mail. 2004h. PRO/AH/EDR> Avian influenza—Eastern Asia (127): Thailand, tigers. Published date: Oct 19, 2004. Archive number: 20041019.2838. Available at http://www.promedmail.org.

ProMED-mail. 2004i. PRO/AD/EDR> Avian influenza—Eastern Asia (128): Thailand, tigers. Published date: October 22, 2004. Archive number: 20041022.2862. Available at http://www.promedmail.org.

ProMED-mail. 2004j. PRO/AD/EDR> Avian influenza, poultry vaccines (08). Published date: March 24, 2004. Archive number: 20040325.0829. Available at http://promedmail.org. Source: New Scientist, 24 Mar 04 [edited]: http://www.newscientist.com/news/news.jsp?id=ns99994810. "Bird vaccination could lead to new strains." Byline: Debora MacKenzie.

ProMED-mail. 2004k (July 16). PRO/AH/EDR> Avian influenza—Eastern Asia (92). Published date: July 16, 2004. Archive number: 20040716.1925. Available at http://www.promedmail.org. Source: The Jakarta Post, 16 July 2004 [edited]: http://www.thejakartapost.com/detailcity.asp?fileid=20040716.G04&i. "IPB, Japan to produce bird flu super vaccine." Byline: Theresia Sufa.

ProMED-mail. 2004l (July 16). PRO/AH/EDR> Avian influenza—Eastern Asia (92). Published date: July 16, 2004. Archive number: 20040716.1925. Available at http://www.promedmail.org. Source: ABC Online [Australia]: 16 July 2004 [edited]: http://www.abc.net.au/news/newsitems/200407/s1155030.htm. "More bird flu outbreaks in Viet Nam."

ProMED-mail. 2004m (July 2). PRO/AH/EDR> Avian influenza—Eastern Asia (83): Viet Nam. Published date: July 2, 2004. Archive number: 20040702.1771. Available at http://www.promedmail.org. Source: Taipei Times: http://www.taipeitimes.com/News/world/archives/2004/07/02/20031773. "Mekong bird flu may be spreading to nearby province."

ProMED-mail. 2004n (July 3). PRO/AH/EDR> Influenza activity update 2003/2004—worldwide. Published date: July 3, 2004. Archive number: 20040703.1776. Available at http://www.promedmail.org.

ProMED-mail. 2004o (August 9). PRO/AH/EDR. Avian influenza—Eastern Asia (103): FAO. Published date: August 9, 2004. Archive number: 20040809.2196. Available at http://www.promedmail.org.

ProMED-mail. 2004p. PRO/AH/EDR> Avian influenza—Belgium ex Thailand: smuggled birds (02): OIE. Published date: October 27, 2004. Archive number: 20041027.2907. Available at http://www.promedmail.org.

ProMED-mail 2004q (July 30). PRO/AH/EDR> Avian influenza—Eastern Asia (100). Published date: July 30, 2004. Archive number: 20040730.2078. Available at http://www.promedmail.org. Source: WHO: http://www.who.int/csr/don/2004_07_30/en/. "Avian influenza—assessment of the current situation."

ProMED-mail. 2004r (July 29). PRO/AH/EDR> Avian influenza—Eastern Asia (99). Published date: July 29, 2004. Archive number: 20040729.2069. Available at http://www.promedmail.org. Source: Sapa-AFP via IOL South Africa, 28 July 2004 [edited]: http://www.iol.co.za/index.php?set_id=1&click_id=31&art_id=qw109099908550B221. "UN to recommend wider use of bird flu vaccine."

ProMED-mail. 2004s. PRO/AD/EDR> Avian influenza, poultry vaccines (08). Published date: March 24, 2004. Archive number: 20040325.0829. Available at http://promedmail.org. Source: New Scientist, 24 Mar 2004 [edited]: http://newscientest.com/news/news.jsp?id=ns99994810. "Bird flue vaccination could lead to new strains."

ProMED-mail. 2004t. PRO/AD/EDR> Avian influenza A/H5N1, migratory birds—Russia (Siberia). Published date: October 28, 2004. Archive number: 20041028.2911. Available at http://promedmail.org.

ProMED-mail. 2004u. (July 30). PRO/AH/EDR> Avian influenza—Eastern Asia (100). Published date: July 30, 2004. Archive number: 20040730.2078. Available at http://www.promedmail.org. Source: WHO: http://www.who.int/csr/don/2004_07_30/en/. "Avian influenza—assessment of the current situation."

ProMED-mail. 2004v (October 25). PRO/AH/EDR> Avian influenza, human—Thailand (08). Published date: October 25, 2004. Archive number: 20041025.2886. Available at http://www.promedmail.org.

ProMED-mail. 2004w. Avian influenza—Eastern Asia (137): Viet Nam. Published date: November 19, 2004. Archive number: 20041119.3103. Available at http://www.promedmail.org.

ProMED-mail. 2005. PRO/AH/EDR> Avian influenza—Eastern Asia (14). Published date: February 1, 2005. Archive number: 20050201.0348. Available at http://www.promedmail.org.

Schoch-Spana M. 2000. Implications of pandemic influenza for bioterrorism response. *Clin Infect Dis.* 31(6):1409–1413.

Shult P. 2004 (June 16). Panel Discussion at the Institute of Medicine Workshop on Pandemic Influenza: Assessing Capabilities for Prevention and Response. Washington, DC: Institute of Medicine Forum on Microbial Threats.

Sibartie D. 2004 (June 17). *Strategies for Preventing and Controlling Avian Influenza and its Transmission Within the Bird and Animal Population.* Presentation at the Institute of Medicine Workshop on Pandemic Influenza: Assessing Capabilities for Prevention and Response. Washington, DC: Institute of Medicine Forum on Microbial Threats.

Simonsen L. 2004 (June 17). *Pandemic Influenza and Mortality: Past Evidence and Projections for the Future.* Presentation at the Institute of Medicine Workshop on Pandemic Influenza: Assessing Capabilities for Prevention and Response. Washington, DC: Institute of Medicine Forum on Microbial Threats.

Slater E. 2004. Industry and government perspective in influenza control. *Texas Heart Institute Journal* 31(1):42–44.

Soebandrio A. 2004 (June 17). *Avian Influenza: Indonesian Experience.* Presentation at the Institute of Medicine Workshop on Pandemic Influenza: Assessing Capabilities for Prevention and Response. Washington, DC: Institute of Medicine Forum on Microbial Threats.

State of California. 2003. State of California Hospital Bioterrorism Preparedness Program: 2003 Implementation Plan. Emergency Medical Services Authority, Department of Health Services, State of California. Pp. 1–6, 35–36.

Stöhr K. 2004 (June 16). *Priority Public Health Interventions Before and During an Influenza Pandemic.* Presentation at the Institute of Medicine Workshop on Pandemic Influenza: Assessing Capabilities for Prevention and Response. Washington, DC: Institute of Medicine Forum on Microbial Threats.

Swayne D. 2004 (June 17). Panel Discussion at the Institute of Medicine Workshop on Pandemic Influenza: Assessing Capabilities for Prevention and Response. Washington, DC: Institute of Medicine Forum on Microbial Threats.

Taubenberger J. 2004 (June 16). *Chasing the Elusive Virus: Preparing for the Future by Examining the Past.* Presentation at the Institute of Medicine Workshop on Pandemic Influenza: Assessing Capabilities for Prevention and Response. Washington, DC: Institute of Medicine Forum on Microbial Threats.

Tompkins SM, Lo C-Y, Tumpey TM, Epstein SL. 2004. Protection against lethal influenza virus challenge by RNA interference in vivo. *Proc Natl Acad Sci USA* 101(23):8682–8686.

Trampuz A, Prabhu RM, Smith TF, Baddour LM. 2004. Avian influenza: A new pandemic threat? *Mayo Clinic Proc.* 79:523-530.

Tran TH, Nguyen TL, Nguyen TD, Luong TS, Pham PM, Nguyen VC, Pham TS, Vo CD, Le TQ, Ngo TT, Dao BK, Le PP, Nguyen TT, Hoang TL, Cao VT, Le TG, Nguyen DT, Le HN, Nguyen KT, Le HS, Le VT, Christiane D, Tran TT, Menno de J, Schultsz C, Cheng P, Lim W, Horby P, Farrar J; World Health Organization International Avian Influenza Investigative Team. 2004. Avian influenza A (H5N1) in 10 patients in Vietnam. *N Engl J Med* 350(12):1179-1188.

Treanor JJ, Hayden FG, Vrooman PS, Barbarash R, Bettis R, Riff D, Singh S, Kinnersley N, Ward P, Mills RG. 2000. Efficacy and safety of the oral neuraminidase inhibitor oseltamivir in treating acute influenza: A randomized controlled trial. U.S. Oral Neuraminidase Study Group. *JAMA* 283(8):1016-1024.

Ungchusak K, Auewarakul P, Dowell SF, Kitphati R, Auwanit W, Puthavathana P, Uiprasertkul M, Boonnak K, Pittayawonganon C, Cox NJ, Zaki SR, Thawatsupha P, Chittaganpitch M, Khontong R, Simmerman JM, Chunsutthiwat S. 2005. Probable person-to-person transmission of avian influenza A (H5N1). *N Engl J Med* 352(4):333-340.

U.S. Department of Commerce. 1976. *Historical Statistics of the United States: Colonial Times to 1970.* Washington, DC: Government Printing Office.

Vastag B. 2002. Experts urge bioterrorism readiness. *JAMA* 285(1):30-32.

Webby RJ, Webster RG. 2003. Are we ready for pandemic influenza? *Science* 302:1519-1522.

Webster R. 2004a (June 17). *A Report from the Field: The 2003/2004 H5N1 Outbreak.* Presentation at the Institute of Medicine Workshop on Pandemic Influenza: Assessing Capabilities for Prevention and Response. Washington, DC: Institute of Medicine Forum on Microbial Threats.

Webster R. 2004b. Wet markets—a continuing source of Severe Acute Respiratory Syndrome and influenza? *Lancet* 363:234-236.

Webster RG. 1998. Influenza: An emerging infectious disease. *Emerg Infect Dis* 4:436-441.

WHO (World Health Organization). 1999. *Influenza Pandemic Plan.* WHO/CDS/CSR/EDC/99.1. [Online]. Available: http://www.who.int/csr/resources/publications/influenza/WHO_CDS_CSR_EDC_99_1/en/ [accessed November 10, 2004].

WHO. 2004a. *WHO Consultation on Priority Public Health Interventions Before and During an Influenza Pandemic.* [Online]. Available: http://www.who.int/csr/disease/avian_influenza/consultation/en/ [accessed November 10, 2004].

WHO. 2004b. Development of a vaccine effective against avian influenza H5N1 infection in humans. *Wkly Epidemiol Rec* 79:25-26.

WHO. 2004c (October 29). *Avian Influenza—Situation in Asia: Altered Role of Domestic Ducks.* [Online]. Available: http://www.who.int/csr/don/2004_10_29/en/print.html [accessed November 10, 2004].

WHO. 2004d. *Cumulative Number of Confirmed Human Cases of Avian Influenza A (H5N1) Since 28 January 2004.* [Online]. Available: http://www.who.int/csr/disease/avian_influenza/country/cases_table_2004_10_25/en/ [accessed November 10, 2004].

1

The Story of Influenza

OVERVIEW

In the early 20th century, science was sufficiently sophisticated to anticipate that influenza, which had twice reached pandemic proportions in the late 19th century, would recur, but was largely powerless to blunt the devastating impact of the 1918 (H1N1) pandemic. Since then, mankind has gained several advantages against the disease: experience of three better characterized pandemics (1918, 1957, and 1968); knowledge of influenza viruses; capacity to design and manufacture vaccines and antiviral drugs to forestall (if not prevent) infection; and molecular technology that may one day pinpoint the viral components that produce virulence, and thereby identify targets for more effective vaccines and drugs.

Yet the world is vulnerable to the next pandemic, perhaps even more than in 1918, when the pace and frequency of global travel was considerably less than today. As the contributors to this chapter demonstrate, there is still much to be learned from past pandemics that can strengthen defenses against future threats. The chapter begins with a review of the events of 1918, the lessons they offer, and the historical and scientific questions they raise. It describes the epidemiology and symptomology of that deadly viral strain, limited efforts toward prevention and treatment, and the resulting social disruption and its exacerbation by the actions of public officials and the media.

The chapter continues with an account of molecular studies underway to determine the origin of the 1918 virus and the source(s) of its exceptional virulence. Clues are being sought by examining viruses preserved in frozen and fixed tissues of victims of the 1918 flu. Characterization of five of the eight RNA segments of the 1918 influenza virus indicates that it was the common ancestor of both subsequent human and swine H1N1 lineages, and experiments testing models of virulence using reverse genetics approaches with 1918 influenza genes have begun in hopes of identifying genetic features that confer virulence in humans.

In a parallel effort, subsequently described, epidemiologists are analyzing death records and serological data to better understand patterns of transmission, morbidity, and mortality in past influenza pandemics. Such findings could inform planning for public health interventions to reduce the incidence of severe outcomes in future pandemics. In particular, these studies reveal a signature change in excess mortality from the elderly to younger age groups, a "pandemic age shift," that occurred with each of the three pandemics of the 20th century. If such a shift could be recognized in incipient pandemics, it might allow sufficient time for the production and distribution of vaccine and antiviral drugs before the worst pandemic impact occurs.

1918 REVISITED:
LESSONS AND SUGGESTIONS FOR FURTHER INQUIRY

John M. Barry

Distinguished Visiting Scholar
Center for Bioenvironmental Research at Tulane and
Xavier Universities

The 1918–1919 influenza pandemic killed more people in absolute numbers than any other disease outbreak in history. A contemporary estimate put the death toll at 21 million, a figure that persists in the media today, but understates the real number. Epidemiologists and scientists have revised that figure several times since then. Each and every revision has been upward. Frank Macfarlane Burnet, who won his Nobel Prize for immunology but who spent most of his life studying influenza, estimated the death toll as probably 50 million, and possibly as high as 100 million. A 2002 epidemiologic study also estimates the deaths at between 50 and 100 million (Johnson and Mueller, 2002).

The world population in 1918 was only 28 percent of today's population. Adjusting for population, a comparable toll today would be 175 to 350 million. By comparison, at this writing AIDS has killed approximately 24 million, and an estimated 40 million more people are infected with the virus.

A letter from a physician at one U.S. Army camp to a colleague puts a more human face on those numbers:

> These men start with what appears to be an ordinary attack of LaGrippe or Influenza, and when brought to the Hosp. they very rapidly develop the most vicious type of Pneumonia that has ever been seen . . . and a few hours later you can begin to see the Cyanosis extending from their ears and spreading all over the face, until it is hard to distinguish the colored men from the white. It is only a matter of a few hours then until death comes. . . . It is horrible. One can stand it to see one, two or twenty men die, but to see these poor devils dropping like flies. . . . We have been averaging about 100 deaths per day. . . . Pneumonia means in about all cases death. . . . We have lost an outrageous number of Nurses and Drs. It takes special trains to carry away the dead. For several days there were no coffins and the bodies piled up something fierce. . . . It beats any sight they ever had in France after a battle. An extra long barracks has been vacated for the use of the Morgue, and it would make any man sit up and take notice to walk down the long lines of dead soldiers all dressed and laid out in double rows. . . . Good By old Pal, God be with you till we meet again (Grist, 1979).

That letter reflected a typical experience in American Army cantonments. The civilian experience was not much better.

In preparing for another pandemic, it is useful to examine events of 1918 for lessons, warnings, and areas for further inquiry.

The Virus Itself

The pandemic in 1918 was hardly the first influenza pandemic, nor was it the only lethal one. Throughout history, there have been influenza pandemics, some of which may have rivaled 1918's lethality. A partial listing of particularly violent outbreaks likely to have been influenza include one in 1510 when a pandemic believed to come from Africa "attacked at once and raged all over Europe not missing a family and scarce a person" (Beveridge, 1977). In 1580, another pandemic started in Asia, then spread to Africa, Europe, and even America (despite the fact that it took 6 weeks to cross the ocean). It was so fierce "that in the space of six weeks it afflicted almost all the nations of Europe, of whom hardly the twentieth person was free of the disease" and some Spanish cities were "nearly entirely depopulated by the disease" (Beveridge, 1977). In 1688, influenza struck England, Ireland, and Virginia; in all these places "the people dyed . . . as in a plague" (Duffy, 1953). A mutated or new virus continued to plague Europe and America again in 1693 and Massachusetts in 1699. "The sickness extended to almost all families. Few or none escaped, and many dyed especially in Boston, and some dyed in a strange or unusual manner, in some families all were sick together, in some towns almost all were sick so that it was a time of disease" (Pettit, 1976). In London in 1847 and 1848, more people died from influenza than from the terrible cholera epidemic of 1832. In 1889 and 1890, a great and violent worldwide pandemic struck again (Beveridge, 1977).

But 1918 seems to have been particularly violent. It began mildly, with a spring wave. In fact, it was so mild that some physicians wonder if this disease actually was influenza. Typically, several Italian doctors argued in separate journal articles that this "febrile disease now widely prevalent in Italy [is] not influenza" (Policlinico, 1918). British doctors echoed that conclusion; a *Lancet* article in July 1918 argued that the spring epidemic was not influenza because the symptoms, though similar to influenza, were "of very short duration and so far absent of relapses or complications" (Little et al., 1918).

Within a few weeks of that *Lancet* article appearing, a second pandemic wave swept around the world. It also initially caused investigators to doubt that the disease was influenza—but this time because it was so virulent. It was followed by a third wave in 1919, and significant disease also struck in 1920. (Victims of the first wave enjoyed significant resistance to the second and third waves, offering compelling evidence that all were caused by the same virus. It is worth noting that the 1889–1890 pandemic also came in waves, but the third wave seemed to be the most lethal.)

The 1918 virus, especially in its second wave, was not only virulent and lethal, but extraordinarily violent. It created a range of symptoms rarely seen with the disease. After H5N1 first appeared in 1997, pathologists reported some findings "not previously described with influenza" (To et al., 2001). In fact, investigators in 1918 described every pathological change seen with H5N1 and more (Jordon, 1927: 266–268).

Symptoms in 1918 were so unusual that initially influenza was misdiagnosed as dengue, cholera, or typhoid. One observer wrote, "One of the most striking of the complications was hemorrhage from mucous membranes, especially from the nose, stomach, and intestine. Bleeding from the ears and petechial hemorrhages in the skin also occurred" (Ireland, 1928: 57). A German investigator recorded "hemorrhages occurring in different parts of the interior of the eye" with great frequency (Thomson and Thomson, 1934b). An American pathologist noted: "Fifty cases of subconjunctival hemorrhage were counted. Twelve had a true hemotypsis, bright red blood with no admixture of mucus. . . . Three cases had intestinal hemorrhage" (Ireland, 1928: 13). The New York City Health Department's chief pathologist said, "Cases with intense pain look and act like cases of dengue . . . hemorrhage from nose or bronchi . . . paresis or paralysis of either cerebral or spinal origin . . . impairment of motion may be severe or mild, permanent or temporary . . . physical and mental depression. Intense and protracted prostration led to hysteria, melancholia, and insanity with suicidal intent" (Jordon, 1927: 265).

The 1918 virus also targeted young adults. In South African cities, those between the ages of 20 and 40 accounted for 60 percent of the deaths (Katzenellenbogen, 1988). In Chicago the deaths among those aged 20 to 40 nearly quintupled deaths of those aged 41 to 60 (Van Hartesveldt, 1992). A Swiss physician "saw no severe case in anyone over 50."[1] In the "registration area" of the United States—those states and cities that kept reliable statistics—the single greatest number of deaths occurred in the cohort aged 25 to 29, the second greatest in those aged 30 to 34, and the third in those aged 20 to 24. More people died in each one of those 5-year groups than the total deaths among all those over age 60, and the combined deaths of those aged 20 to 34 more than doubled the deaths of all those over 50 (U.S. Bureau of the Census, 1921). The single group most likely to die if infected were pregnant women. In 13 studies of hospitalized pregnant women during the 1918 pandemic, the death rate ranged from 23 to 71 percent (Jordon, 1927: 273). Of the pregnant women who survived, 26 percent lost the child (Harris, 1919). (As far back as 1557, people connected influenza with miscarriage and the death of pregnant women.)

The case mortality rate varied widely. An overall figure is impossible to obtain, or even estimate reliably, because no solid information about total cases exists. In U.S. Army camps where reasonably reliable statistics were kept, case mortality often exceeded 5 percent, and in some circumstances exceeded 10 percent. In the British Army in India, case mortality for white troops was 9.6 percent, for Indian troops 21.9 percent.

In isolated human populations, the virus killed at even higher rates. In the Fiji islands, it killed 14 percent of the entire population in 16 days. In Labrador and Alaska, it killed at least one-third of the entire native population (Jordon, 1927; Rice, 1988).

But perhaps most disturbing and most relevant for today is the fact that a significant minority—and in some subgroups of the population a majority—of deaths came directly from the virus, not from secondary bacterial pneumonias.

In 1918, pathologists were intimately familiar with the condition of lungs of victims of bacterial pneumonia at autopsy. But the viral pneumonias caused by the influenza pandemic were so violent that many investigators said the only lungs they had seen that resembled them were from victims of poison gas.

---

[1] *Correspondenz-Blatt für Schweizer Aerzte*, Basel, 11/5/18. 48, #40, "influenza epidemic," E. bircher, p. 1338, quoted in *JAMA* 71(23):1946.

Then, the Army called them "atypical pneumonias." Today we would call this atypical pneumonia Acute Respiratory Distress Syndrome (ARDS). The Army's pneumonia board judged that "more than half" of all the deaths among soldiers came from this atypical pneumonia (Ireland, 1928).

One cannot extrapolate from this directly to the civilian population. Army figures represent a special case both in terms of demographics and environment, including overcrowded barracks.

Even so, the fact that ARDS likely caused more than half the deaths among young adults sends a warning. ARDS mortality rates today range from 40 to 60 percent, even with support in modern intensive care units (ICUs). In a pandemic, ICUs would be quickly overwhelmed, representing a major challenge for public health planners.

Treatment and Prevention in 1918

Physicians tried everything they knew, everything they had ever heard of, from the ancient art of bleeding patients, to administering oxygen, to developing new vaccines and sera (chiefly against what we now call Hemophilus influenzae—a name derived from the fact that it was originally considered the etiological agent—and several types of pneumococci). Only one therapeutic measure, transfusing blood from recovered patients to new victims, showed any hint of success.

George Whipple, later a Nobel laureate, studied numerous vaccines and sera and found them "without therapeutic benefit." But of some vaccines he said, "The statistical evidence, so far as it goes, indicates a probability . . . [of] some prophylactic value."[2] Some bacterial vaccines may have prevented particular secondary pneumonias.

Meanwhile, the public used home remedies of every description. None showed any evidence of effect.

Some nonmedical interventions did succeed. Total isolation, cutting a community off from the outside world, did work if done early enough. Gunnison, Colorado, a town that was a rail center and was large enough to have a college, succeeded in isolating itself. So did Fairbanks, Alaska. American Samoa escaped without a single case, while a few miles away in Western Samoa, 22 percent of the entire population died.

More interestingly—and perhaps importantly—an Army study found that isolating both individual victims and entire commands that contained infected soldiers "failed when and where [these measures] were carelessly

---

[2]*JAMA* 71(16):1317 current comment, Vaccines in influenza.

applied," but "did some good . . . when and where they were rigidly carried out" (Soper, undated draft report).

Even if isolation only slowed the virus, it had some value. One of the more interesting epidemiologic findings in 1918 was that the later in the second wave someone got sick, the less likely he or she was to die, and the more mild the illness was likely to be.

This was true in terms of how late in the second wave the virus struck a given area, and, more curiously, it was also true within an area. That is, cities struck later tended to suffer less, and individuals in a given city struck later also tended to suffer less. Thus west coast American cities, hit later, had lower death rates than east coast cities, and Australia, which was not hit by the second wave until 1919, had the lowest death rate of any developed country.

Again, more curiously, someone who got sick 4 days into an outbreak in one place was more likely to develop a viral pneumonia that progressed to ARDS than someone who got sick 4 weeks into the outbreak in the same place. They were also more likely to develop a secondary bacterial pneumonia, and to die from it.

The best data on this comes from the U.S. Army. Of the Army's 20 largest cantonments, in the first five affected, roughly 20 percent of all soldiers with influenza developed pneumonia. Of those, 37.3 percent died (Soper, 1918; undated draft report).

In the last five camps affected—on average 3 weeks later—only 7.1 percent of influenza victims developed pneumonia. Only 17.8 percent of the soldiers who developed pneumonia died (Soper, 1918).

Inside each camp the same trend held true. Soldiers struck down early died at much higher rates than soldiers in the same camp struck down late.

Similarly, the first cities struck—Boston, Baltimore, Pittsburgh, Philadelphia, Louisville, New York, New Orleans, and smaller cities hit at the same time—all suffered grievously. But in those same places, the people struck by influenza later in the epidemic were not becoming as ill, and were not dying at the same rate, as those struck in the first 2 to 3 weeks.

Cities struck later in the epidemic also usually had lower mortality rates. One of the most careful epidemiologic studies of the epidemic was conducted in Connecticut. The investigator noted that "one factor that appeared to affect the mortality rate was proximity in time to the original outbreak at New London, the point at which the disease was first introduced into Connecticut. . . . The virus was most virulent or most readily communicable when it first reached the state, and thereafter became generally attenuated" (Thompson and Thompson, 1934a: 215).

The same pattern held true throughout the country and the world. It was not a rigid predictor. The virus was never completely consistent. But places hit later tended to suffer less.

One obvious hypothesis that might explain this phenomenon is that medical care improved as health care workers learned how to cope with the disease. But this hypothesis collapses upon examination. In a given city, as the epidemic proceeded, medical care disintegrated. Doctors and nurses were overworked and sick themselves, and victims—possibly even a majority of victims—received no care at all late in an epidemic.

Even in Army camps, where one could expect communication between physicians from one camp to the next, there seemed to be no improvements in medical care that could account for the different mortality rates. A distinguished investigator specifically looked for evidence of improved care or better preventive measures in Army camps and found none.

A second obvious explanatory hypothesis, that the most vulnerable people were struck first, also fails. For that hypothesis to be true, Americans on the east coast had to have been more vulnerable than those on the west coast, and Americans and western Europeans had to have been more vulnerable than Australians.

But another hypothesis, although entirely speculative, may be worth exploring. If one steps back and looks at the entire United States, it seems that people across the country infected with the virus in September and early to mid-October suffered the most severe attacks. Those infected later, in whatever part of the country they were, suffered less.

At the peak of the pandemic, then, the virus seemed to still be mutating rapidly, virtually with each passage through humans, and it was mutating toward a less lethal form.

We do know that after a mild spring wave, after a certain number of passages through humans, a lethal virus evolved. Possibly after additional passages it became less virulent. This makes sense particularly if the virus was immature when it erupted in September, if it entered the human population only a few months before the lethal wave.

This hypothesis may suggest some areas for investigation.

Social Disruption and Public Health Lessons

In the United States, national and local government and public health authorities badly mishandled the epidemic, offering a useful case study.

The context is important. Every country engaged in World War I tried to control public perception. To avoid hurting morale, even in the nonlethal first wave the press in countries fighting in the war did not mention the outbreak. (But Spain was not at war and its press wrote about it, so the pandemic became known as the Spanish flu).

The United States was no different. In 1917 California Senator Hiram Johnson made the since-famous observation that "The first casualty when war comes is truth." The U.S. government passed a law that made it punishable by 20 years in jail to "utter, print, write or publish any disloyal, profane, scurrilous, or abusive language about the government of the United States."

One could go to jail for cursing or criticizing the government, even if what one said was true. A Congressman was jailed. Simultaneously, the government mounted a massive propaganda effort. An architect of that effort said, "Truth and falsehood are arbitrary terms. . . . There is nothing in experience to tell us that one is always preferable to the other. . . . The force of an idea lies in its inspirational value. It matters very little if it is true or false" (Vaughn, 1980).

The combination of rigid control and disregard for truth had dangerous consequences. Focusing on the shortest term, local officials almost universally told half-truths or outright lies to avoid damaging morale and the war effort. They were assisted—not challenged—by the press, which although not censored in a technical sense cooperated fully with the government's propaganda machine.

Routinely, as influenza approached a city or town—one could watch it march from place to place—local officials initially told the public not to worry, that public health officials would prevent the disease from striking them. When influenza first appeared, officials routinely insisted at first it was only ordinary influenza, not the Spanish flu. As the epidemic exploded, officials almost daily assured the public that the worst was over.

This pattern repeated itself again and again. Chicago offers one example: Its public health commissioner said he'd do "nothing to interfere with the morale of the community. . . . It is our duty to keep the people from fear. Worry kills more people than the epidemic" (Robertson, 1918).

That idea—"Fear kills more than the disease"—became a mantra nationally and in city after city. As *Literary Digest,* one of the largest circulation periodicals in the country, advised, "Fear is our first enemy" (Van Hartesveldt, 1992).

In Philadelphia, when the public health commissioner closed all schools, houses of worship, theaters, and other public gathering places, one newspaper went so far as to say that this order was "not a public health measure" and reiterated that "there is no cause for panic or alarm."

But as people heard these reassurances, they could see neighbors, friends, and spouses dying horrible deaths.

In Chicago, the Cook County Hospital mortality rate of all influenza admissions—not just those who developed pneumonia—was 39.8 percent (Keeton and Cusman, 1918). In Philadelphia, bodies remained uncollected in homes for days, until eventually open trucks and even horse-drawn carts were sent down city streets and people were told to bring out the dead. The bodies were stacked without coffins and buried in cemeteries in mass graves dug by steam shovels.

This horrific disconnect between reassurances and reality destroyed the credibility of those in authority. People felt they had no one to turn to, no one to rely on, no one to trust.

Ultimately society depends on trust. Without it, society began to come apart. Normally in 1918 America, when someone was ill, neighbors helped. That did not happen during the pandemic. Typically, the head of one city's volunteer effort, frustrated after repeated pleas for help yielded nothing, turned bitter and contemptuous:

> Hundreds of women who are content to sit back had delightful dreams of themselves in the roles of angels of mercy, had the unfathomable vanity to imagine that they were capable of great sacrifice. Nothing seems to rouse them now. They have been told that there are families in which every member is ill, in which the children are actually starving because there is no one to give them food. The death rate is so high and they still hold back.[3]

That attitude persisted outside of cities as well. In rural Kentucky, the Red Cross reported "people starving to death not from lack of food but because the well were panic stricken and would not go near the sick" (An Account of the Influenza Epidemic, 1919).

As the pressure from the virus continued, an internal Red Cross report concluded, "A fear and panic of the influenza, akin to the terror of the Middle Ages regarding the Black Plague, [has] been prevalent in many parts of the country" (The Mobilization of the American National Red Cross, 1920). Similarly, Victor Vaughan, a sober scientist not given to overstatement, worried, "If the epidemic continues its mathematical rate of acceleration, civilization could easily . . . disappear . . . from the face of the earth within a matter of a few more weeks" (Collier, 1974).

Of course, the disease generated fear independent of anything officials did or did not do, but the false reassurances given by the authorities and the media systematically destroyed trust. That magnified the fear and turned it into panic and terror.

It is worth noting that this terror, at least in paralyzing form, did not seem to materialize in the few places where authorities told the truth.

One lesson is clear from this experience: In handling any crisis, it is absolutely crucial to retain credibility. Giving false reassurance is the worst thing one can do. If I may speculate, let me suggest that almost as bad as outright lying is holding information so closely that people think officials know more than they say.

---

[3]October 16, 1918, minutes of Philadelphia General Hospital Woman's Advisory Council.

The Site of Origin

It is very possible that we will never know with certainty where the 1918 virus crossed into man. In the 1920s and 1930s, outstanding investigators in several countries launched massive reviews of evidence searching for the site of origin. They could not definitively answer the question. But they were unanimous in believing that no known outbreak in China could, as one investigator said, "be reasonably regarded as the true forerunner" of the epidemic.

They considered the most likely sites of origin to be France and the United States, and most agreed with Macfarlane Burnet, who concluded that the evidence was "strongly suggestive" that the 1918 influenza pandemic began in the United States, and that its spread was "intimately related to war conditions and especially the arrival of American troops in France" (Burnet and Clark, 1942).

My own research also makes me think that the United States was the most likely site of origin. The unearthing of previously unknown epidemiologic evidence has led me to advance my own hypothesis that the pandemic began in rural Kansas and traveled with draftees to what is now Fort Riley.

But whether the pandemic began in France or the United States is not really important. What does matter is that the pandemic most likely did **not** begin in Asia.

This has important implications for modern surveillance efforts. Although Asia's population density and the close proximity of humans and animals there makes the region particularly dangerous, the evidence of 1918—confirmed by the H7N7 outbreak in Europe of 2003—demonstrates the need for surveillance worldwide.

Something else should be addressed regarding surveillance. A physician now active in public health who received his medical degree in Honduras in 1986 says that he and his colleagues were taught that there was no difference between a cold and influenza. He believes physicians in Central America and possibly elsewhere in the world routinely ignore influenza. Clearly, if we are to have an adequate surveillance system, physicians need to be alert to the disease.

Data

Outstanding laboratory investigators have made enormous progress over the years in understanding the virus and developing effective antiviral drugs as well as new technologies to make vaccines. But one area remains in which investigators have lagged behind—in applying modern insights and statistical methods to old data.

To use an analogy, a similar situation is found in the flooding of the Sacramento River, one of the few rivers in the country where flood control is the direct responsibility of the U.S. Army Corps of Engineers. The Corps has as powerful computers as anyone, but in a recent 10-year period, the Sacramento River experienced a 100-year flood three times, devastating parts of California—despite the fact that each time the Corps raised the standard for a 100-year flood. The point is not that the river exceeded the 100-year level three times in 10 years. Random chance could account for that. The point is that it did so even though the Corps changed the definition of a 100-year flood. A senior Corps official confessed that the Corps simply did not have enough data to know what a 100-year flood was.

We may be in a similar situation with influenza. We have had only three pandemics in the 20th century. That is not a good base on which to build models. Indeed, the Centers for Disease Control and Prevention's model of what would happen in the United States should another pandemic strike predicts that the most likely death toll would fall between 89,000 and 207,000. Yet the actual death tolls of two of the three pandemics fell well outside the predicted range. Adjusted for population, 1968 deaths were somewhat fewer than the best case scenario, and 1918 nearly 800 percent worse than the worst case. (In 1918, antibiotics would likely have lessened this gap, but the increased population of those with impaired immune systems would somewhat balance that benefit, and increase deaths.)

In addition, we have not taken advantage of the data that we do have. Several presentations at this conference demonstrate that fact—some on the plus side, by deriving findings of value by reviewing records from 1918, but also on the negative side, by making certain assumptions about 1918 that conflict with actual data.

A careful review of old data would also prove valuable. Studying 1889 (and enough data can be found, possibly from earlier pandemics as well), 1918, 1957, and 1968 might tell us whether each followed the same patterns, which in turn could help us to devise strategies for the use of antivirals and vaccines.

The Next Pandemic

Virtually every expert on influenza believes another pandemic is nearly inevitable, that it will kill millions of people, and that it could kill tens of millions—and a virus like 1918, or H5N1, might kill a hundred million or more—and that it could cause economic and social disruption on a massive scale. This disruption itself could kill as well.

Given those facts, every laboratory investigator and every public health official involved with the disease has two tasks: first, to do his or her work, and second, to make political leaders aware of the risk. The preparedness effort needs resources. Only the political process can allocate them.

CHASING THE ELUSIVE 1918 VIRUS: PREPARING FOR THE FUTURE BY EXAMINING THE PAST

Jeffery K. Taubenberger[4]

Department of Molecular Pathology
Armed Forces Institute of Pathology

Introduction

Influenza A viruses are negative strand RNA viruses of the genus *Orthomyxoviridae*. They continually circulate in humans in yearly epidemics (mainly in the winter in temperate climates) and antigenically novel virus strains emerge sporadically as pandemic viruses (Cox and Subbarao, 2000). In the United States, influenza is estimated to kill 30,000 people in an average year (Simonsen et al., 2000; Thompson et al., 2003). Every few years, a more severe influenza epidemic occurs, causing a boost in the annual number of deaths past the average, with 10,000 to 15,000 additional deaths. Occasionally, and unpredictably, influenza sweeps the world, infecting 20 to 40 percent of the population in a single year. In these pandemic years, the numbers of deaths can be dramatically above average. In 1957–1958, a pandemic was estimated to cause 66,000 excess deaths in the United States (Simonsen et al., 1998). In 1918, the worst pandemic in recorded history was associated with approximately 675,000 total deaths in the United States (U.S. Department of Commerce, 1976) and killed at least 40 million people worldwide (Crosby, 1989; Patterson and Pyle, 1991; Johnson and Mueller, 2002).

Influenza A viruses constantly evolve by the mechanisms of antigenic drift and shift (Webster et al., 1992). Consequently they should be considered emerging infectious disease agents, perhaps "continually" emerging pathogens. The importance of predicting the emergence of new circulating influenza virus strains for subsequent annual vaccine development cannot be underestimated (Gensheimer et al., 1999). Pandemic influenza viruses have emerged three times in this century: in 1918 ("Spanish" influenza, H1N1), in 1957 ("Asian" influenza, H2N2), and in 1968 ("Hong Kong" influenza, H3N2) (Cox and Subbarao, 2000; Webby and Webster, 2003). Recent circulation of highly pathogenic avian H5N1 viruses in Asia from 1997 to 2004 has caused a small number of human deaths (Claas et al., 1998; Subbarao et al., 1998; Tran et al., 2004; Peiris et al., 2004). How and

---

[4]This work has been partially supported by National Institutes of Health grants, and previously by grants from the Veterans Administration and the American Registry of Pathology, and by the Armed Forces Institute of Pathology.

when novel influenza viruses emerge as pandemic virus strains and how they cause disease is still not understood.

Studying the extent to which the 1918 influenza was like other pandemics may help us to understand how pandemic influenzas emerge and cause disease in general. On the other hand, if we determine what made the 1918 influenza different from other pandemics, we may use the lessons of 1918 to predict the magnitude of public health risks a new pandemic virus might pose.

Origin of Pandemic Influenza Viruses

The predominant natural reservoir of influenza viruses is thought to be wild waterfowl (Webster et al., 1992). Periodically, genetic material from avian virus strains is transferred to virus strains infectious to humans by a process called reassortment. Human influenza virus strains with recently acquired avian surface and internal protein-encoding RNA segments were responsible for the pandemic influenza outbreaks in 1957 and 1968 (Scholtissek et al., 1978a; Kawaoka et al., 1989). The change in the hemagglutinin subtype or the hemagglutinin (HA) and the neuraminidase (NA) subtype is referred to as antigenic shift. Because pigs can be infected with both avian and human virus strains, and various reassortants have been isolated from pigs, they have been proposed as an intermediary in this process (Scholtissek, 1994; Ludwig et al., 1995). Until recently there was only limited evidence that a wholly avian influenza virus could directly infect humans, but in 1997 18 people were infected with avian H5N1 influenza viruses in Hong Kong, and 6 died of complications after infection (Claas et al., 1998; Subbarao et al., 1998; Scholtissek, 1994; Ludwig et al., 1995). Although these viruses were very poorly transmissible or non-transmissible (Claas et al., 1998; Subbarao et al., 1998; Scholtissek, 1994; Ludwig et al., 1995; Katz et al., 1999), their isolation from infected patients indicates that humans can be infected with wholly avian influenza virus strains. In 2003–2004, H5N1 outbreaks in poultry have become widespread in Asia (Tran et al., 2004), and at least 32 people have died of complications of infection in Vietnam and Thailand (World Health Organization, 2004). In 2003, a highly pathogenic H7N7 outbreak occurred in poultry farms in The Netherlands. This virus caused infections (predominantly conjunctivitis) in 86 poultry handlers and 3 secondary contacts. One of the infected individuals died of pneumonia (Fouchier et al., 2004; Koopmans et al., 2004; World Health Organization, 2004). In 2004, an H7N3 influenza outbreak in poultry in Canada also resulted in the infection of a single individual (World Health Organization, 2004), and a patient in New York was reported to be sick following infection with an H7N2 virus (Lipsman, 2004). Therefore, it may not be necessary to invoke swine as the intermediary in the formation of a pandemic virus strain because reassortment between an avian and a human influenza virus could take place directly in humans.

While reassortment involving genes encoding surface proteins appears to be a critical event for the production of a pandemic virus, a significant amount of data exists to suggest that influenza viruses must also acquire specific adaptations to spread and replicate efficiently in a new host. Among other features, there must be functional HA receptor binding and interaction between viral and host proteins (Weis et al., 1988). Defining the minimal adaptive changes needed to allow a reassortant virus to function in humans is essential to understanding how pandemic viruses emerge.

Once a new virus strain has acquired the changes that allow it to spread in humans, virulence is affected by the presence of novel surface protein(s) that allow the virus to infect an immunologically naïve population (Kilbourne, 1977). This was the case in 1957 and 1968 and was almost certainly the case in 1918. While immunological novelty may explain much of the virulence of the 1918 influenza, it is likely that additional genetic features contributed to its exceptional lethality. Unfortunately not enough is known about how genetic features of influenza viruses affect virulence. The degree of illness caused by a particular virus strain, or virulence, is complex and involves host factors like immune status, and viral factors like host adaptation, transmissibility, tissue tropism, or viral replication efficiency. The genetic basis for each of these features is not yet fully characterized, but is most likely polygenic in nature (Kilbourne, 1977).

Prior to the analyses on the 1918 virus described in this review, only two pandemic influenza virus strains were available for molecular analysis: the H2N2 virus strain from 1957 and the H3N2 virus strain from 1968. The 1957 pandemic resulted from the emergence of a reassortant influenza virus in which both HA and NA had been replaced by gene segment closely related to those in avian virus strains (Scholtissek et al., 1978b; Schafer et al., 1993; Webster et al., 1995). The 1968 pandemic followed with the emergence of a virus strain in which the H2 subtype HA gene was exchanged with an avian-derived H3 HA RNA segment (Scholtissek et al., 1978b; Webster et al., 1995), while retaining the N2 gene derived in 1957. More recently it has been shown that the PB1 gene was replaced in both the 1957 and the 1968 pandemic virus strains, also with a likely avian derivation in both cases (Kawaoka et al., 1989). The remaining five RNA segments encoding the PA, PB2, nucleoprotein, matrix and non-structural proteins, all were preserved from the H1N1 virus strains circulating before 1957. These segments were likely the direct descendants of the genes present in the 1918 virus. Because only the 1957 and 1968 influenza pandemic virus strains have been available for sequence analysis, it is not clear what changes are necessary for the emergence of a virus strain with pandemic potential. Sequence analysis of the 1918 influenza virus allows us potentially to address the genetic basis of virulence and human adaptation.

Historical Background

The influenza pandemic of 1918 was exceptional in both breadth and depth. Outbreaks of the disease swept not only North America and Europe, but also spread as far as the Alaskan wilderness and the most remote islands of the Pacific. It has been estimated that one-third of the world's population may have been clinically infected during the pandemic (Frost, 1920; Burnet and Clark, 1942). The disease was also exceptionally severe, with mortality rates among the infected of more than 2.5 percent, compared to less than 0.1 percent in other influenza epidemics (Marks and Beatty, 1976; Rosenau and Last, 1980). Total mortality attributable to the 1918 pandemic was probably around 40 million (Crosby, 1989; Johnson and Mueller, 2002; Patterson and Pyle, 1991).

Unlike most subsequent influenza virus strains that have developed in Asia, the "first wave" or "spring wave" of the 1918 pandemic seemingly arose in the United States in March 1918 (Barry, 2004; Crosby, 1989; Jordan, 1927). However, the near simultaneous appearance of influenza in March–April 1918 in North America, Europe, and Asia makes definitive assignment of a geographic point of origin difficult (Jordan, 1927). It is possible that a mutation or reassortment occurred in the late summer of 1918, resulting in significantly enhanced virulence. The main wave of the global pandemic, the "fall wave" or "second wave," occurred in September–November 1918. In many places, there was yet another severe wave of influenza in early 1919 (Jordan, 1927).

Three extensive outbreaks of influenza within 1 year is unusual, and may point to unique features of the 1918 virus that could be revealed in its sequence. Interpandemic influenza outbreaks generally occur in a single annual wave in the late winter. The severity of annual outbreaks is affected by antigenic drift, with an antigenically modified virus strain emerging every 2 to 3 years. Even in pandemic influenza, while the normal late winter seasonality may be violated, the successive occurrence of distinct waves within a year is unusual. The 1890 pandemic began in the late spring of 1889 and took several months to spread throughout the world, peaking in northern Europe and the United States late in 1889 or early 1890. The second wave peaked in spring 1891 (over a year after the first wave) and the third wave in early 1892 (Jordan, 1927). As in 1918, subsequent waves seemed to produce more severe illness so that the peak mortality was reached in the third wave of the pandemic. The three waves, however, were spread over more than 3 years, in contrast to less than 1 year in 1918. It is unclear what gave the 1918 virus this unusual ability to generate repeated waves of illness. Perhaps the surface proteins of the virus drifted more rapidly than other influenza virus strains, or perhaps the virus had an unusually effective mechanism for evading the human immune system.

The influenza epidemic of 1918 killed an estimated 675,000 Americans, including 43,000 servicemen mobilized for World War I (Crosby, 1989). The impact was so profound as to depress average life expectancy in the United States by more than 10 years (Grove and Hetzel, 1968) (Figure 1-1) and may have played a significant role in ending the World War I conflict (Crosby, 1989; Ludendorff, 1919).

Many individuals who died during the pandemic succumbed to secondary bacterial pneumonia (Jordan, 1927; LeCount, 1919; Wolbach, 1919) because no antibiotics were available in 1918. However, a subset died rapidly after the onset of symptoms often with either massive acute pulmonary hemorrhage or pulmonary edema, often in less than 5 days (LeCount, 1919; Winternitz et al., 1920; Wolbach, 1919). In the hundreds of autopsies performed in 1918, the primary pathologic findings were confined to the respiratory tree and death was due to pneumonia and respiratory failure (Winternitz et al., 1920). These findings are consistent with infection by a well-adapted influenza virus capable of rapid replication throughout the entire respiratory tree (Reid and Taubenberger, 1999; Taubenberger et al.,

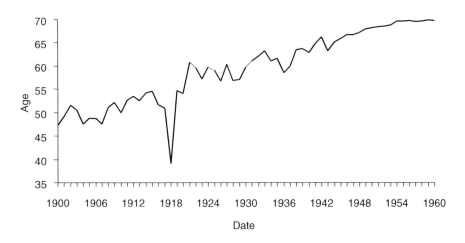

FIGURE 1-1 Life expectancy in the United States, 1900–1960, showing the impact of the 1918 influenza pandemic.
SOURCES: U.S. Department of Commerce (1976); Grove and Hetzel (1968); Linder and Grove (1943).

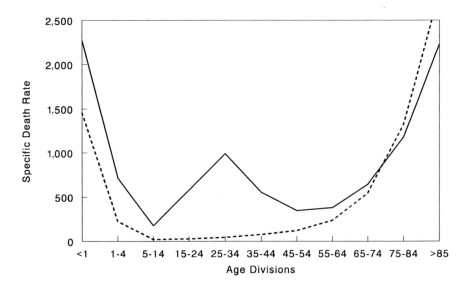

FIGURE 1-2 Influenza and pneumonia mortality by age, United States. Influenza and pneumonia specific mortality by age, including an average of the interpandemic years 1911–1915 (dashed line), and the pandemic year 1918 (solid line). Specific death rate is per 100,000 of the population in each age division.
SOURCES: U.S. Department of Commerce (1976); Grove and Hetzel (1968); Linder and Grove (1943).

2000). There was no clinical or pathological evidence for systemic circulation of the virus (Winternitz et al., 1920).

Furthermore, in the 1918 pandemic most deaths occurred among young adults, a group that usually has a very low death rate from influenza. Influenza and pneumonia death rates for 15- to 34-year-olds were more than 20 times higher in 1918 than in previous years (Linder and Grove, 1943; Simonsen et al., 1998) (Figure 1-2). The 1918 pandemic is also unique among influenza pandemics in that absolute risk of influenza mortality was higher in those younger than age 65 than in those older than 65. Strikingly, persons less than 65 years old accounted for more than 99 percent of all excess influenza-related deaths in 1918–1919 (Simonsen et al., 1998). In contrast, the less-than-65 age group accounted for only 36 percent of all excess influenza-related mortality in the 1957 H2N2 pandemic and 48 percent in the 1968 H3N2 pandemic. Overall, nearly half of the influenza-related deaths in the 1918 influenza pandemic were young adults aged 20 to 40 (Simonsen et al., 1998) (Figure 1-2). Why this particular age group suffered such extreme mortality is not fully understood (see below).

The 1918 influenza had another unique feature: the simultaneous infection of both humans and swine. Interestingly, swine influenza was first recognized as a clinical entity in that species in the fall of 1918 (Koen, 1919) concurrently with the spread of the second wave of the pandemic in humans (Dorset et al., 1922–1923). Investigators were impressed by clinical and pathological similarities of human and swine influenza in 1918 (Koen, 1919; Murray and Biester, 1930). An extensive review by the veterinarian W.W. Dimoch of the diseases of swine published in August 1918 makes no mention of any swine disease resembling influenza (Dimoch, 1918–1919). Thus, contemporary investigators were convinced that influenza virus had not circulated as an epizootic disease in swine before 1918 and that the virus spread from humans to pigs because of the appearance of illness in pigs after the first wave of the 1918 influenza in humans (Shope and Lewis, 1931).

Thereafter the disease became widespread among swine herds in the U.S. midwest. The epizootic of 1919–1920 was as extensive as in 1918–1919. The disease then appeared among swine in the midwest every year, leading to Shope's isolation of the first influenza virus in 1930, A/swine/Iowa/30 (Shope and Lewis, 1931), 3 years before the isolation of the first human influenza virus, A/WS/33 by Smith, Andrewes, and Laidlaw (Smith et al., 1933). Classical swine viruses have continued to circulate not only in North American pigs, but also in swine populations in Europe and Asia (Brown et al., 1995; Kupradinun et al., 1991; Nerome et al., 1982).

During the fall and winter of 1918–1919, severe influenza-like outbreaks were noted not only in swine in the United States, but also in Europe and China (Beveridge, 1977; Chun, 1919; Koen, 1919). Since 1918 there have been many examples of both H1N1 and H3N2 human influenza A virus strains becoming established in swine (Brown et al., 1998; Castrucci et al., 1993; Zhou et al., 2000), while swine influenza A virus strains have been isolated only sporadically from humans (Gaydos et al., 1977; Woods et al., 1981).

The unusual severity of the 1918 pandemic and the exceptionally high mortality it caused among young adults have stimulated great interest in the influenza virus strain responsible for the 1918 outbreak (Crosby, 1989; Kolata, 1999; Monto et al., 1997). Because the first human and swine influenza A viruses were not isolated until the early 1930s (Shope and Lewis, 1931; Smith et al., 1933), characterization of the 1918 virus strain previously has had to rely on indirect evidence (Kanegae et al., 1994; Shope, 1958).

Serology and Epidemiology of the 1918 Influenza Virus

Analyses of antibody titers of 1918 influenza survivors from the late 1930s suggested correctly that the 1918 virus strain was an H1N1-subtype

76 THE THREAT OF PANDEMIC INFLUENZA

influenza A virus, closely related to what is now known as "classic swine" influenza virus (Dowdle, 1999; Philip and Lackman, 1962; Shope, 1936). The relationship to swine influenza is also reflected in the simultaneous influenza outbreaks in humans and pigs around the world (Beveridge, 1977; Chun, 1919; Koen, 1919). Although historical accounts described above suggest that the virus spread from humans to pigs in the fall of 1918, the relationship of these two species in the development of the 1918 influenza has not been resolved.

Which influenza A subtype(s) circulated before the 1918 pandemic is not known for certain. In a recent review of the existing archaeoserologic and epidemiologic data, Walter Dowdle concluded that an H3-subtype influenza A virus strain circulated from the 1889–1891 pandemic to 1918, when it was replaced by the novel H1N1 virus strain of the 1918 pandemic (Dowdle, 1999).

It is reasonable to conclude that the 1918 virus strain must have contained a hemagglutinin gene encoding a novel subtype such that large portions of the population did not have protective immunity (Kilbourne, 1977; Reid and Taubenberger, 1999). In fact, epidemiological data collected between 1900 and 1918 on influenza prevalence by age in the population provide good evidence for the emergence of an antigenically novel influenza virus in 1918 (Jordan, 1927). Jordan showed that from 1900 to 1917, the 5 to 15 age group accounted for 11 percent of total influenza cases in this series while the >65 age group similarly accounted for 6 percent of influenza cases. In 1918 the 5- to 15-year-old group jumped to 25 percent of influenza cases, compatible with exposure to an antigenically novel virus strain. The >65 age group only accounted for 0.6 percent of the influenza cases in 1918. It is likely that this age group accounted for a significantly lower percentage of influenza cases because younger people were so susceptible to the novel virus strain (as seen in the 1957 pandemic [Ministry of Health, 1960; Simonsen et al., 1998]), but it is also possible that this age group had pre-existing H1 antibodies. Further evidence for pre-existing H1 immunity can be derived from the age-adjusted mortality data in Figure 1-2. Those individuals >75 years had a lower influenza and pneumonia case mortality rate in 1918 than they had for the prepandemic period of 1911–1917.

When 1918 influenza case rates by age (Jordan, 1927) are superimposed on the familiar "W"-shaped mortality curve (seen in Figure 1-2), a different perspective emerges (Figure 1-3). As shown, those <35 years of age in 1918 accounted for a disproportionately high influenza incidence by age. Interestingly, the 5 to 14 age group accounted for a large fraction of 1918 influenza cases, but had an extremely low case mortality rate compared to other age groups (Figure 1-3). Why this age group had such a low case fatality rate cannot yet be fully explained. Conversely, why the 25 to 34 age

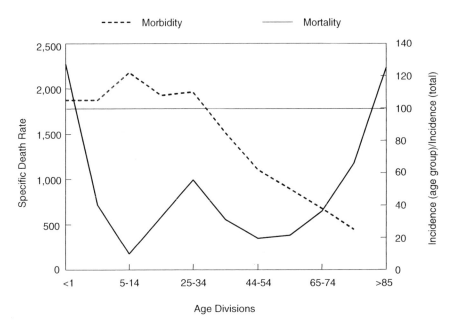

FIGURE 1-3 Influenza and pneumonia mortality by age (solid line), with influenza morbidity by age (dashed line) superimposed. Influenza and pneumonia mortality by age as in Figure 1-2. Specific death rate per age group, left ordinal axis. Influenza morbidity presented as ratio of incidence in persons of each group to incidence in persons of all ages (=100), right ordinal axis. Horizontal line at 100 (right ordinal axis) represents average influenza incidence in the total population. SOURCES: Taubenberger et al. (2001); adapted from Jordan (1927).

group had such a high influenza and pneumonia mortality rate in 1918 remains enigmatic, but it is one of the truly unique features of the 1918 influenza pandemic.

One theory that may explain these data concerns the possibility that the virus had an intrinsically high virulence that was only tempered in those patients who had been born before 1889. It can be speculated that the virus circulating prior to 1889 was an H1-like virus strain that provided partial protection against the 1918 virus strain (Ministry of Health, 1960; Simonsen et al., 1998; Taubenberger et al., 2001). Short of this cross-protection in patients older than 29 years of age, the pandemic of 1918 might have been even more devastating (Zamarin and Palese, 2004). A second possibility remains that the high mortality of young adults in the 20 to 40 age group may have been a consequence of immune enhancement in this age group. Currently, however, the absence of pre-1918 human influenza samples and the lack of pre-1918 sera samples for analysis makes it impossible to test this hypothesis.

Thus, it seems clear that the H1N1 virus of the 1918 pandemic contained an antigenically novel hemagglutinin to which most humans and swine were susceptible in 1918. Given the severity of the pandemic, it is also reasonable to suggest that the other dominant surface protein, NA, also would have been replaced by antigenic shift before the start of the pandemic (Reid and Taubenberger, 1999; Taubenberger et al., 2000). In fact, sequence and phylogenetic analyses suggest that the genes encoding these two surface proteins were derived from an avian-like influenza virus shortly before the start of the 1918 pandemic and that the precursor virus did not circulate widely in either humans or swine before 1918 (Fanning et al., 2002; Reid et al., 1999, 2000) (Figure 1-4). It is currently unclear what other influenza gene segments were novel in the 1918 pandemic virus in comparison to the previously circulating virus strain. It is possible that sequence and phylogenetic analyses of the gene segments of the 1918 virus may help elucidate this question.

Genetic Characterization of the 1918 Virus

Sequence and Functional Analysis of the Hemagglutinin and Neuraminidase Gene Segments

Samples of frozen and fixed lung tissue from five second-wave influenza victims (dating from September 1918 to February 1919) have been used to examine directly the genetic structure of the 1918 influenza virus. Two of the cases analyzed were U.S. Army soldiers who died in September 1918, one in Camp Upton, New York, and the other in Fort Jackson, South Carolina. The available material consists of formalin-fixed, paraffin-embedded autopsy tissue, hematoxylin and eosin-stained microscopic sections, and the clinical histories of these patients. A third sample was obtained from an Alaskan Inuit woman who had been interred in permafrost in Brevig Mission, Alaska, since her death from influenza in November 1918. The influenza virus sequences derived from these three cases have been called A/South Carolina/1/18 (H1N1), A/New York/1/18 (H1N1), and A/Brevig

FIGURE 1-4 Phylogenetic tree of the influenza virus hemagglutinin gene segment. Amino acid changes in three lineages of the influenza virus hemagglutinin protein segment, HA1. The tree shows the numbers of unambiguous changes between these sequences, with branch lengths being proportional to number of changes. SOURCE: Reid et al. (1999).

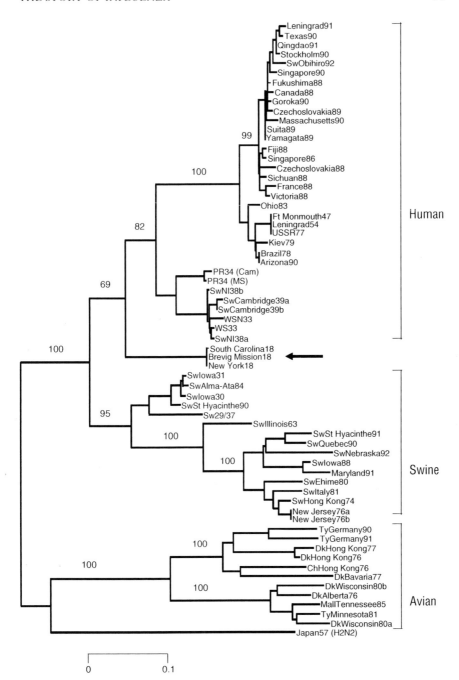

Mission/1/18 (H1N1), respectively. To date, five RNA segment sequences have been published (Basler et al., 2001; Reid et al., 1999, 2000, 2002, 2004). More recently, the HA sequences of two additional fixed autopsy cases of 1918 influenza victims from the Royal London Hospital were determined (Reid et al., 2003). The HA sequences from these five cases show >99 percent sequence identity, but differ at amino acid residue 225 (see below).

The sequence of the 1918 HA is most closely related to that of the A/swine/Iowa/30 virus. However, despite this similarity the sequence has many avian features. Of the 41 amino acids that have been shown to be targets of the immune system and subject to antigenic drift pressure in humans, 37 match the avian sequence consensus, suggesting there was little immunologic pressure on the HA protein before the fall of 1918 (Reid et al., 1999). Another mechanism by which influenza viruses evade the human immune system is the acquisition of glycosylation sites to mask antigenic epitopes. The HAs from modern H1N1 viruses have up to five glycosylation sites in addition to the four found in all avian HAs. The HA of the 1918 virus has only the four conserved avian sites (Reid et al., 1999).

Influenza virus infection requires binding of the HA protein to sialic acid receptors on the host cell surface. The HA receptor binding site consists of a subset of amino acids that are invariant in all avian HAs, but vary in mammalian-adapted HAs. Human-adapted influenza viruses preferentially bind sialic acid receptors with $\alpha(2\text{-}6)$ linkages. Those viral strains adapted to birds preferentially bind $\alpha(2\text{-}3)$ linked sugars (Gambaryan et al., 1997; Matrosovich et al., 1997; Weis et al., 1988). To shift from the proposed avian-adapted receptor-binding site configuration (with a preference for $\alpha(2\text{-}3)$ sialic acids) to that of swine H1s (which can bind both $\alpha(2\text{-}3)$ and $\alpha(2\text{-}6)$) requires only one amino acid change, E190D. The HA sequences of all five 1918 cases have the E190D change (Reid et al., 2003). In fact, the critical amino acids in the receptor-binding site of two of the 1918 cases are identical to that of the A/swine/Iowa/30 HA. The other three 1918 cases have an additional change from the avian consensus, G225D. Because swine viruses with the same receptor site as A/swine/Iowa/30 bind both avian- and mammalian-type receptors (Gambaryan et al., 1997), A/New York/1/18 virus probably also had the capacity to bind both. The change at residue 190 may represent the minimal change necessary to allow an avian H1-subtype HA to bind mammalian-type receptors (Reid et al., 1999, 2003; Stevens et al., 2004; Gamblin et al., 2004; Glaser et al., 2004), a critical step in host adaptation.

The crystal structure analysis of the 1918 HA (Stevens et al., 2004; Gamblin et al., 2004) suggests that the overall structure of the receptor binding site is akin to that of an avian H5 HA in terms of its having a narrower pocket than that identified for the human H3 HA (Wilson et al.,

1981). This provides an additional clue for the avian derivation of the 1918 HA. The four antigenic sites that have been identified for another H1 HA, the A/PR/8/34 virus HA (Caton et al., 1982), also appear to be the major antigenic determinants on the 1918 HA. The X-ray analyses suggest that these sites are exposed on the 1918 HA and thus they could be readily recognized by the human immune system.

The principal biological role of NA is the cleavage of the terminal sialic acid residues that are receptors for the virus's HA protein (Palese and Compans, 1976). The active site of the enzyme consists of 15 invariant amino acids that are conserved in the 1918 NA. The functional NA protein is configured as a homotetramer in which the active sites are found on a terminal knob carried on a thin stalk (Colman et al., 1983). Some early human virus strains have short (11-16 amino acids) deletions in the stalk region, as do many virus strains isolated from chickens. The 1918 NA has a full-length stalk and has only the glycosylation sites shared by avian N1 virus strains (Schulze, 1997). Although the antigenic sites on human-adapted N1 neuraminidases have not been definitively mapped, it is possible to align the N1 sequences with N2 subtype NAs and examine the N2 antigenic sites for evidence of drift in N1. There are 22 amino acids on the N2 protein that may function in antigenic epitopes (Colman et al., 1983). The 1918 NA matches the avian consensus at 21 of these sites (Reid et al., 2000). This finding suggests that the 1918 NA, like the 1918 HA, had not circulated long in humans before the pandemic and very possibly had an avian origin (Reid and Taubenberger, 2003).

Neither the 1918 HA nor NA genes have obvious genetic features that can be related directly to virulence. Two known mutations that can dramatically affect the virulence of influenza virus strains have been described. For viral activation, HA must be cleaved into two pieces, HA1 and HA2, by a host protease (Lazarowitz and Choppin, 1975; Rott et al., 1995). Some avian H5 and H7 subtype viruses acquire a mutation that involves the addition of one or more basic amino acids to the cleavage site, allowing HA activation by ubiquitous proteases (Kawaoka and Webster, 1988; Webster and Rott, 1987). Infection with such a pantropic virus strain can cause systemic disease in birds with high mortality. This mutation was not observed in the 1918 virus (Reid et al., 1999; Taubenberger et al., 1997).

The second mutation with a significant effect on virulence through pantropism has been identified in the NA gene of two mouse-adapted influenza virus strains, A/WSN/33 and A/NWS/33. Mutations at a single codon (N146R or N146Y, leading to the loss of a glycosylation site) appear, like the HA cleavage site mutation, to allow the virus to replicate in many tissues outside the respiratory tract (Li et al., 1993). This mutation was also not observed in the NA of the 1918 virus (Reid et al., 2000).

Therefore, neither surface protein-encoding gene has known mutations that would allow the 1918 virus to become pantropic. Because clinical and pathological findings in 1918 showed no evidence of replication outside the respiratory system (Winternitz et al., 1920; Wolbach, 1919), mutations allowing the 1918 virus to replicate systemically would not have been expected. However, the relationship of other structural features of these proteins (aside from their presumed antigenic novelty) to virulence remains unknown. In their overall structural and functional characteristics, the 1918 HA and NA are avian-like, but they also have mammalian-adapted characteristics.

Interestingly, recombinant influenza viruses containing the 1918 HA and NA and up to three additional genes derived from the 1918 virus (the other genes being derived from the A/WSN/33 virus) were all highly virulent in mice (Tumpey et al., 2004). Furthermore, expression microarray analysis performed on whole lung tissue of mice infected with the 1918 HA/NA recombinant showed increased upregulation of genes involved in apoptosis, tissue injury, and oxidative damage (Kash et al., 2004). These findings were unusual because the viruses with the 1918 genes had not been adapted to mice. The completion of the sequence of the entire genome of the 1918 virus and the reconstruction and characterization of viruses with 1918 genes under appropriate biosafety conditions will shed more light on these findings and should allow a definitive examination of this explanation.

Antigenic analysis of recombinant viruses possessing the 1918 HA and NA by hemagglutination inhibition tests using ferret and chicken antisera suggested a close relationship with the A/swine/Iowa/30 virus and H1N1 viruses isolated in the 1930s (Tumpey et al., 2004), further supporting data of Shope from the 1930s (Shope, 1936). Interestingly, when mice were immunized with different H1N1 virus strains, challenge studies using the 1918-like viruses revealed partial protection by this treatment, suggesting that current vaccination strategies are adequate against a 1918-like virus (Tumpey et al., 2004). In fact, the data may even allow us to suggest that the human population, having experienced a long period of exposure to H1N1 viruses, may be partially protected against a 1918-like virus (Tumpey et al., 2004).

Because virulence (in the immunologically naïve person) has not yet been mapped to particular sequence motifs of the 1918 HA and NA genes, what can gene sequencing tell us about the origin of the 1918 virus? The best approach to analyzing the relationships among influenza viruses is phylogenetics, whereby hypothetical family trees are constructed that take available sequence data and use them to make assumptions about the ancestral relationships between current and historical influenza virus strains (Fitch et al., 1991; Gammelin et al., 1990; Scholtissek et al., 1993) (Figure 1-5). Because influenza viruses possess eight discrete RNA segments that can move independently between virus strains by the process of

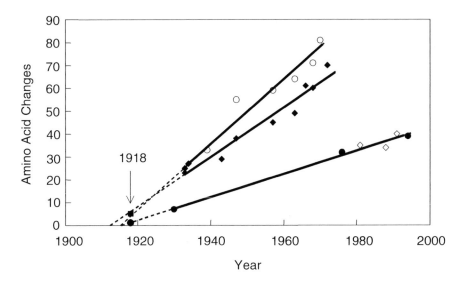

FIGURE 1-5 Change in hemagglutinin (HA) and neuraminidase (NA) proteins over time. The number of amino acid changes from a hypothetical ancestor was plotted versus the date of viral isolation for viruses isolated from 1930 to 1993. Open circles, human HA; closed diamonds, human NA; closed circles, swine HA; open diamonds, swine NA. Regression lines were drawn, extrapolated to the x-intercept and then the 1918 data points, closed square, 1918 HA; closed circle, 1918 NA were added to the graph (arrow).
SOURCES: Reid et al. (1999, 2000); Taubenberger et al. (2000).

reassortment, these evolutionary studies must be performed independently for each gene segment.

A comparison of the complete 1918 HA (Figure 1-5) and NA genes with those of numerous human, swine, and avian sequences demonstrates the following: Phylogenetic analyses based on HA nucleotide changes (either total or synonymous) or HA amino acid changes always place the 1918 HA with the mammalian viruses, not with the avian viruses (Reid et al., 1999). In fact, both synonymous and nonsynonymous changes place the 1918 HA in the human clade. Phylogenetic analyses of total or synonymous NA nucleotide changes also place the 1918 NA sequence with the mammalian viruses, but analysis of nonsynonymous changes or amino acid changes places the 1918 NA with the avian viruses (Reid et al., 2000). Because the 1918 HA and NA have avian features and most analyses place HA and NA near the root of the mammalian clade (close to an ancestor of the avian genes), it is likely that both genes emerged from an avian-like influenza reservoir just prior to 1918 (Reid et al., 1999, 2000, 2003; Fanning and

Taubenberger, 1999; Fanning et al., 2000) (Figure 1-4). Clearly, by 1918 the virus had acquired enough mammalian-adaptive changes to function as a human pandemic virus and to form a stable lineage in swine.

Sequence and Functional Analysis of the Non-Structural Gene Segment

The complete coding sequence of the 1918 non-structural (NS) segment was completed (Basler et al., 2001). The functions of the two proteins, NS1 and NS2 (NEP), encoded by overlapping reading frames (Lamb and Lai, 1980) of the NS segment, are still being elucidated (O'Neill et al., 1998; Li et al., 1998; Garcia-Sastre et al., 1998; Garcia-Sastre, 2002; Krug et al., 2003). The NS1 protein has been shown to prevent type I interferon (IFN) production by preventing activation of the latent transcription factors IRF-3 (Talon et al., 2000) and NF-κB (Wang et al., 2000). One of the distinctive clinical characteristics of the 1918 influenza was its ability to produce rapid and extensive damage to both the upper and lower respiratory epithelium (Winternitz et al., 1920). Such a clinical course suggests a virus that replicated to a high titer and spread quickly from cell to cell. Thus, an NS1 protein that was especially effective at blocking the type I IFN system might have contributed to the exceptional virulence of the 1918 virus strain (Garcia-Sastre et al., 1998; Talon et al., 2000; Wang et al., 2000). To address this possibility, transfectant A/WSN/33 influenza viruses were constructed with the 1918 NS1 gene or with the entire 1918 NS segment (coding for both NS1 and NS2 [NEP] proteins) (Basler et al., 2001). In both cases, viruses containing 1918 NS genes were attenuated in mice compared to wild-type A/WSN/33 controls. The attenuation demonstrates that NS1 is critical for the virulence of A/WSN/33 in mice. On the other hand, transcriptional profiling (microarray analysis) of infected human lung epithelial cells showed that a virus with the 1918 NS1 gene was more effective at blocking the expression of IFN-regulated genes than the isogenic parental mouse-adapted A/WSN/33 virus (Geiss et al., 2002), suggesting that the 1918 NS1 contributes virulence characteristics in human cells, but not murine ones. The 1918 NS1 protein varies from that of the WSN virus at 10 amino acid positions. The amino acid differences between the 1918 and A/WSN/33 NS segments may be important in the adaptation of the latter virus strain to mice and likely account for the observed differences in virulence in these experiments. Recently, a single amino acid change (D92E) in the NS1 protein was associated with increased virulence of the 1997 Hong Kong H5N1 viruses in a swine model (Seo et al., 2002). This amino acid change was not found in the 1918 NS1 protein.

Sequence and Functional Analysis of the Matrix Gene Segment

The coding region of influenza A RNA segment 7 from the 1918 pandemic virus, consisting of the open reading frames of the two matrix genes, M1 and M2, has been sequenced (Reid et al., 2002). Although this segment is highly conserved among influenza virus strains, the 1918 sequence does not match any previously sequenced influenza virus strains. The 1918 sequence matches the consensus over the M1 RNA-binding domains and nuclear localization signal and the highly conserved transmembrane domain of M2. Amino acid changes that correlate with high yield and pathogenicity in animal models were not found in the 1918 virus strain.

Influenza A virus RNA segment 7 encodes two proteins, the matrix proteins M1 and M2. The M1 mRNA is colinear with the viral RNA, while the M2 mRNA is encoded by a spliced transcript (Lamb and Krug, 2001). The proteins encoded by these mRNAs share their initial 9 amino acids and also have a stretch of 14 amino acids in overlapping reading frames. The M1 protein is a highly conserved 252-amino-acid protein. It is the most abundant protein in the viral particle, lining the inner layer of the viral membrane and contacting the ribonucleoprotein (RNP) core. M1 has been shown to have several functions (Lamb and Krug, 2001), including regulation of nuclear export of vRNPs, both permitting the transport of vRNP particles into the nucleus upon infection and preventing newly exported vRNP particles from reentering the nucleus. The 97-amino-acid M2 protein is a homotetrameric integral membrane protein that exhibits ion-channel activity and is the target of the drug amantadine (Hay et al., 1985). The ion-channel activity of M2 is important both during virion uncoating and during viral budding (Lamb and Krug, 2001).

Five amino acid sites have been identified in the transmembrane region of the M2 protein that are involved in resistance to the antiviral drug amantadine: sites 26, 27, 30, 31, and 34 (Holsinger et al., 1994). The 1918 influenza M2 sequence is identical at these positions to that of the amantadine-sensitive influenza virus strains. Thus, it was predicted that the M2 protein of the 1918 influenza virus would be sensitive to amantadine. This was recently demonstrated experimentally. A recombinant virus possessing the 1918 matrix segment was inhibited effectively both in tissue culture and in vivo by the M2 ion-channel inhibitors amantadine and rimantadine (Tumpey et al., 2002).

The phylogenetic analyses suggest that the 1918 matrix genes, while more avian-like than those of other mammalian influenza viruses, were mammalian adapted (Reid et al., 2002). For example, the extracellular domain of the M2 protein contains four amino acids that differ consistently between the avian and mammalian clades (M2 residues #14, 16, 18, and 20). The 1918 sequence matches the mammalian sequence at all four of these residues (Reid et al., 2002), suggesting that the matrix segment may have been circulating in human virus strains for at least several years before 1918.

Sequence and Functional Analysis of the Nucleoprotein Gene Segment

The nucleoprotein gene (NP) of the 1918 pandemic influenza A virus has been amplified and sequenced from archival material (Reid et al., 2004). The NP gene is known to be involved in many aspects of viral function and to interact with host proteins, thereby playing a role in host specificity (Portela and Digard, 2002). NP is highly conserved, with a maximum amino acid difference of 11 percent among virus strains, probably because it must bind to multiple proteins, both viral and cellular. Numerous studies suggest that NP is a major determinant of host specificity (Scholtissek et al., 1978a, 1985). The 1918 NP amino acid sequence differs at only six amino acids from avian consensus sequences, consistent with reassortment from an avian source shortly before 1918. However, the 1918 NP nucleotide sequence has more than 170 differences from avian consensus sequences, suggesting substantial evolutionary distance from known avian sequences. Both the 1918 NP gene and protein sequences fall within the mammalian clade upon phylogenetic analysis.

Phylogenetic analyses of NP sequences from many virus strains result in trees with two main branches, one consisting of mammalian-adapted virus strains and one of avian-adapted virus strains (Gammelin et al., 1990; Gorman et al., 1991; Shu et al., 1993). The NP gene segment was not replaced in the pandemics of 1957 and 1968, so it is likely that the sequences in the mammalian clade are descended from the 1918 NP segment. The mammalian branches, unlike the avian branch, show a slow but steady accumulation of changes over time. Extrapolation of the rate of change along the human branch back to a putative common ancestor suggests that this NP entered the mammalian lineage sometime after 1900 (Gammelin et al., 1990; Gorman et al., 1991; Shu et al., 1993). Separate analyses of synonymous and nonsynonymous substitutions also placed the 1918 virus NP gene in the mammalian clade (Reid et al., 2004). When synonymous substitutions were analyzed, the 1918 virus gene was placed within and near the root of swine viruses. When nonsynonymous viruses were analyzed, the 1918 virus gene was placed within and near the root of the human viruses.

The evolutionary distance of the 1918 NP from avian and mammalian sequences was examined using several different parameters. There are at least three possibilities for the origin of the 1918 NP gene segment (Reid et al., 2004). First, it could have been retained from the previously circulating human virus, as was the case with the 1957 and 1968 pandemic virus strains, whose NP segments are descendants of the 1918 NP. The large number of nucleotide changes from the avian consensus and the placement of the 1918 sequence in the mammalian clade are consistent with this hypothesis. Neighbor-joining analyses of nonsynonymous nucleotide sequences or of amino acid sequences place the 1918 sequence within and near the root of the human clade. The 1918 NP has only a few amino acid differences from most bird virus strains, but this consistent group of amino acid changes is shared by the 1918 NP and its subsequent mammalian descendants and is not found in any birds, resulting in the 1918 sequence being placed outside the avian clade (Reid et al., 2004). One or more of these amino acid substitutions may be important for adaptation of the protein to humans. However, the very small number of amino acid differences from the avian consensus argues for recent introduction from birds— 80 years after 1918, the NP genes of human influenza virus strains have accumulated more than 30 additional amino acid differences from the avian consensus (a rate of 2.3 amino acid changes per year). Thus it seems unlikely that the 1918 NP, with only six amino acid differences from the avian consensus, could have been in humans for many years before 1918. This conclusion is supported by the regression analysis that suggests that the progenitor of the 1918 virus probably entered the human population around 1915 (Reid et al., 2004).

A second possible origin for the 1918 NP segment is direct reassortment from an avian virus. The small number of amino acid differences between 1918 and the avian consensus supports this hypothesis. While 1918 varies at many nucleotides from the nearest avian virus strain, avian virus strains are quite diverse at the nucleotide level. Synonymous/nonsynonymous ratios between 1918 and avian virus strains are similar to the ratios between avian virus strains, opening the possibility that avian virus strains may exist that are more closely related to 1918. The great evolutionary distance between the 1918 sequence and the avian consensus suggests that no avian virus strain similar to those in the currently identified clades could have provided the 1918 virus strain with its NP segment.

A final possibility is that the 1918 gene segment was acquired shortly before 1918 from a source not currently represented in the database of influenza sequences. There may be a currently unknown influenza host that, while similar to currently characterized avian virus strains at the amino acid level, is quite different at the nucleotide level. It is possible that such a host was the source of the 1918 NP segment (Reid et al., 2004).

Future Work

Five of the eight RNA segments of the 1918 influenza virus have been sequenced and analyzed. Their characterization has shed light on the origin of the virus and strongly supports the hypothesis that the 1918 virus was the common ancestor of both subsequent human and swine H1N1 lineages. Sequence analysis of the genes to date offers no definitive clue as to the exceptional virulence of the 1918 virus strain. Thus, experiments testing models of virulence using reverse genetics approaches with 1918 influenza genes have begun.

In future work it is hoped that the 1918 pandemic virus strain can be placed in the context of influenza virus strains that preceded it and followed it. The direct precursor of the pandemic virus, the first or "spring" wave virus strain, lacked the exceptional virulence of the fall wave virus strain. Identification of an influenza RNA-positive case from the first wave would have tremendous value in deciphering the genetic basis for virulence by allowing differences in the sequences to be highlighted. Identification of pre-1918 human influenza RNA samples would clarify which gene segments were novel in the 1918 virus.

In many respects, the 1918 influenza pandemic was similar to other influenza pandemics. In its epidemiology, disease course, and pathology, the pandemic generally was different in degree but not in kind from previous and subsequent pandemics. Furthermore, laboratory experiments using recombinant influenza viruses containing genes from the 1918 virus suggest that the 1918 and 1918-like viruses would be as sensitive to the Food and Drug Administration-approved anti-influenza drugs rimantadine and oseltamivir as other virus strains (Tumpey et al., 2002). However, there are some characteristics of the pandemic that appear to be unique: Mortality was exceptionally high, ranging from 5 to 20 times higher than normal. Clinically and pathologically, the high mortality appears to be the result of a higher proportion of severe and complicated infections of the respiratory tract, not with systemic infection or involvement of organ systems outside the influenza virus's normal targets. The mortality was concentrated in an unusually young age group. Finally, the waves of influenza activity followed each other unusually rapidly, resulting in three major outbreaks within a year's time. Each of these unique characteristics may find their explanation in genetic features of the 1918 virus. The challenge will be in determining the links between the biological capabilities of the virus and the known history of the pandemic.

Research Agenda for the Future

The work on the 1918 influenza virus, especially its origin, has led to the support of more comprehensive influenza virus surveillance and genomics initiatives for both human and animal influenza A viruses. We believe significant advancement in the understanding of influenza biology and ecology can be made by the generation of full genomic sequences of a large number of influenza viruses from different hosts. In conclusion, some of the questions that need to be addressed in pandemic influenza include the following:

- Can an entire avian influenza virus adapt directly in a human, or is reassortment necessary to generate a pandemic strain?
- Does adaptation of an avian influenza virus to humans require an intermediate host?
- Can all possible subtypes of avian influenza virus reassort to form functional human pandemic strains, or are there biological limitations to particular HA and NA subtypes?
- A novel HA seems to be required for a pandemic strain; what about the other gene segments?
- Can genetic changes be mapped to "virulence"?
- Can features of virulence be separated from the host in question? Can the viral genetic component of human virulence be modeled in experimental animal or in vitro systems?
- What molecular changes are necessary for avian strains to adapt to mammals, and to humans in particular?
- Can host-adaptive changes (genetic fingerprints) be used to trace the evolution of a pandemic strain through intermediate hosts?

Unless we make progress in understanding these and other issues involving the complex ecology and biology of influenza viruses, we will face the risk of revisiting the past in our future.

PANDEMIC INFLUENZA AND MORTALITY: PAST EVIDENCE AND PROJECTIONS FOR THE FUTURE[5]

L. Simonsen,[6] D.R. Olson,[7] C. Viboud,[8] E. Heiman,[6] R.J. Taylor,[9] M.A. Miller,[8] and T.A. Reichert[10]

[5]This work was partially supported by a research grant from the National Vaccine Program Office, Unmet Needs. We thank Steven S. Morse and David S. Fedson for their support of this research activity, and our many international colleagues who supplied mortality data for the Multinational Influenza Seasonal Mortality Study (MISMS) network.
[6]National Institute of Allergy and Infectious Diseases, National Institutes of Health (NIH), Bethesda, MD.
[7]Columbia University, New York, NY.
[8]Fogarty International Center (FIC), NIH, Bethesda, MD.
[9]Under contract to National Institute of Allergy and Infectious Diseases, NIH, Bethesda, MD.
[10]Entropy Research Institute, NJ, under contract to FIC, NIH, Bethesda, MD.

SUMMARY

Pandemic influenza is often thought of as a tornado—a sudden disaster that arrives with little warning and does its worst in a relatively short time. Only three of these calamities occurred in the twentieth century. Their mortality impact ranged from devastating (the 1918 "Spanish" A(H1N1) influenza) to moderate (the 1957 Asian A(H2N2) pandemic) to mild (the 1968 "Hong Kong" A(H3N2) virus). In this paper we review the "pandemic age shift," a signature change of mortality impact from the elderly to younger age groups that has occurred during each of these pandemics. We also suggest that the "tornado" paradigm may not be completely apt, in that past pandemics have given epidemiologic warning signs of their arrival, and generally play out over several years.

For the 1918 Spanish influenza pandemic, a new study by Olson et al. documents substantial mortality impact during a pandemic "herald wave" in early spring of 1918 in New York City, and a general lack of increased pandemic mortality in those over 45 years of age. For the 1957 pandemic, a classic study documented that the emerging H2N2 influenza virus caused substantial excess mortality during the first three seasons it was in circulation. The 1968 pandemic mortality impact was only "smoldering" in Europe during the first season and did not break into open flame until the next season, during which the majority of mortality impact occurred. Although mortality caused by the 1968 pandemic virus was unimpressive relative to surrounding severe epidemics, the age shift signature sets it apart. Furthermore, antibodies to H3-like antigens—the result of exposure to these antigens in childhood prior to 1892—relatively protected people aged 77 years and older.

Because our experience with pandemic influenza is so limited, it is difficult to predict the mortality impact of future pandemics except to say that the likely range is wide (from ~20 to ~500 deaths per 100,000 population) and that those under 65 years of age will account for a high proportion of the deaths. It may be helpful to think of pandemic mortality impact as the sum of influenza-related deaths that occur over several seasons dominated by the emerging virus until the pandemic age shift pattern gives way to "business as usual," which typically occurs after a decade or less.

The good news from epidemiological studies for pandemic preparedness planning is that past pandemics gave significant warning signs of their arrival. In 1918, a pandemic herald wave occurred 6 months or more before the majority of mortality impact the following fall. The Asian H2N2 influenza virus was characterized by early summer, 1957, but significant mortality in the United States did not occur until October. In 1968, the pandemic wave of mortality in Europe crested a full year after the pandemic strain first arrived. Furthermore, in both the 1957 and 1968 pandemics, much of the total impact occurred as a series of smaller "twisters" in the first several seasons after its emergence, before the total population had been affected. These facts suggest that there may well be sufficient time for production and distribution of vaccine and antiviral drugs to prevent much of the mortality impact of the next pandemic, and that these medical interventions will continue to play an important role in limiting "pandemic" mortality for years after the pandemic season. Finally, the pandemic age shift documented for all pandemics studied begs the crucial question of who should be given first priority for vaccine and antivirals, should these be in short supply in the early phase of a pandemic.

The Charge: Using Lessons from Past Pandemics to Help Project the Impact of Future Pandemics

In the case of pandemics, we are planning for the equivalent of a tornado . . . rare and completely unpredictable until the last minute, when a "weather watch" (e.g., pandemic alert) appears on the TV screen (Kilbourne, 1997).

The lesson of the history of pandemics appears to be that at least the initial attack may sometimes occur with gentleness and thus may afford a substantial breathing space for the preparation and use of specific vaccine (Stuart-Harris, 1970).

Why worry about pandemics of the past? Three influenza pandemics occurred in the twentieth century, and the patterns and magnitude of pandemic mortality are the only impact data available for all three of these events (Table 1-1). We believe, therefore, that continued epidemiological

TABLE 1-1 Mortality Impact in the Three Pandemics of the Twentieth Century in the United States

	Antigenic Shift (Pandemic Event)	Number of Excess Deaths in the Pandemic Season (All-Cause Deaths)	Total Excess Mortality Rate per 100,000 Population (Crude) (All-Cause Deaths)
1918–1919 A(H1N1)	H + N (All novel virus?)	~ 500,000	530
1957–1958 A(H2N2)	H + N	~ 60,000	40
1968–1969 A(H3N2)	H only	~ 40,000	18

analyses of historic mortality data and sero-archaeology—the study of stored serum samples to uncover when specific influenza antigens were circulating—can expand our understanding of pandemic mortality patterns and severity, and that such studies will greatly aid public health planning for pandemic influenza.

In this review, we present the story of pandemic influenza as seen through the lens of epidemiology. For the 1968 pandemic we present data comparing the mortality impact internationally—and highlight the still un-explained finding of "smoldering" pandemic activity in Europe. We review more recent efforts to characterize the signature "age shift" of pandemic influenza and highlight the value of sero-archaeology as a tool to under-stand what we call "the virtues of antigenic sin"—protection derived from exposure in childhood to influenza H-antigens that are recycled in later pandemic viruses. We revisit a classic study of the 1957 pandemic that analyzes age-specific mortality data from the United States, which shows that most of the mortality was spread over three seasons; we also compare the age-specific mortality impact in the United States to that in Japan. For the 1918 pandemic, we present a study of newly uncovered mortality data from New York City that tells a fetching story about a herald wave and the sparing of the elderly (Olson et al., 2004).

These efforts to study the epidemiology of past pandemic impact on mortality are akin to the efforts by virologists who, in the interest of pre-dicting the future, are hard at work identifying and studying preserved human and animal virus specimens from the 1918 Spanish flu pandemic (Reid and Taubenberger, 2003). But instead of molecular clues to viral pathogenicity and recombination, mortality data provides some important insights into how the pandemic evolves over time, and which age groups are at highest risk for severe outcomes. First, a future pandemic may not appear as a completely unpredictable "tornado" that hits hard the first season and leaves little time for production and distribution of vaccines and antivirals. It is certainly true that, like a tornado, no one can predict precisely when a new pandemic strain might emerge. However, studies of past pandemics show that the next pandemic may well not do its worst in the first season. Instead, historical evidence shows that there can be herald waves or smolder-ing activity during the first season in which the pandemic influenza virus emerges, suggesting that the preparation time for pandemic vaccines and antivirals might be longer than a few months. Second, pandemic impact cannot be discussed without speaking of age. During a pandemic, the younger population is at substantially increased risk relative to non-pandemic influenza seasons; in some pandemics, this sparing of the elderly may occur as a consequence of antigen recycling. The pandemic age shift has important consequences for thinking about how best to protect the population and minimize years of life lost to future pandemic influenza.

The Pandemic Age Shift: A Signature of Pandemic Mortality Impact

It has previously been demonstrated that all three pandemics of this century were characterized by a shift in the age distribution of deaths (Simonsen et al., 1998). The younger population (in that study, persons under 65 years of age) experienced a sharply elevated mortality risk and accounted for a markedly increased fraction of all influenza-related deaths. As we will discuss below, the 1968 pandemic age shift pattern was exacerbated by the protection of the very elderly by virtue of their experience with H3 antigens as children (Simonsen et al., 2003). For the 1968 pandemic, then, the observed age shift was due to a combination of increased risk among the young and decreased risk among the elderly (Simonsen et al., 2003).

During the 1957 A(H2N2) Asian pandemic in the United States, nearly 40 percent of all influenza-related deaths occurred in the younger population under 65 years of age. The proportion of deaths among people under age 65 that occurred during A(H2N2) epidemics dropped to 5 percent by 1968, when circulation of this virus ceased. In the 1968 A(H3N2) pandemic, this proportion was approximately 50 percent, but declined to less than 10 percent over the next decade (Figure 1-6) (Simonsen et al., 2003).

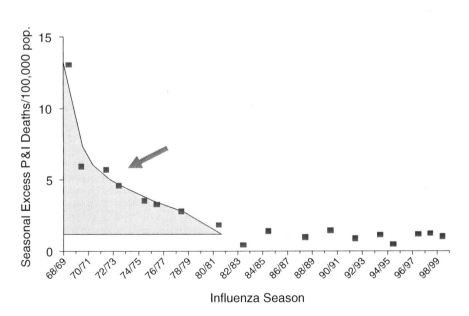

FIGURE 1-6 A pandemic "decade": Seasonal excess pneumonia and influenza (P&I) mortality rates for A(H3N2)-dominated seasons remained elevated for a decade after 1968 in persons aged 45–64 years, United States, 1968–1999.

The age shift in mortality was even more pronounced in the 1918 A(H1N1) Spanish influenza pandemic (Collins, 1931; Simonsen, 1998; Olson et al., 2004).

The 1968 Hong Kong Pandemic: Some New Observations

The Unimpressive Impact of the 1968 Pandemic on Mortality in the United States

The 1968 pandemic is the only one known in which a shift in the hemagglutinin antigen was not accompanied by a shift in the neuramini-dase antigen. Perhaps for that reason, the 1968 pandemic mortality impact was not particularly severe compared to the severe epidemic in 1967–1968 (the last A(H2N2) epidemic), as well as two severe H3N2 epidemics in 1975–1976 and 1980–1981 (Table 1-2). People aged 75 years and older were far less likely to die of influenza during the pandemic than during these three surrounding epidemics, whereas people aged 45–64 years were at nearly three-fold elevated risk. Despite the differences in *relative* risk among age groups in different years, the *absolute* risk of dying of influenza during the pandemic was about 3 times higher for the elderly than for the younger age group (Table 1-2).

TABLE 1-2 The Age-Specific Impact of the 1968 Pandemic in the United States*: Comparison to Surrounding Severe Epidemics

	Excess All-Cause (and P&I) Deaths/100,000 Population		
	All Ages	75+ Years of Age	45–64 Years of Age
1967–1968 A/H2N2 epidemic	18 [6.3]	349 [107]	14 [3.6]
1968–1969 A/H3N2 pandemic	19 [9.1]	131 [79]	37 [13.0]
1975–1976 A/H3N2 epidemic	8 [6.5]	222 [113]	5 [3.2]
1980–1981 A/H3N2 epidemic	23 [4.3]	316 [70]	15 [1.8]

*Winter-seasonal excess mortality rates (crude rates, unpublished data, Simonsen et al.) estimated by applying a Serfling (Serfling, 1963) model to U.S. monthly mortality data from 1967–1982.

Virtues of Antigenic Sin: The Sparing of the Elderly

Sero-archaeological studies have demonstrated that the majority of the very elderly had H3 antibodies before they were exposed to the 1968 A(H3N2) pandemic virus (Dowdle, 1999; Marine and Workman, 1969). These antibodies were remnants of the immune response to exposure to H3N? viruses that circulated before 1891 (Marine and Workman, 1969); thus, the 1968 pandemic virus apparently contained an H3 antigen "recycled" after 77 years of absence. Marine and Workman hypothesized that the pre-existing anti-H3 antibodies were the result of "original antigenic sin" (Davenport et al., 1953)—childhood exposure to H3 antigens—and that these antibodies might have protected the elderly during the 1968 A(H3N2) pandemic (Marine and Workman, 1969). We recently confirmed this hypothesis when we used U.S. national mortality data to demonstrate that people over the age of 77 were, in fact, protected from influenza-related mortality during the 1968 pandemic, compared to surrounding severe non-pandemic seasons (Simonsen et al., 2003). Even so, the absolute risk of dying from 1968 pandemic influenza was always highest among the very elderly, although this risk was likely significantly lower than it would have been without the protection provided by the anti-H3 antibodies still present in this age group. Figure 1-7 shows the several-fold increase in

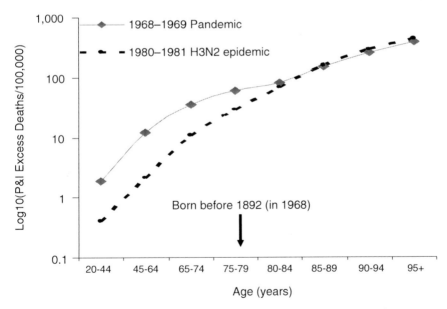

FIGURE 1-7 Evidence of protection of the very elderly by "virtues of antigenic sin": Age-specific excess P&I mortality rates for the 1968 pandemic compared to the 1980–1981 season.

pneumonia and influenza (P&I) mortality rates during the 1968 pandemic among younger age groups in the United States compared to the 1980–1981 season, and the absence of any such increase among the very elderly.

These findings have significant implications for both pandemic planning and the prioritization of high-risk groups for vaccination in the scenario of vaccine shortage. Indeed, if one wishes to minimize the number of years-of-life-lost should vaccine be in short supply, then it would be more effective to immunize the middle aged and younger elderly than the very elderly.

The European 1968 Experience: A "Smoldering" Pattern

The 1968 pandemic experience in Europe was different from that of the United States. It began with the rapid spread of a new virus, which reached Europe about 2 months after its emergence in Hong Kong (Cockburn et al., 1969). But influenza activity remained curiously weak in the wave that occurred during the 1968–1969 winter in Europe (Assaad et al., 1973; Stuart-Harris, 1970). At the same time, influenza-related mortality and morbidity increased substantially in the United States, especially among the young (Housworth and Spoon, 1971). More surprising, a much more severe wave occurred in the United Kingdom during the winter of 1969–1970, although no change in the circulating strain had been identified (Miller et al., 1971). We revisited the pandemic experience in the United States and the United Kingdom by extending the analysis of mortality data from both countries (Figure 1-8) to better describe and possibly explain the geographical differences.

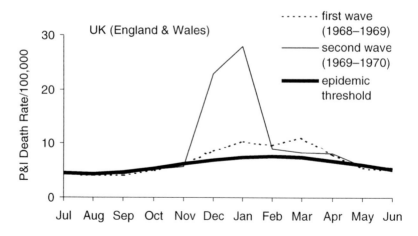

FIGURE 1-8 Monthly pneumonia and influenza (P&I) mortality rate during the first two waves of the 1968 pandemic (A/H3N2) in the United Kingdom. Epidemic threshold determined by a spline-Serfling regression model.

TABLE 1-3 Comparison of the Relative Impact* of the First Two Waves of A/H3N2 Viruses and the Age Distribution of Influenza Deaths in the United States and United Kingdom, 1968–1970

A/H3N2 Pandemic seasons	USA (population: 205 million)		UK (England and Wales) (population: 48 million)	
	Relative impact of each wave [derived from excess P&I mortality rate/100,000 (all ages)]	Proportion of excess P&I deaths in persons under 65 years of age	Relative impact of each wave [derived from excess P&I mortality rate/100,000 (all ages)]	Proportion of excess P&I deaths in persons under 65 years of age
1968/1969 (1st wave)	70%	38%	22%	20%
1969/1970 (2nd wave)	30%	37%	78%	25%
Total pandemic impact (sum of 2 seasons)	100%	38%	100%	24%

*All figures are standardized with regard to the 1969 population of England and Wales and based on a Serfling regression "spline" model applied to monthly data.
SOURCE: Viboud et al. (2004).

In both countries, we studied the age distribution of mortality rates associated with the first and second pandemic waves of A/H3N2, which occurred during the winters of 1968–1969 and 1969–1970 (Table 1-3). Consistent with the epidemiologic signature of a pandemic (Simonsen et al., 1998), a mortality shift towards younger age groups was observed simultaneously in both the United States and United Kingdom. The shift in the first pandemic wave (1968/1969) in the United Kingdom was not quite as definitive, but was nonetheless above the background of preceding epidemic seasons. In both countries, the proportion of deaths in younger age groups was highly elevated in the second wave. This age shift is consistent with the fact that virus surveillance systems reported widespread circulation of A(H3N2) in both countries during both seasons (Miller et al., 1971; Housworth and Spoon, 1971).

Because pneumonia mortality rates throughout the year were more than two-fold higher in the United Kingdom than in the United States during the 1950s and 1960s (Langmuir and Housworth, 1969; WHO, 1971), direct comparison of the *absolute* excess P&I mortality impact of the two pandemic waves is less revealing than their *relative* impact. In the United States, the first wave (1968–1969) accounted for 70 percent of the pandemic deaths, and the second season accounted for the remaining 30 percent. In the United Kingdom, however, the proportions were reversed: the first wave accounted for only 22 percent of UK pandemic deaths, whereas the remaining 78 percent occurred in the second (Table 1-3). Given that circulation of the pandemic virus is well-documented, we use the term "smoldering pandemic" to characterize the first wave in the United Kingdom—the pandemic started slowly, but built to a more destructive conflagration in the second season. We are currently studying other countries, and it thus far appears that the UK pattern describes the typical "European" 1968 pandemic experience (Stuart-Harris, 1970), while the U.S. pattern appears to represent the North American experience (Viboud et al., 2004).

The impact of a novel influenza virus is thought to decrease over time as immunity increases in the population (Cox and Subbarao, 2000; Miller et al., 1971). The European 1968 pandemic pattern, with its smoldering delay, did not fit this pattern, however. More than 30 years later, the reasons for the "smoldering waves" and the differences between North America and Europe are not clear (Nguyen-Van-Tam and Hampson, 2003). It is possible that in Europe only, a high level of immunity to neuraminidase N2 protected the population during the first A/H3N2 wave (Stuart-Harris, 1970). Such immunity would have been acquired through past exposure to A/H2N2 viruses. The "immunity" hypothesis is supported by a high rate of asymptomatic illnesses reported during the first pandemic wave in Europe (Miller et al., 1971; Sohier and Henry, 1969). Alternatively, the different patterns may be due to minor genetic differences in the A/H3N2 viruses that circulated on the two continents. This hypothesis is difficult to address because only a very limited number of influenza A(H3N2) genetic sequences from the 1968–1970 period are available in the public domain. A new influenza genomics initiative recently funded by the National Institute of Allergy and Infectious Diseases (NIAID) should help change this situation, however. Under this program the Institute for Genomic Research (TIGR) will sequence qualified and properly prepared influenza virus samples for investigators (http://www.niaid.nih.gov/dmid/genomes/mscs/projects.htm). This initiative should encourage scientists everywhere to dig out old isolates sitting quietly in laboratory freezers, so that their complete sequences can be placed in GenBank for all to use.

From the perspective of pandemic planning, the smoldering European 1968 pandemic experience is encouraging, in that a repeat of this pattern in a future pandemic might allow the production and distribution of pandemic vaccines to occur in time to prevent a great many deaths. Indeed, had an effective pandemic vaccine become available in Europe even a full year after the emergence of A(H3N2) viruses in 1968, the majority of deaths associated with this pandemic might have been prevented. Whether smoldering patterns will occur in future pandemics is, of course, not known.

The 1957 Asian Pandemic: Impact Over Several Seasons

The 1957 influenza pandemic, which claimed the lives of more than one million people worldwide, has long been an unofficial model scenario for a future pandemic in the United States. In order to increase the utility of this model for pandemic planners, we have recently begun to compare the well-characterized mortality patterns observed in the United States during the pandemic (Serfling et al., 1967) with those of other countries.

The U.S. Experience: Three Waves Between 1957 and 1963

The Asian H2N2 influenza virus is thought to have first emerged in China in February or March 1957. It reached the United States in early summer, at which time it caused sporadic outbreaks (Jordan, 1958a; Dunn, 1958). However, a measurable impact on U.S. mortality did not occur until October (Serfling et al., 1967). Moreover, each of the first three seasons dominated by the emerging A(H2N2) virus—1957–1958, 1959–1960 and 1962–1963—resulted in roughly equivalent spikes in excess P&I mortality rates in the U.S. population (Serfling et al., 1967) (Table 1-4). These observations suggest that the second twentieth century pandemic did not strike in a sudden, overwhelming onslaught. Instead, measurable mortality impact occurred 4 to 6 months after the virus had begun to circulate and was isolated.

Serfling's analyses of the U.S. data also revealed that of all the deaths that occurred among age groups 45 years or younger during the first three serious H2N2 seasons, the majority occurred in the pandemic season of 1957–1958. Conversely, those 45 years and older felt the majority of the mortality impact in the next two A(H2N2)-dominated seasons, 1959–1960 and 1962–1963. For example, 71 percent of the excess deaths among 15–19 year olds in all three seasons occurred during the pandemic 1957–1958 season, while for people aged 75 and older only 33 percent of excess deaths occurred in the pandemic season (Table 1-4). These differences in age-related mortality patterns closely reflected differences in age-specific attack rates of the influenza virus, which were available from the Cleveland Family Study (Jordan et al., 1958a) and Tecumseh, Michigan (Hennessy et al., 1964). Indeed, the attack rate among school children was very high (72.9 percent) in 1957–1958 (Jordan et al., 1958b), but far lower in 1959–1960 and 1962–1963 (Hennessy et al., 1964). It was considered possible that the lower 1957–1958 attack rates left a larger proportion of susceptible people among older cohorts during the subsequent seasons (Hennessy et al., 1964). In summary, the bulk of A(H2N2) infection and mortality among younger age groups occurred in 1957/1958; much less occurred in the subsequent seasons, during which these younger age groups were probably protected by immunity gained through their first encounter with A(H2N2) viruses. However, for the middle aged and elderly, the "pandemic" impact was almost evenly divided between the first three seasons dominated by A(H2N2) viruses (Serfling et al., 1967).

To investigate whether this age-specific mortality pattern also describes the international experience, we set out to develop a methodology for

TABLE 1-4 Relative Impact of First Three "Waves" of A(H2N2) Influenza in the United States, 1957–1963 (modified from data in Serfling et al., 1967)

	Excess P&I Mortality Rate/100,000 Population in the United States and the [Proportional Contribution to the Total for Three Seasons]		
Pandemic	All Ages	School Children 5–14 Years of Age	Elderly 75+ Years of Age
1957/1958	10.6 [44%]	1.5 [75%]	97 [33%]
1959/1960	7.4 [30%]	0.3 [15%]	102 [35%]
1962/1963	6.3 [26%]	0.2 [10%]	94 [32%]
Total pandemic impact (sum of 3 seasons)	24.3 [100%]	2.0 [100%]	293 [100%]

TABLE 1-5 Relative impact of first 3 "waves" of A(H2N2) influenza in JAPAN, 1957–1963 (data from Heiman et al., unpublished)

Pandemic	Excess P&I Mortality Rate/100,000 Population in Japan and the [Proportional Contribution to the Total for Three Seasons]		
	All Ages	School Children 5–14 Years of Age	Elderly 75+ Years of Age
1957/1958	1.8 [44%]	1.9 [79%]	29 [36%]
1959/1960	0.9 [30%]	0.2 [8%]	18 [22%]
1962/1963	1.3 [26%]	0.3 [13%]	34 [42%]
Total pandemic impact (sum of 3 seasons)	4.0 [100%]	2.4 [100%]	81 [100%]

measuring pandemic mortality burden based on annual mortality data (Heiman et al., unpublished). Annual age-specific P&I mortality data were provided by WHO for the United States and Japan. We estimated the pandemic excess mortality in 1957 and 1958 by subtracting as background the number of deaths in surrounding years when there was little or no influenza A activity. We validated this approach by comparing these U.S. age-specific excess mortality estimates with those generated using actual seasonal data (Serfling et al., 1967). We found that for Japan, the age pattern of relative impact over the first seasons was very similar to that observed in the United States (Table 1-5). Also, in contrast to the United States where there was no measurable increase in influenza-related mortality until October, P&I mortality in Japan was elevated in the early summer of 1957 (Reichert et al., 2001).

The 1918 Spanish Influenza Pandemic Revisited: Evidence for a Severe Herald Wave and Protection of the Elderly in New York City

The exact time and place that the 1918 pandemic virus originated has never been conclusively determined. Public health investigators recognized almost immediately that the so-called Spanish influenza, which spread across Europe in the late spring and summer of 1918 and exploded globally in the autumn and winter of 1918/1919, probably did not originate in Spain (Low, 1920). Reports of influenza epidemics in U.S. military training camps in spring 1918, however, led some to identify the central United States as the "presumptive primary focus" of the pandemic (Vaughn, 1921).

Although this hypothesis has been cited many times over the years, it has never been subject to rigorous reexamination. Moreover, an old analysis of regional urban U.S. mortality statistics showed that excess mortality increased in several Atlantic seaboard cities in the spring of 1918, especially in New York City, suggesting that perhaps the pandemic strain might already have been spreading in this region (Frost, 1919).

To investigate whether and when the characteristic age shift occurred in influenza seasons preceding the 1918–1919 pandemic season in the United States, age-stratified excess deaths in New York City were analyzed (Olson et al., 2004). Comparison of all-cause mortality data for people over and under age 45 indicated that a shift in age-specific excess mortality happened very early in 1918, in the midst of an ongoing influenza season. This pattern is consistent with the arrival of the pandemic virus in New York City at about this time, and the subsequent occurrence of a pandemic herald wave from February to April 1918 (Figure 1-9, Table 1-6).

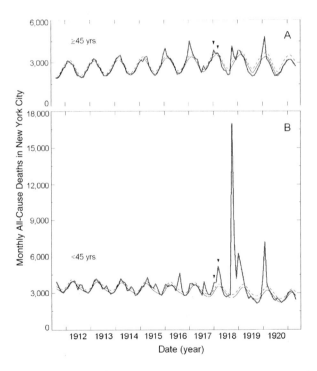

FIGURE 1-9 Monthly all-cause deaths in New York City by age. Classic Serfling model estimates of baseline mortality and 95 percent confidence limits were calculated for under-45 [B] and 45-and-over [A] all-cause deaths. The seasonal pattern indicates that the 1917–1918 influenza season (arrowheads) showed two periods with distinct age-specific peaks. (Figure modified from Olson et al., 2004.)

TABLE 1-6 Age-Specific Mortality Impact of the 1918–1919 A(H1N1) Pandemic in New York City (Population: 5 million) and During the "Herald Wave" in Early 1918 (modified from Olson et al., 2004)

Age Groups (years of age)	Pre-Herald Wave January 1918 All-Cause Excess Mortality Rate/100,000 Population	Herald Wave February–April 1918 All-Cause Excess Mortality Rate/100,000 Population	Major Pandemic September 1918–March 1919 All-Cause Excess Mortality Rate/100,000 Population
<5	84	230	720
5–14	2	21	190
15–24	5	64	580
25–44	7	38	760
45–64	18	14	210
65+	190	95	150
All ages	21	56	530

The New York City data also demonstrate that mortality among people aged 45 and older during the 1918–1919 pandemic influenza season was no worse than in surrounding years. For people under age 45, however, the 1918–1919 influenza season was very bad—people in this age group were far more likely to die of influenza than in previous years. Indeed, the age groups at highest *absolute* risk of dying during the 1918–1919 A(H1N1) pandemic were young children and young and middle-aged adults (Table 1-6).

These findings suggest that the early 1918 pandemic herald wave was spreading as early as February 1918, 6–7 months before the beginning of the explosive 1918–1919 pandemic. Relative to preceding influenza epidemic seasons, both the herald and pandemic waves caused proportionally more mortality in younger age groups but less mortality among those over 45 years of age, possibly as the result of recycling of an H1-like antigen from half a century earlier (Olson et al., 2004).

Conclusion: Lessons from Pandemics Past for Pandemics Still to Come

Epidemiologic studies of past pandemics offer at least three important insights into what we can expect when the next influenza pandemic occurs. We believe these observations can help to guide pandemic detection and preparedness planning.

1. Mortality impact is difficult to predict, but a shift to younger ages is highly likely. Because our experience with pandemic influenza is so limited (N = 3), it is difficult to predict the mortality impact of a future pandemic. One can say, however, that the likely range is wide (from ~20 to ~500 deaths per 100,000 people) and that people under 65 years of age will account for a high proportion of these death.

2. Pandemic mortality impact is not always "tornado-like." Pandemic influenza is not always like a sudden storm, followed by a return to clear skies. Instead, mortality rates can remain elevated for several years—during which time an effective vaccine would be in high demand. For example, in the 1957 pandemic worldwide, and in the 1968 pandemic in North America, much of the pandemic mortality impact occurred in a series of smaller but still severe twisters in subsequent years. This seems well explained by attack rates: The pattern of cumulative age-specific mortality impact during the first waves mirrored the age-specific attack rates, at least for the 1957 pandemic (Serfling et al., 1967). Thus, the majority of middle-aged and elderly people—age groups that account for most of the cumulative pandemic mortality—were only affected by the emerging strain during the second or third season after its emergence.

3. Often there is a warning. For the 1918 pandemic, a herald wave that caused substantial mortality occurred at least 6 months before the major force of the pandemic hit in September. The 1957 pandemic virus had been characterized in Asia by the spring and was known to be circulating in the United States as early as June—months before the pandemic mortality impact began. For the 1968 pandemic, the majority of European deaths occurred after a 1-year delay. Thus, in all three pandemics, some form of warning was available.

Although mortality data are useful to characterize the patterns and impact of past pandemics, in most countries such data would not be available to allow timely detection of mortality age shifts to reveal pandemic activity. Instead, influenza virus surveillance efforts are most likely to provide the first warning of a future pandemic. And because younger people are disproportionately infected by pandemic strains when these first emerge, focusing pandemic virus surveillance efforts on isolates from children and young adults with severe outcomes of upper respiratory diseases would help to ensure that pandemic activity is detected as quickly as possible.

The idea that the next pandemic may not do all or even most of its damage in the first season is certainly good news for preparedness planning. In all three pandemics in the twentieth century, the majority of associated deaths occurred 6 months to a year *after* the pandemic virus first emerged. This suggests that intense and timely surveillance of both age-specific mortality and new influenza viruses could provide sufficient time for production and distribution of vaccines and antivirals to prevent much, if not most, of the mortality impact. Moreover, these medical interventions are likely to continue to play an important role for many years after the pandemic season. One should also note that the 1957 and 1968 pandemics tended to respect normal seasonality patterns, giving one hemisphere of the world an extra 6 months to prepare.

Finally, the existence of the pandemic age shift documented for all pandemics studied raises a crucial question: Who should get vaccines and antivirals first if these are in short supply, younger people or the elderly? If a future pandemic were to be like the severe 1918/1919 pandemic, in which young and middle-aged adults were the age groups at highest absolute risk of dying, then younger people should clearly get priority. But if a future pandemic were like the 1957 or the 1968 pandemics, the answer would not be so obvious. In those years, young and middle-aged adults were facing the most dramatic risk increase relative to non-pandemic influenza, yet they remained at a lower absolute risk than the elderly. The situation would be made more complex if the pandemic virus were to contain a recycled influenza antigen. In this instance, elderly age groups with prior exposure to similar antigens might be at less risk than in preceding non-pandemic seasons.

Of course, with or without recycling, a pattern like those seen in 1957 or 1968 would result in the elderly having a higher absolute risk of death.

If the metric used to measure effectiveness of vaccination were "numbers of deaths prevented," then perhaps the elderly should be given priority— assuming they can produce an adequate antibody response to the pandemic vaccine. But if the concern is to minimize the years-of-life-lost, then the vaccine may be better used in young and middle-aged adults. This point was illustrated in a paper that sought to determine vaccination priorities by age and risk status; when basing priority on "returns due to vaccination," an endpoint that is heavily influenced by years of life lost, the young and middle aged rose to the top of the priority list (Meltzer et al., 1999). Other authors have proposed that children be given priority to receive pandemic vaccine (Stuart-Harris, 1970; Longini et al., 1978; Reichert et al., 2001) and antivirals (Longini et al., 2004) in order to reduce transmission in the community and thereby indirectly reduce influenza impact among the elderly. The 2004 U.S. Pandemic Influenza Preparedness and Response Plan developed by the National Vaccine Program Office has not yet defined such priority groups (DHHS, 2004:24).

Given the very different proposals for how to best employ pandemic vaccines and antivirals should a shortage occur, we urge that a framework for determining priority groups be developed immediately. Such a scheme should be agreed on beforehand and be flexible enough to adapt to the likely level of disaster at hand. Any such an assessment would depend on rapid interpretation of early data on transmissibility and case fatality in the pandemic epicenter.

Will the next pandemic be 1918-like or 1957/1968-like? That is the question.

REFERENCES

An Account of the Influenza Epidemic in Perry County, Kentucky. 1919. 8/14/19, NA, RG 200, Box 689.

Assaad F, Cockburn WC, Sundaresan TK. 1973. Use of excess mortality from respiratory diseases in the study of influenza. *Bull World Health Organ* 49(3):219–233.

Barry JM. 2004. *The Great Influenza: The Epic Story of the Deadliest Plague in History.* New York: Viking Press. P. 560.

Basler CF, Reid AH, Dybing JK, Janczewski TA, Fanning TG, Zheng H, Salvatore M, Perdue ML, Swayne DE, Garcia-Sastre A, Palese P, Taubenberger JK. 2001. Sequence of the 1918 pandemic influenza virus nonstructural gene (NS) segment and characterization of recombinant viruses bearing the 1918 NS genes. *Proc Natl Acad Sci USA* 98:2746–2751.

Beveridge W. 1977. *Influenza: The Last Great Plague, an Unfinished Story of Discovery.* New York: Prodist.

Brown IH, Chakraverty P, Harris PA, Alexander DJ. 1995. Disease outbreaks in pigs in Great Britain due to an influenza A virus of H1N2 subtype. *Vet Rec* 136:328–329.

Brown IH, Harris PA, McCauley JW, Alexander DJ. 1998. Multiple genetic reassortment of avian and human influenza A viruses in European pigs, resulting in the emergence of an H1N2 virus of novel genotype. *J Gen Virol* 79:2947–2955.

Burnet F, Clark E. 1942. *Influenza: A Survey of the Last 50 Years in the Light of Modern Work on the Virus of Epidemic Influenza.* Melbourne, Australia: Macmillan.

Castrucci MR, Donatelli I, Sidoli L, Barigazzi G, Kawaoka Y, Webster RG. 1993. Genetic reassortment between avian and human influenza A viruses in Italian pigs. *Virology* 193:503–506.

Caton AJ, Brownlee GG, Yewdell JW, Gerhard W. 1982. The antigenic structure of the influenza virus A/PR/8/34 hemagglutinin (H1 subtype). *Cell* 31:417–427.

Chun J. 1919. Influenza: Including its infection among pigs. *National Medical Journal* (of China) 5:34–44.

Claas EC, Osterhaus AD, van Beek R, De Jong JC, Rimmelzwaan GF, Senne DA, Krauss S, Shortridge KF, Webster RG. 1998. Human influenza A H5N1 virus related to a highly pathogenic avian influenza virus. *Lancet* 351:472–477.

Cockburn WC, Delon PJ, Ferreira W. 1969. Origin and progress of the 1968-69 Hong Kong influenza epidemic. *Bull World Health Organ* 41(3):345–348.

Collier R. 1974. *The Plague of the Spanish Lady.* London, England: Macmillan. P. 266.

Collins S. 1931. Age and sex incidence of influenza and pneumonia morbidity and mortality in the epidemic of 1928-29 with comparative data for the epidemic of 1918-19. *Pub Health Rep* 46:1909–1937.

Colman PM, Varghese JN, Laver WG. 1983. Structure of the catalytic and antigenic sites in influenza virus neuraminidase. *Nature* 303:41–44.

Cox NJ, Subbarao K. 2000. Global epidemiology of influenza: Past and present. *Annu Rev Med* 51:407–421.

Crosby A. 1989. *America's Forgotten Pandemic.* Cambridge, England: Cambridge University Press.

Davenport FM, Hennesey AV, Francis T. 1953. Epidemiologic and immunologic significance of age distribution of antibody to antigenic variants of influenza virus. *J Exp Med* 99:641–656.

DHHS (Department of Health and Human Services). 2004. Pandemic Influenza Response and Preparedness Plan. [Online]. Available: http://www.hhs.gov/nvpo/pandemicplan/ [accessed December 17, 2004].

Dimoch WW. 1918–1919. Diseases of swine. *J Am Vet Med Assn* 54:321–340.

Dorset M, McBryde CN, Niles WB. 1922–1923. Remarks on "Hog" flu. *J Am Vet Med Assn* 62:162–171.

Dowdle WR. 1999. Influenza A virus recycling revisited. *Bull World Health Organ* 77:820–828.

Duffy J. 1953. *Epidemics in Colonial America.* Baton Rouge, LA: LSU Press. Pp. 187–188.

Dunn FL. 1958. Pandemic influenza in 1957: Review of international spread of new Asian strain. *JAMA* 166(10):1140–1148.

Fanning TG, Taubenberger JK. 1999. Phylogenetically important regions of the influenza A H1 hemagglutinin protein. *Virus Res* 65:33–42.

Fanning TG, Reid AH, Taubenberger JK. 2000. Influenza A virus neuraminidase: Regions of the protein potentially involved in virus-host interactions. *Virology* 276:417–423.

Fanning TG, Slemons RD, Reid AH, Janczewski TA, Dean J, Taubenberger JK. 2002. 1917 avian influenza virus sequences suggest that the 1918 pandemic virus did not acquire its hemagglutinin directly from birds. *J Virol* 76:7860–7862.

Fitch W, Leiter J, Li X, Palese P. 1991. Positive Darwinian evolution in human influenza A viruses. *Proc Natl Acad Sci USA* 88:4270–4274.

Fouchier RA, Schneeberger PM, Rozendaal FW, Broekman JM, Kemink SA, Munster V, Kuiken T, Rimmelzwaan GF, Schutten M, Van Doornum GJ, Koch G, Bosman A, Koopmans M, Osterhaus AD. 2004. Avian influenza A virus (H7N7) associated with human conjunctivitis and a fatal case of acute respiratory distress syndrome. *Proc Natl Acad Sci USA* 101:1356–1361.

Frost W. 1920. Statistics of influenza morbidity. *Pub Health Rep* 35:584–597.

Frost WH. 1919. The epidemiology of influenza. *JAMA* 70:313–318.

Gambaryan AS, Tuzikov AB, Piskarev VE, Yamnikova SS, Lvov DK, Robertson JS, Bovin NV, Matrosovich MN. 1997. Specification of receptor-binding phenotypes of influenza virus isolates from different hosts using synthetic sialylglycopolymers: Non-egg-adapted human H1 and H3 influenza A and influenza B viruses share a common high binding affinity for 6'-Sialyl(N-acetyllactosamine). *Virology* 232:345–350.

Gamblin SJ, Haire LF, Russell RJ, Stevens DJ, Xiao B, Ha Y, Vasisht N, Steinhauer DA, Daniels RS, Elliot A, Wiley DC, Skehel JJ. 2004. The structure and receptor binding properties of the 1918 influenza hemagglutinin. *Science* 303:1838–1842.

Gammelin M, Altmuller A, Reinhardt U, Mandler J, Harley VR, Hudson PJ, Fitch WM, Scholtissek C. 1990. Phylogenetic analysis of nucleoproteins suggests that human influenza A viruses emerged from a 19th-century avian ancestor. *Mol Biol Evol* 7:194–200.

Garcia-Sastre A. 2002. Mechanisms of inhibition of the host interferon alpha/beta-mediated antiviral responses by viruses. *Microbes Infect* 4:647–655.

Garcia-Sastre A, Egorov A, Matassov D, Brandt S, Levy DE, Durbin JE, Palese P, Muster T. 1998. Influenza A virus lacking the NS1 gene replicates in interferon-deficient systems. *Virology* 252:324–330.

Gaydos JC, Hodder RA, Top FH Jr, Soden VJ, Allen RG, Bartley JD, Zabkar JH, Nowosiwsky T, Russell PK. Swine influenza A at Fort Dix, New Jersey (January–February 1976). Case finding and clinical study of cases. *J Infect Dis* 136:S356–S362.

Geiss GK, Salvatore M, Tumpey TM, Carter VS, Wang X, Basler CF, Taubenberger JK, Bumgarner RE, Palese P, Katze MG, Garcia-Sastre A. 2002. Cellular transcriptional profiling in influenza A virus-infected lung epithelial cells: The role of the nonstructural NS1 protein in the evasion of the host innate defense and its potential contribution to pandemic influenza. *Proc Natl Acad Sci USA* 99:10736–10741.

Gensheimer KF, Fukuda K, Brammer L, Cox N, Patriarca PA, Strikas RA. 1999. Preparing for pandemic influenza: The need for enhanced surveillance. *Emerg Infect Dis* 5:297–299.

Glaser L, Zamarin D, Taubenberger JK, Palese P. 2004 (submitted). A Single Amino Acid Substitution in the 1918 Influenza Virus Hemagglutinin Changes the Receptor Binding Specificity.

Gorman OT, Bean WJ, Kawaoka Y, Donatelli I, Guo YJ, Webster RG. 1991. Evolution of influenza A virus nucleoprotein genes: Implications for the origins of H1N1 human and classical swine viruses. *J Virol* 65:3704–3714.

Grist NR. 1979. Pandemic influenza 1918. *Brit Med J* 2(6203):1632–1633.

Grove RD, Hetzel AM. 1968. *Vital Statistics Rates in the United States: 1940–1960.* Washington, DC: National Center for Health Statistics. Government Printing Office.

Harris J. 1919. Influenza occurring in pregnant women: A statistical study of 130 cases. *JAMA* 72(14):978–980.

Hay A, Wolstenholme A, Skehel J, Smith M. 1985. The molecular basis of the specific anti-influenza action of amantadine. *EMBO J* 4:3021–3024.

Hennessy AV, Davenport FM, Horton RJ, Napier JA, Francis T Jr. 1964. Asian influenza: Occurrence and recurrence, a community and family study. *Mil Med* 129:38–50.

Holsinger LJ, Nichani D, Pinto LH, Lamb RA. 1994. Influenza A virus M2 ion channel protein: A structure-function analysis. *J Virol* 68:1551–1563.

Housworth WJ, Spoon MM. 1971. The age distribution of excess mortality during A2 Hong Kong influenza epidemics compared with earlier A2 outbreaks. *Am J Epidemiol* 94:348–350.

Ireland MW, ed. 1928. Medical Department of the United States Army in the World War. *Commun Dis* 9:61.

Johnson NP, Mueller J. 2002. Updating the accounts: Global mortality of the 1918–1920 "Spanish" influenza pandemic. *Bull Hist Med* 76:105–115.

Jordan E. 1927. *Epidemic Influenza: A survey*. Chicago, IL: American Medical Association.

Jordan WS, Badger GF, Dingle JH. 1958a. A study of illness in a group of Cleveland families. XVI. The epidemiology of influenza, 1948-1953. *Am J Hyg* 68:169–189.

Jordan WS, Denny FW, Badger GF, Curtiss C, Dingle JH, Oseasohn R, Stevens DA. 1958b. A study of illness in a group of Cleveland families. XVII. The occurrence of Asian influenza. *Am J Hyg* 68:190–212.

Kanegae Y, Sugita S, Sortridge K, Yoshioka Y, Nerome K. 1994. Origin and evolutionary pathways of the H1 hemagglutinin gene of avian, swine and human influenza viruses: Cocirculation of two distinct lineages of swine viruses. *Arch Virol* 134:17–28.

Kash JC, Basler CF, Garcia-Sastre A, Carter V, Billharz R, Swayne DE, Przygodzki RM, Taubenberger JK, Katze MG, Tumpey TM. 2004. Global host immune response: Pathogenesis and transcriptional profiling of type A influenza viruses expressing the hemagglutinin and neuraminidase genes from the 1918 pandemic virus. *J Virol* 78(17):9499–9511.

Katz JM, Lim W, Bridges CB, Rowe T, Hu-Primmer J, Lu X, Abernathy RA, Clarke M, Conn L, Kwong H, Lee M, Au G, Ho YY, Mak KH, Cox NJ, Fukuda K. 1999. Antibody response in individuals infected with avian influenza A (H5N1) viruses and detection of anti-H5 antibody among household and social contacts. *J Infect Dis* 180:1763–1770.

Katzenellenbogen JM. 1988. The 1918 influenza epidemic in Mamre. *S Afr Med J* 74(7):362–364.

Kawaoka Y, Webster RG. 1988. Molecular mechanism of acquisition of virulence in influenza virus in nature. *Microb Pathog* 5:311–318.

Kawaoka Y, Krauss S, Webster RG. 1989. Avian-to-human transmission of the PB1 gene of influenza A viruses in the 1957 and 1968 pandemics. *J Virol* 63:4603–4608.

Keeton R, Cusman AB. 1918. The influenza epidemic in Chicago. *JAMA* 71(24):1963. (Note: The 39.8 percent corrects an earlier report in *JAMA* by Nuzum on 11/9/18, p. 1562.)

Kilbourne E. 1977. Influenza pandemics in perspective. *JAMA* 237:1225–1228.

Kilbourne ED. 1997. Perspectives on pandemics: A research agenda. *J Infect Dis* 176(Suppl 1):S29–S31.

Koen JS. 1919. A practical method for field diagnoses of swine diseases. *Am J Vet Med* 14:468–470.

Kolata GB. 1999. *Flu: The Story of the Great Influenza Pandemic of 1918 and the Search for the Virus That Caused It*. New York: Farrar Straus & Giroux.

Koopmans M, Wilbrink B, Conyn M, Natrop G, van der Nat H, Vennema H, Meijer A, van Steenbergen J, Fouchier R, Osterhaus A, Bosman A. 2004. Transmission of H7N7 avian influenza A virus to human beings during a large outbreak in commercial poultry farms in the Netherlands. *Lancet* 363:587–593.

Krug RM, Yuan W, Noah DL, Latham AG. 2003. Intracellular warfare between human influenza viruses and human cells: The roles of the viral NS1 protein. *Virology* 309:181–189.

Kupradinun S, Peanpijit P, Bhodhikosoom C, Yoshioka Y, Endo A, Nerome K. 1991. The first isolation of swine H1N1 influenza viruses from pigs in Thailand. *Arch Virol* 118:289–297.

Lamb R, Krug R. 2001. Orthomyxoviridae: The viruses and their replication. In: Knipe D, Howley P, eds. *Fields Virology*. Vol. 1. Philadelphia, PA: Lippincott Williams & Wilkins. Pp. 1487–1531.

Lamb RA, Lai CJ. 1980. Sequence of interrupted and uninterrupted mRNAs and cloned DNA coding for the two overlapping nonstructural proteins of influenza virus. *Cell* 21:475–485.

Langmuir AD, Housworth J. 1969. A critical evaluation of influenza surveillance. *Bull World Health Organ* 41:393–398.

Lazarowitz SG, Choppin PW. 1975. Enhancement of the infectivity of influenza A and B viruses by proteolytic cleavage of the hemagglutinin polypeptide. *Virology* 68:440–454.

LeCount ER. 1919. The pathologic anatomy of influenza bronchopneumonia. *JAMA* 72: 650–652.

Li S, Schulman J, Itamura S, Palese P. 1993. Glycosylation of neuraminidase determines the neurovirulence of influenza A/WSN/33 virus. *J Virol* 67:6667–6673.

Li Y, Yamakita Y, Krug R. 1998. Regulation of a nuclear export signal by an adjacent inhibitory sequence: The effector domain of the influenza virus NS1 protein. *Proc Natl Acad Sci USA* 95:4864–4869.

Linder FE, Grove RD. 1943. *Vital Statistics Rates in the United States: 1900–1940.* Washington, DC: National Office of Vital Statistics. Government Printing Office.

Lipsman J. 2004. *H7N2 Avian Influenza Identified in Westchester Resident.* New York: Westchester County Department of Health.

Little TR, Garofalo CJ, Williams PA. 1918. B. influenzae and present epidemic. *Lancet* 2:4950.

Longini IM, Ackerman E, Elveback LR. 1978. An optimization model for influenza A epidemics. *Math Biosci* 38:141–157.

Longini IM, Halloran ME, Nizam A, Yang Y. 2004. Containing pandemic influenza with antiviral agents. *Am J Epidemiol* 159:623–633.

Low RB. 1920. In: *Reports on Public Health and Medical Subjects.* No. 4. London, England: Her Majesty's Stationery Office.

Ludendorff E. 1919. *Meine Kriegserinnerungen 1914–1918.* Berlin, Germany: Ernst Siegfried Mittler und Sohn Verlagsbuchhandlung. P. 514.

Ludwig S, Stitz L, Planz O, Van H, Fitch WM, Scholtissek C. 1995. European swine virus as a possible source for the next influenza pandemic? *Virology* 212:551–561.

Marine WM, Workman WM. 1969. Hong Kong influenza immunologic recapitulation. *Am J Epidemiol* 90:406–415.

Marks G, Beatty WK. 1976. *Epidemics.* New York: Scribner.

Matrosovich MN, Gambaryan AS, Teneberg S, Piskarev VE, Yamnikova SS, Lvov DK, Robertson JS, Karlsson KA. 1997. Avian influenza A viruses differ from human viruses by recognition of sialyloigosaccharides and gangliosides and by a higher conservation of the HA receptor-binding site. *Virology* 233:224–234.

Meltzer MI, Cox NJ, Fukuda K. 1999. The economic impact of pandemic influenza in the United States: Priorities for intervention. *Emerg Infect Dis* 5:659–671.

Miller DL, Pereira MS, Clarke M. 1971. Epidemiology of the Hong Kong-68 variant of influenza A2 in Britain. *Br Med J* 1:475–479.

Ministry of Health, United Kingdom. 1960. The influenza epidemic in England and Wales, 1957–1958. In: *Reports on Public Health and Medical Subjects.* Vol. 100. London, England: Ministry of Health.

Monto AS, Iacuzio DA, La Montagne JR. 1997. Pandemic influenza: Confronting a reemergent threat. *J Infect Dis* 176:S1–S3.

Murray C, Biester HE. 1930. Swine influenza. *J Am Vet Med Assn* 76:349–355.

Nerome K, Ishida M, Oya A, Oda K. 1982. The possible origin H1N1 (Hsw1N1) virus in the swine population of Japan and antigenic analysis of the isolates. *J Gen Virol* 62:171–175.

Nguyen-Van-Tam JS, Hampson AW. 2003. The epidemiology and clinical impact of pandemic influenza. *Vaccine* 21:1762–1768.

Olson DR, Simonsen L, Edleson PJ, Morse SS. 2004. In: *4th International Conference on Emerging Infectious Diseases.* Atlanta, GA.

O'Neill RE, Talon J, Palese P. 1998. The influenza virus NEP (NS2 protein) mediates the nuclear export of viral ribonucleoproteins. *EMBO* 17:288–296.

Palese P, Compans RW. 1976. Inhibition of influenza virus replication in tissue culture by 2-deoxy-2,3-dehydro-N-trifluoroacetylneuraminic acid (FANA): Mechanism of action. *J Gen Virol* 33:159–163.

Patterson KD, Pyle GF. 1991. The geography and mortality of the 1918 influenza pandemic. *Bull Hist Med* 65:4–21.

Peiris JS, Yu WC, Leung CW, Cheung CY, Ng WF, Nicholls JM, Ng TK, Chan KH, Lai ST, Lim WL, Yuen KY, Guan Y. 2004. Re-emergence of fatal human influenza A subtype H5N1 disease. *Lancet* 363:617–619.

Pettit DA. 1976. *A Cruel Wind: America Experiences the Pandemic Influenza, 1918–1920.* P. 32. PhD dissertation, University of New Hampshire.

Philip RN, Lackman DB. 1962. Observations on the present distribution of influenza A/swine antibodies among Alaskan natives relative to the occurrence of influenza in 1918–1919. *Am J Hyg* 75:322–334.

Policlinico. 1918, 6/30/18, 25(26), quoted in *JAMA* 71(9):780.

Portela A, Digard P. 2002. The influenza virus nucleoprotein: A multifunctional RNA-binding protein pivotal to virus replication. *J Gen Virol* 83:723–734.

Reichert TA, Sugaya N, Fedson DS, Glezen WP, Simonsen L, Tashiro M. 2001. The Japanese experience of vaccinating school children against influenza. *N Engl J Med* 344:889–896.

Reid AH, Taubenberger JK. 1999. The 1918 flu and other influenza pandemics: "Over there" and back again. *Lab Invest* 79:95–101.

Reid AH, Taubenberger JK. 2003. The origin of the 1918 pandemic influenza virus: A continuing enigma. *J Gen Virol* 84:2285–2292.

Reid AH, Fanning TG, Hultin JV, Taubenberger JK. 1999. Origin and evolution of the 1918 "Spanish" influenza virus hemagglutinin gene. *Proc Natl Acad Sci USA* 96:1651–1656.

Reid AH, Fanning TG, Janczewski TA, Taubenberger JK. 2000. Characterization of the 1918 "Spanish" influenza virus neuraminidase gene. *Proc Natl Acad Sci USA* 97:6785–6790.

Reid AH, Fanning TG, Janczewski TA, McCall S, Taubenberger JK. 2002. Characterization of the 1918 "Spanish" influenza virus matrix gene segment. *J Virol* 76:10717–10723.

Reid AH, Janczewski TA, Lourens RM, Elliot AJ, Daniels RS, Berry CL, Oxford JS, Taubenberger JK. 2003. 1918 influenza pandemic caused by highly conserved viruses with two receptor-binding variants. *Emerg Infect Dis* 9(10):1249–1253.

Reid AH, Fanning TG, Janczewski TA, Lourens R, Taubenberger JK. 2004. Novel origin of the 1918 pandemic influenza virus nucleoprotein gene segment. *J Virol* 78(22):12462–12470.

Rice G. 1988. *Black November.* Wellington, New Zealand: Allen and Unwin. P. 140.

Robertson JD. 1918. *Report of an Epidemic of Influenza in Chicago Occurring During the Fall of 1918.* Chicago, IL: Department of Health.

Rosenau MJ, Last JM. 1980. *Maxcy-Rosenau Preventative Medicine and Public Health.* New York: Appleton-Century-Crofts.

Rott R, Klenk HD, Nagai Y, Tashiro M. 1995. Influenza viruses, cell enzymes, and pathogenicity. *Am J Respir Crit Care Med* 152:S16–S19.

Schafer JR, Kawaoka Y, Bean WJ, Suss J, Senne D, Webster RG. 1993. Origin of the pandemic 1957 H2 influenza A virus and the persistence of its possible progenitors in the avian reservoir. *Virology* 194:781–788.

Scholtissek C. 1994. Source for influenza pandemics. *Eur J Epidemiol* 10:455–458.

Scholtissek C, Koennecke I, Rott R. 1978a. Host range recombinants of fowl plague (influenza A) virus. *Virology* 91:79–85.

Scholtissek C, Rohde W, Von Hoyningen V, Rott R. 1978b. On the origin of the human influenza virus subtypes H2N2 and H3N2. *Virology* 87:13–20.

Scholtissek C, Burger H, Kistner O, Shortridge KF. 1985. The nucleoprotein as a possible major factor in determining host specificity of influenza H3N2 viruses. *Virology* 147:287–294.

Scholtissek C, Ludwig S, Fitch W. 1993. Analysis of influenza A virus nucleoproteins for the assessment of molecular genetic mechanisms leading to new phylogenetic virus lineages. *Arch Virol* 131:237–250.

Schulze IT. 1997. Effects of glycosylation on the properties and functions of influenza virus hemagglutinin. *J Infect Dis* 176(Suppl 1):S24–S28.

Seo SH, Hoffmann E, Webster RG. 2002. Lethal H5N1 influenza viruses escape host antiviral cytokine responses. *Nat Med* 8:950–954.

Serfling R. 1963. Methods for current statistical analysis of excess pneumonia-influenza deaths. *Pub Health Rep* 78:494–506.

Serfling RE, Sherman IL, Houseworth WJ. 1967. Excess pneumonia-influenza mortality by age and sex in three major influenza A2 epidemics, United States, 1957-58, 1960 and 1963. *Am J Epidemiol* 86:433–441.

Shope R. 1958. Influenza: History, epidemiology, and speculation. *Pub Health Rep* 73: 165–178.

Shope RE. 1936. The incidence of neutralizing antibodies for swine influenza virus in the sera of human beings of different ages. *J Exp Med* 63:669–684.

Shope RE, Lewis PA. 1931. Swine influenza: Experimental transmission and pathology. *J Exp Med* 54:349–359.

Shu L, Bean W, Webster R. 1993. Analysis of the evolution and variation of the human influenza A virus nucleoprotein gene from 1933 to 1990. *J Virol* 67:2723–2729.

Simonsen L, Clarke MJ, Schonberger LB, Arden NH, Cox NJ, Fukuda K. 1998. Pandemic versus epidemic influenza mortality: A pattern of changing age distribution. *J Infect Dis* 178:53–60.

Simonsen L, Fukuda K, Schonberger LB, Cox NJ. 2000. The impact of influenza epidemics on hospitalizations. *J Infect Dis* 181:831–837.

Simonsen L, Reichert TA, Miller M. 2003. In: Kawaoka Y, ed. *Options for the Control of Influenza V.* International Congress Series 1263. Vol. ICS 1265. Okinawa, Japan: Elsevier. Pp. 791–794.

Smith W, Andrewes C, Laidlaw P. 1933. A virus obtained from influenza patients. *Lancet* 225:66–68.

Sohier R, Henry M. 1969. Epidemiological data on Hong Kong influenza in France. *Bull World Health Organ* 41:402–404.

Soper G. 1918, November 8. The influenza-pneumonia pandemic in the American Army camps, September and October 1918. *Science* 454.

Soper G. undated. *The Influenza Pandemic in the Camps.* Undated draft report. Sanitation Corps, NA, RG 112, Box 394.

Stevens J, Corper AL, Basler CF, Taubenberger JK, Palese P, Wilson IA. 2004. Structure of the uncleaved human H1 hemagglutinin from the extinct 1918 influenza virus. *Science* 303:1866–1870.

Stuart-Harris CH. 1970. Pandemic influenza: An unresolved problem in prevention. *J Infect Dis* 122:108–115.

Subbarao K, Klimov A, Katz J, Regnery H, Lim W, Hall H, Perdue M, Swayne D, Bender C, Huang J, Hemphill M, Rowe T, Shaw M, Xu X, Fukuda K, Cox N. 1998. Characterization of an avian influenza A (H5N1) virus isolated from a child with a fatal respiratory illness. *Science* 279:393–396.

Talon J, Horvath CM, Polley R, Basler CF, Muster T, Palese P, Garcia-Sastre A. 2000. Activation of interferon regulatory factor 3 is inhibited by the influenza A virus NS1 protein. *J Virol* 74:7989–7996.

Taubenberger JK, Reid AH, Krafft AE, Bijwaard KE, Fanning TG. 1997. Initial genetic characterization of the 1918 "Spanish" influenza virus. *Science* 275:1793–1796.

Taubenberger J, Reid A, Fanning T. 2000. The 1918 influenza virus: A killer comes into view. *Virology* 274:241–245.

Taubenberger JK, Reid AH, Janczewski TA, Fanning TG. 2001. Integrating historical, clinical and molecular genetic data in order to explain the origin and virulence of the 1918 Spanish influenza virus. *Philos Trans R Soc Lond B Biol Sci* 356:1829–1839.

The Mobilization of the American National Red Cross During the Influenza Pandemic 1918–1919. 1920. Geneva, Switzerland. P. 24.

Thomson D, Thomson R. 1934a. *Annals of the Pickett-Thomson Research Laboratory*. Volume IX, *Influenza*. Baltimore, MD: Williams and Wilkens.

Thomson D, Thomson R. 1934b. *Annals of the Pickett-Thomson Research Laboratory*. Volume X, *Influenza*. Baltimore, MD: Williams and Wilkens.

Thompson WW, Shay DK, Weintraub E, Brammer L, Cox N, Anderson LJ, Fukuda K. 2003. Mortality associated with influenza and respiratory syncytial virus in the United States. *JAMA* 289:179–186.

To KF, Chan PK, Chan KF, Lee WK, Lam WY, Wong KF, Tang NL, Tsang DN, Sung RY, Buckley TA, Tam JS, Cheng AF. 2001. Pathology of fatal human infection associated with avian influenza A H5N1 virus. *J Med Virol* 63(3):242–246.

Tran TH, Nguyen TL, Nguyen TD, Luong TS, Pham PM, Nguyen VC, Pham TS, Vo CD, Le TQ, Ngo TT, Dao BK, Le PP, Nguyen TT, Hoang TL, Cao VT, Le TG, Nguyen DT, Le HN, Nguyen KT, Le HS, Le VT, Christiane D, Tran TT, Menno de J, Schultsz C, Cheng P, Lim W, Horby P, Farrar J; World Health Organization International Avian Influenza Investigative Team. 2004. Avian influenza A (H5N1) in 10 patients in Vietnam. *N Engl J Med* 350:1179–1188.

Tumpey TM, Garcia-Sastre A, Mikulasova A, Taubenberger JK, Swayne DE, Palese P, Basler CF. 2002. Existing antivirals are effective against influenza viruses with genes from the 1918 pandemic virus. *Proc Natl Acad Sci USA* 99:13849–13854.

Tumpey TM, Garcia-Sastre A, Taubenberger JK, Palese P, Swayne DE, Basler CF. 2004. Pathogenicity and immunogenicity of influenza viruses with genes from the 1918 pandemic virus. *Proc Natl Acad Sci USA* 101(9):3166–3171.

U.S. Bureau of the Census. 1921. *Mortality Statistics*. Washington, DC: Government Printing Office. P. 30.

U.S. Department of Commerce. 1976. *Historical Statistics of the United States: Colonial Times to 1970*. Washington, DC: Government Printing Office.

Van Hartesveldt FR. 1992. *The 1918–1919 Pandemic of Influenza: The Urban Impact in the Western World*. Lewiston, NY: Edwin Mellen Press. Pp. 121, 144.

Vaughn S. 1980. *Holding Fast the Line: Democracy, Nationalism, and the Committee on Public Information*. Chapel Hill, NC: University of North Carolina Press.

Vaughn WT. 1921. Influenza: An epidemiological study. *Am J Hyg* Monograph No. 1.

Viboud C, Grais RF, Lafont BAP, Miller MA, Simonsen L. 2004. Multi-national impact of the 1968 Hong-Kong influenza pandemic: Evidence for a smoldering pandemic. Submitted.

Wang X, Li M, Zheng H, Muster T, Palese P, Beg AA, Garcia-Sastre A. 2000. Influenza A virus NS1 protein prevents activation of NF-kappaB and induction of alpha/beta interferon. *J Virol* 74:11566–11573.

Webby RJ, Webster RG. 2003. Are we ready for pandemic influenza? *Science* 302:1519–1522.

Webster R, Rott R. 1987. Influenza virus A pathogenicity: The pivotal role of hemagglutinin. *Cell* 50:665–666.

Webster RG, Bean WJ, Gorman OT, Chambers TM, Kawaoka Y. 1992. Evolution and ecology of influenza A viruses. *Microbiol Rev* 56:152–179.

Webster RG, Sharp GB, Claas EC. 1995. Interspecies transmission of influenza viruses. *Am J Respir Crit Care Med* 152:S25–S30.

Weis W, Brown JH, Cusack S, Paulson JC, Skehel JJ, Wiley DC. 1988. Structure of the influenza virus haemagglutinin complexed with its receptor, sialic acid. *Nature* 333:426–431.

WHO (World Health Organization). 1971. *Stat Bull* 52:8–11.

WHO. 2004. *Avian Influenza A(H7) Human Infections in Canada.* [Online]. Available: http://www.who.int/csr/don/2004_04_05/en/ [accessed December 17, 2004].

Wilson IA, Skehel JJ, Wiley DC. 1981. Structure of the haemagglutinin membrane glycoprotein of influenza virus at 3 A resolution. *Nature* 289:366–373.

Winternitz MC, Wason IM, McNamara FP. 1920. *The Pathology of Influenza.* New Haven, CT: Yale University Press.

Wolbach SB. 1919. Comments on the pathology and bacteriology of fatal influenza cases, as observed at Camp Devens, Mass. *Johns Hopkins Hospital Bulletin* 30:104.

Woods GT, Schnurrenberger PR, Martin RJ, Tompkins WA. 1981. Swine influenza virus in swine and man in Illinois. *J Occup Med* 23:263–267.

Zamarin D, Palese P. 2004 (in press). Influenza virus: Lessons learned. In: Kowalski JB, Morissey JB, eds. *International Kilmer Conference Proceedings.* Champlain, NY: Polyscience Publications.

Zhou NN, Senne DA, Landgraf JS, Swenson SL, Erickson G, Rossow K, Liu L, Yoon KJ, Krauss S, Webster RG. 2000. Emergence of H3N2 reassortant influenza A viruses in North American pigs. *Vet Microbiol* 74:47–58.

2

Today's Pandemic Threat: H5N1 Influenza

OVERVIEW

There is particular pressure to recognize and heed the lessons of past influenza pandemics in the shadow of the worrisome 2003–2004 flu season. An early-onset, severe form of influenza A (H3N2) made headlines when it claimed the lives of several children in the United States in late 2003. As a result, stronger than usual demand for annual flu inactivated vaccine outstripped the vaccine supply, of which 10 to 20 percent typically goes unused. Because statistics on pediatric flu deaths had not been collected previously, it is unknown if the 2003–2004 season witnessed a significant change in mortality patterns.

Then, even more alarmingly, 34 human cases of H5N1 avian influenza—a highly pathogenic flu that has ravaged poultry stocks in several Asian countries—were confirmed in Thailand and Vietnam. Twenty-three (68 percent) of these patients, mostly children and young adults, had died of the disease by early 2004. Another six confirmed human deaths occurred in Vietnam during a resurgence of the epidemic during the summer of 2004, as this report was being prepared (ProMED-mail, 2004a,b). Thailand has confirmed another four deaths (ProMED-mail, 2004c,d), with one case possibly having been transmitted from human to human (ProMED-mail, 2004e).

The past decade has seen increasingly frequent and severe outbreaks of highly pathogenic avian influenza, as described in the Summary and Assessment. The current ongoing epidemic of H5N1 avian influenza in Asia is unprecedented in its scale, in its spread, and in the economic losses it has caused. Tens of millions of birds died of influenza and hundreds of millions were culled to protect humans.

The chapter begins with a reconstruction of the descent of the virus that infected and killed humans in Thailand and Vietnam during the winter of 2003–2004 from the H5N1 virus first known to have infected humans (in Hong Kong in 1997). These findings indicate that domestic ducks in southern China played a central role in the generation and maintenance of H5N1 and that wild birds spread the virus across Asia, to the point where it is now endemic in the region—an ecological niche from which it now presents a long-term pandemic threat to humans.

The chapter continues with descriptions of the approach taken by two countries most severely affected by the H5N1 epidemic: Thailand and Vietnam. Each country's circumstances and their handling of the epidemic—beyond the use of common, time-tested strategies for detecting and stamping-out of infection—were unique, as illustrated in these contributions. The diversity of these responses, and their resulting outcomes, offer important lessons for the control of future avian flu outbreaks—a key protection against a human pandemic.

GENESIS OF A HIGHLY PATHOGENIC AND POTENTIALLY PANDEMIC H5N1 INFLUENZA VIRUS IN EASTERN ASIA[1,2,3]

K.S. Li,[4] Y. Guan,[1,5] J. Wang,[1,2] G.J.D. Smith,[1,2]
K.M. Xu,[1,2] L. Duan,[1,2] A.P. Rahardjo,[6]
P. Puthavathana,[7] C. Buranathai,[8] T.D. Nguyen,[9]
A.T.S. Estoepangestie,[3] A. Chaisingh,[5] P. Auewarakul,[4]
H.T. Long,[10] N.T.H. Hanh,[7] R.J. Webby,[11]
L.L.M. Poon,[2] H. Chen,[1,2] K.F. Shortridge,[1,2] K.Y. Yuen,[2]
R.G. Webster, J.S.M. Peiris[1,2]

[1]Correspondence and requests for materials should be addressed to Y. Guan (yguan@hkucc.hku.hk). The sequences reported in this paper have been deposited in GenBank under accession numbers AY651320–AY651758.

[2]We acknowledge K. Stöhr and the World Health Organization for facilitating the study; L.J. Zhang, C.L. Cheung, and Y.H.C. Leung for technical assistance; N. Ng and colleagues for provision of computing facilities; and T.M. Ellis, K. Dyrting, W. Wong, P. Li, and C. Li of the Department of Agriculture, Fisheries and Conservation of Hong Kong for their support of field work, and W. Lim, for virus isolates. We also thank S. Naron for editorial assistance. These studies were supported by a grant from the National Institutes of Health, a grant from

A highly pathogenic avian influenza virus, H5N1, caused disease outbreaks in poultry in China and seven other east Asian countries between late 2003 and early 2004; the same virus was fatal to humans in Thailand and Vietnam (WHO, 2004a). Here we demonstrate a series of genetic reassortment events traceable to the precursor of the H5N1 viruses that caused the initial human outbreak in Hong Kong in 1997 (Claas et al., 1998; Guan et al., 1999; Xu et al., 1999) and subsequent avian outbreaks in 2001 and 2002 (Guan et al., 2002, 2004). These events gave rise to a dominant H5N1 genotype (Z) in chickens and ducks that was responsible for the regional outbreak in 2003–04. Our findings indicate that domestic ducks in southern China had a central role in the generation and maintenance of this virus, and that wild birds may have contributed to the increasingly wide spread of the virus in Asia. Our results suggest that H5N1 viruses with pandemic potential have become endemic in the region and are not easily eradicable. These developments pose a threat to public and veterinary health in the region and potentially the world, and suggest that long-term control measures are required.

The Asian outbreak of highly pathogenic avian influenza H5N1 disease in poultry in 2003 and 2004 was unprecedented in its geographical extent, and its transmission to humans was an ominous sign (WHO, 2004a). To trace the ecological and genetic origins of these outbreaks, we compared H5N1 viruses recently isolated from poultry in Indonesia, Thailand, and Vietnam as well as from humans in Thailand and Vietnam with 253 H5N1 isolates obtained during prospective surveillance of live poultry markets in Hong Kong and in Guangdong, Hunan, and Yunnan provinces, China, from 2000 to 2004 (Figure 2-1). Results of this surveillance are summarized

The Wellcome Trust, the Ellison Foundation, the Li Ka Shing Foundation, and grants from the Research Grants Council of Hong Kong.

[3]The authors declare that they have no competing financial interests.

[4]Joint Influenza Research Centre (SUMC & HKU), Shantou University Medical College, Shantou, Guangdong 515031, China.

[5]Department of Microbiology, The University of Hong Kong, Queen Mary Hospital, Hong Kong SAR, China.

[6]Fakultas Kedokteran Hewan, Universitas Airlangga, Surabaya 60115, Indonesia.

[7]Department of Microbiology, Sriraj Hospital, Bangkok 10700, Thailand.

[8]Department of Livestock Development, National Institute of Animal Health, Bangkok 10900, Thailand.

[9]Department of Virology, National Institute of Veterinary Research, Ministry of Agriculture and Rural Development, Hanoi, Vietnam.

[10]Virology Department, National Institute of Hygiene and Epidemiology, Hanoi, Vietnam.

[11]Virology Division, Department of Infectious Diseases, St. Jude Children's Research Hospital, Memphis, TN 38105.

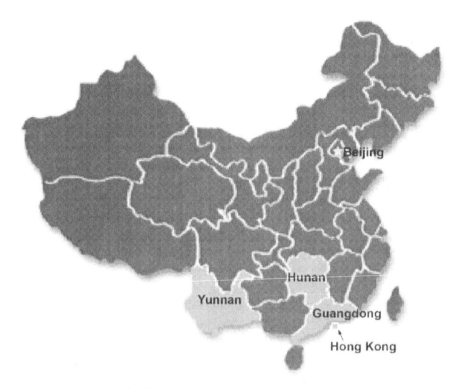

FIGURE 2-1 Map of China showing Hong Kong and Guangdong, Hunan, and Yunnan provinces, where influenza surveillance was conducted.

in Table 2-1. Since 2001, H5N1 viruses have continued to circulate in mainland China with a seasonal pattern, peaking from October to March, when the mean temperature is below 20°C (Figure 2-2). The survival and viability of influenza A virus are known to increase at lower environmental temperatures (Shortridge et al., 1998). H5N1 viruses were isolated exclusively from aquatic poultry during 2000; however, from 2001 onwards they were isolated from both aquatic and terrestrial poultry, although the rate of isolation remained greatest in ducks.

The genes of the virus isolates that encode the surface antigens haemagglutinin (HA) and neuraminidase (NA) were derived from the Goose/Guangdong/1/96 (*Gs/Gd*)-like lineage. Six genes, which encode internal viral proteins, arose from many other sources through reassortment and served as the basis for assignment to different genotypes (Figure 2-3). By 2001, six H5N1 reassortants (genotypes *A*, *B*, *C*, *D*, *E*, and X_0) had been isolated from aquatic and, for the first time since 1997, terrestrial poultry (Guan et al., 1999, 2002). From 2002 onwards, eight new H5N1 genotypes (V, W, X_1, X_2, X_3, Y, Z, and Z^+) were detected. Genotypes A, C, D and E and their common precursor Gs/Gd were no longer found, suggesting that later genotypes had acquired a survival advantage by means of adaptation. At least nine genotypes of H5N1 viruses continued to circulate in southern China in 2002. All genotypes, except for Gs/Gd and X_0–X_3, had a five-amino-acid deletion (position 80–84) in the NS1 protein. Similarly, viruses isolated in 2002 and later, except for genotypes B, W, and Z^+, had a 20-amino-acid deletion in the stalk of the NA molecule (position 49–68). Deletion in the NA stalk may be associated with adaptation of influenza viruses to land-based poultry (Matrosovich et al., 1999).

Since January 2002, genotype Z, which contains both the NA and NS1 deletions, has become the dominant H5N1 virus in southern China (Table 2-1 and Figure 2-3). In February 2003, human H5N1 disease was diagnosed for the first time since December 1997. The human isolates (A/HK/212/03 and A/HK/213/03) had the same gene constellation as genotype Z, but lacked the NA stalk deletion, and were designated genotype Z^+ (Figure 2-3) (Guan et al., 2004). Sixty-two H5N1 virus isolates from 2003 were genetically sequenced and 60 of them belonged to genotype Z (Table 2-1). All of the viruses that caused outbreaks in Indonesia, Thailand, and Vietnam in late 2003 and early 2004 (Hien et al., 2004; WHO, 2004a) were genotype Z viruses (Figure 2-4).

Although all viruses tested derived their HA genes from Gs/Gd-like viruses, the Z and Z^+ genotypes, as well as the single known isolate of genotype V (Ck/ST/4231/03), formed a distinct sublineage (2002/04-V, Z, Z^+; 81% bootstrap support) that included viruses from Hong Kong; Guangdong, Hunan, and Yunnan provinces of mainland China; Indonesia; Thailand; and Vietnam (Figure 2-4a). Within this sublineage, viruses isolated from humans and poultry in Thailand and Vietnam formed a separate group (96% bootstrap) most closely related to H5N1 viruses isolated from poultry and wild birds in Hong Kong (genotypes Z and Z^+). Viruses isolated in Indonesia formed a separate group related to those isolated in Yunnan (Figure 2-4a).

Phylogenetic relationships of the other seven gene segments were broadly consistent with those of the HA gene (Figure 2-4b; see also Supplementary Figs 1 and 2).[12] The M and NS genes were closest to those of influenza viruses of diverse subtypes isolated from ducks in southern China, suggesting that aquatic avian viruses were the gene donors for these new reassortants (Figure 2-4b; see also Supplementary Fig. 2).[12] Bi-directional transmission of influenza virus between terrestrial and aquatic poultry gave

---

[12]Supporting online material, http://www.nature.com/nature/journal/v430/n6996/suppinfo/nature02746.html.

TABLE 2-1 Analysis of H5N1 Influenza viruses isolated from poultry in Hong Kong and mainland China during 2000–04

	2000		2001	
	Aquatic	Terrestrial	Aquatic	Terrestrial
Sampling				
Hong Kong				
H5N1-Positive/ total tested	33/533	0/8,256	37/606	36/16,116
Non-H5N1 isolates	16	715	11	983
Mainland China				
H5N1-Positive/ total tested	0/445	0/1,891	38/2,579	10/3,197
Non-H5N1 isolates	122	143	468	290
Total number sampled	11,125		22,498	
Genetic Analysis				
Hong Kong				
Number of viruses analysed (genotypes detected)	11 (9Gs/Gd; 2C)	—	13 (4B, 9C)	24 (13A, 4B, 4C, 1D, 2E)
Mainland China				
Number of viruses analysed (genotypes detected)	—	—	7 (2B, 5X_0)	1 (1X_0)
Number of Genotypes	2		6	

Faecal droppings from apparently healthy poultry in live poultry markets in Hong Kong (2000–04), Guangdong (2000–04) and Hunan and Yunnan (2002–04) provinces were sampled monthly for influenza virus isolation. For each month that H5N1 virus was identified, one

rise to new H9N2 reassortants (Li et al., 2003), and a similar mechanism may generate novel H5N1 reassortants.

It is notable that in the short time since its emergence in 2002, genotype Z has replaced genotypes A–E, X, and Y to become dominant in both aquatic and terrestrial poultry in this region (Table 2-1). To define the genetic stability of this new gene constellation, we analysed the rates of non-synonymous (K_a) and synonymous (K_s) nucleotide substitutions in six internal gene segments of genotype Z viruses isolated in 2002–04. A K_a/K_s ratio >1 suggests evidence of positive natural selection (Presgraves et al., 2003). Of these internal genes, the M2 gene was under positive selection pressure in late 2002 to early 2003, but under less selection pressure in late 2003 to early 2004. The NS1 and NS2 genes, acquired in late 2000, were also under positive selection pressure (Supplementary Table 1).[12] These

2002		2003		2004	
Aquatic	Terrestrial	Aquatic	Terrestrial	Aquatic	Terrestrial
14/578	323/14,691	4/3,694	112/12,146	1/756	0/1,807
10	369	12	288	0	20
73/4,539	8/4,059	297/7,209	50/10,308	152/1152	26/1,673
507	297	301	361	22	75
23,867		33,357		5,388	
12 (1B, 8Z, 3Z⁺)	100 (7B, $8X_0$, $2X_1$, $3X_2$, $1X_3$, 10Y, 69Z)	4 (4Z)	38 (37Z, 1Z⁺)	1 (1Z)	—
10 (3B, 5Z, 2W)	7 (7Z)	11 (11Z)	9 (8Z, 1V)	3 (3Z)	2 (2Z)
9		3		1	

isolate was selected from each type of infected poultry for sequencing. During H5N1 disease outbreaks, additional isolates were sequenced. Of a total of 96,235 samples, 253 H5N1 virus isolates were genetically sequenced and analysed.

findings suggest that the gene constellation of genotype Z viruses has not yet fully adapted to poultry, and this raises the possibility that they may continue to evolve through mutation or reassortment to achieve greater viral fitness (Webster et al., 1992).

The presence of residue Asp 31 in the M2 protein invariably confers resistance to the amantadines (Scholtissek et al., 1998), a group of antiviral drugs used for treatment of human influenza. Sequence analysis revealed that Asp 31 was present in all avian and human genotype Z viruses isolated in Thailand and Vietnam, but in only one of six viruses isolated from poultry in Indonesia. Asp 31 was also observed in some genotype B, Y, and Z⁺ viruses. The distribution of this mutation in different virus genotypes suggests that it was independently acquired rather than having descended from a single lineage of amantadine-resistant M2 genes (Figure 2-4b).

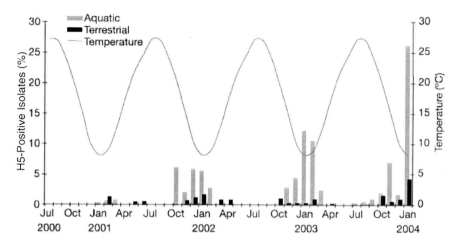

FIGURE 2-2 Seasonality of the isolation of avian H5N1 viruses from domestic poultry in mainland China during July 2000 to January 2004 (see Table 2-1). The mean monthly temperature in southern China (approximated from the monthly average temperatures of the cities Changsha, Kunming, and Xiamen) is shown for reference.

FIGURE 2-3 The genotypes of H5N1 influenza virus reassortants from eastern Asia. The eight gene segments are (horizontal bars starting at the top downwards): *PB2*, *PB1*, *PA*, *HA*, *NP*, *NA*, *M*, and *NS*. Each colour represents a virus lineage (red indicates origin from Gs/Gd/1/96). Genotypes (indicated by letters) were defined by gene phylogeny: a distinct phylogenetic lineage with bootstrap support ≥70% (≥50% for *M*, *NP*, and *PA* genes) indicated a common origin. Genotypes *A*, *B*, and *C* were reassortants of Gs/Gd/1/96 and one or more aquatic avian viruses. Genotype *D* was created when the *NP* gene of genotype *C* was replaced by that of a Dk/HK/Y280/97-like virus (H9N2 subtype). Genotype *E* was created when the *NP* gene of genotype *C* was replaced by that of another avian virus. Further reassortment of genotype *E* with other aquatic avian influenza viruses gave rise to the genotypes X_0–X_3, distinguished by the sources of their *PB2*, *PA*, and *NS* genes. Genotype *W* differs from genotype *B* only in its *PB2*, *NP*, and *M* genes. Further reassortment of genotype *A* or *B* with other aquatic avian viruses gave rise to genotypes *V*, *Y*, *Z*, and *Z+*. Alternatively, genotype *V* may have resulted from reassortment of genotype *Z* with other aquatic avian viruses.

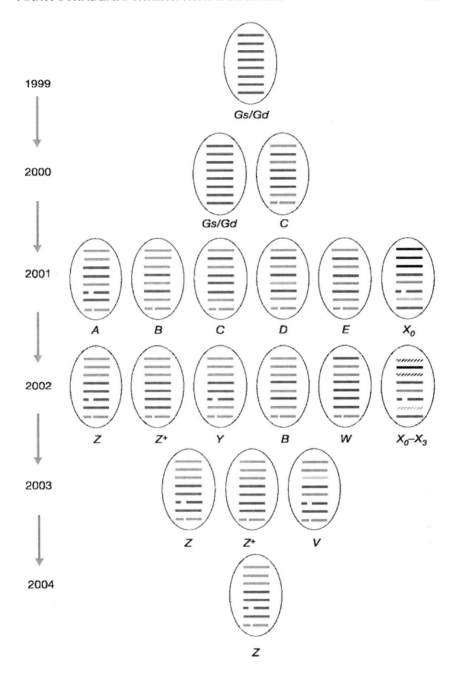

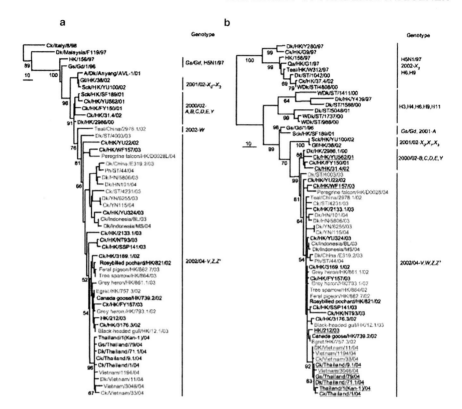

FIGURE 2-4 Phylogenetic relationships of the haemagglutinin (a) and matrix protein (b) genes of representative influenza A viruses isolated in southeastern Asia, including 2 of 6 from Indonesia, 5 of 8 from Thailand, and 4 of 12 from Vietnam. Trees were generated by using maximum parsimony in the PAUP* program (Swofford, 2001) (neighbor-joining analysis with the Tamura–Nei γ-model, implemented in the MEGA program [Kumar et al., 2001], revealed the same relationships). Numbers below branches indicate bootstrap values from 1,000 replicates. Only bootstrap values that define important groups have been included owing to space constraints. Analysis was based on nucleotides 1–1012 (1,012 bp) of the *HA* gene and 90–945 (856 bp) of the *M* gene. The HA tree was rooted to A/tern/South Africa/61 and the M tree to A/equine/Prague/1/56. Scale bar, 10 nucleotide changes. Green text indicates viruses isolated from wild birds in Hong Kong; pink text indicates viruses from smuggled birds in China; and other colours show the country of origin of isolates from the late 2003 to early 2004 H5N1 outbreak. Underlined viruses have the amantadine-resistance mutation (Ser31Asn) in the M2 ion channel. Ck, chicken; Dk, duck; Gd, Guangdong; Gf, Guinea fowl; Gs, goose; HK, Hong Kong; HN, Hunan; Qa, quail; SCk, silky chicken; ST, Shantou; WDk, wild duck; YN, Yunnan.

NOTE: For color figure, please see original figure. Available at: http://www.nature.com.

Mutations Ser64Ala and Glu66Ala in the M2 protein were also observed in genotype Z and Z^+ viruses from highly pathogenic avian influenza H5N1 outbreaks in Kowloon and Penfold parks in Hong Kong in December 2002, from viruses isolated from humans in Hong Kong in February 2003, and from viruses isolated in Thailand and Vietnam in 2003–04. The remaining genotype Z viruses, including those isolated from Indonesia and mainland China in 2003–04, maintained Ser 64 in the M2 protein. Residue Ser 64 is the predominant site of post-translational phosphorylation in the M2 protein (Holsinger et al., 1995; Thomas et al., 1998). The mutation Ser64Ala induces no significant change in ion-channel activity (Holsinger et al., 1995), and phosphorylation of the cytoplasmic tail does not affect intracellular transport of M2 protein or viral assembly (Thomas et al., 1998). Therefore, the biological role of phosphorylation at position 64 of M2 is still unclear. The biological significance of residue 66 of the M2 ion channel has not been reported.

The molecular determinants of H5N1 transmission to humans in Vietnam and Thailand in 2004 are unclear. In H5N1 viruses recently isolated from humans and poultry in Thailand and Vietnam, amino acid residues at the receptor-binding pocket of HA1—that is, positions Gln 222 and Gly 224 (positions 226 and 228 for H3 influenza numbering)—retain configurations (2,3-NeuAcGal linkages) predicted to have affinity for avian cell-surface receptors (Ha et al., 2001). The substitution Ser227Asn, identified in viruses isolated from two patients with H5N1 influenza after visiting Fujian Province, China, in 2003 (Guan et al., 2004), was not seen in any other H5N1 viruses. Other amino acid residues relevant to receptor binding (residues 91, 130–134, 149, 151, 179, 186, 190–191, 220–225) were identical to those of A/HK/156/97 and Gs/Gd-like viruses (Claas et al., 1998), with the exception of A/Vietnam/3046/04, which had an Ala134Val mutation.

The HA molecules of most genotype Z viruses isolated since late 2002 in Hong Kong, of two out of six isolates from Indonesia, and of all isolates from Thailand, Vietnam, and Yunnan Province in late 2003 and early 2004 had acquired a potential N-linked glycosylation site at positions 154–156. Glycosylation at this site, adjacent to the receptor-binding (Claas et al., 1998) and antigenic sites (Kaverin et al., 2002) at the globular tip of the H5 influenza HA molecule (Supplementary Fig. 3),[13] is capable of altering the receptor-binding profile (Iwatsuki-Horimoto et al., 2004) and may help the virus to evade the host antibody response.

Lys 627 in the PB2 protein has been associated with increased virulence of H5N1 viruses in mice (Hatta et al., 2001) and of H7N7 viruses in

---

[13]Supporting online material, http://www.nature.com/nature/journal/v430/n6996/suppinfo/nature02746.html.

humans (Fouchier et al., 2004). Three out of four H5N1 human virus isolates from Vietnam had this mutation, but the human virus from Thailand did not, nor did any other avian influenza viruses tested. No recent H5N1 viruses characterized in this study had Glu 92 in the NS1 protein, which is reportedly associated with increased virulence in pigs (Seo et al., 2002).

The apparently simultaneous occurrence of H5N1 outbreaks across eastern Asia remains unexplained, but the presence of H5N1 viruses in dead migratory birds suggests that wild bird populations may be involved. In Hong Kong between late 2002 and the time of this report, genotype Z⁺ H5N1 virus was isolated from a dead little egret (*Egretta garzetta*), and genotype Z viruses were isolated from two dead grey herons (*Ardea cinerea*), a black-headed gull (*Larus ridibundus*), a feral pigeon (*Columba livia*), a tree sparrow (*Passer montanus*), and a peregrine falcon (*Falco peregrinus*). In the gene phylogenies, the H5N1 viruses isolated from wild birds have either an out-group or sister-group relation to recent Thailand and Vietnam H5N1 isolates (Figure 2-4; see also Supplementary Figs 1 and 2).[13] The timing and distribution of the H5N1 infection in poultry in China from 2001 onwards (Figure 2-2) coincides with the general period of winter bird migration to southern China; however, it is not known whether the H5N1 virus has become established in wild bird populations. The potential role of wild birds in the maintenance and spread of H5N1 viruses must be considered in strategies for regional control.

H5N1 virus is now endemic in poultry in Asia (Table 2-1) and has gained an entrenched ecological niche from which to present a long-term pandemic threat to humans. At present, these viruses are poorly transmitted from poultry to humans, and there is no conclusive evidence of human-to-human transmission. However, continued, extensive exposure of the human population to H5N1 viruses increases the likelihood that the viruses will acquire the necessary characteristics for efficient human-to-human transmission through genetic mutation or reassortment with a prevailing human influenza A virus. Furthermore, contemporary human H3N2 influenza viruses are now endemic in pigs in southern China (Peiris et al., 2001) and can reassort with avian H5N1 viruses in this 'intermediate host.' Therefore, it is imperative that outbreaks of H5N1 disease in poultry in Asia are rapidly and sustainably controlled. The seasonality of the disease in poultry, together with the control measures already implemented, are likely to reduce temporarily the frequency of H5N1 influenza outbreaks and the probability of human infection. However, complacency would be

---

[13]Supporting online material, http://www.nature.com/nature/journal/v430/n6996/suppinfo/ nature02746.html.

unwise. Governments in the region face an endemic and recurrent problem that presents a serious threat to human health. Although other countries in the region have been affected, Hong Kong has remained remarkably free of H5N1 outbreaks in poultry in 2004, thanks to preventive measures implemented over the past few years (Sims et al., 2003).

Methods

Surveillance, Virus Isolation and Characterization

Faecal droppings from apparently healthy poultry in live poultry markets in Hong Kong and in Guangdong, Hunan, and Yunnan provinces were sampled monthly for influenza virus isolation. Methods used for virus isolation and characterization have been previously described (Guan et al., 2000). In addition to systematic surveillance in the poultry markets, sick or dead poultry from markets and farms in Hong Kong were similarly studied. This analysis included representative H5N1 viruses isolated from birds in Vietnam (n = 8), Thailand (n = 7), and Indonesia (n = 6), and from humans in Vietnam (n = 4) and Thailand (n = 1) during the 2003–2004 H5N1 outbreak.

Genetic Analysis

All sequences were edited with the Staden software package and aligned with ClustalX. Phylogenetic trees were generated using PAUP* version 4.0 (Swofford, 2001) and MEGA version 2.1 (Kumar et al., 2001). K_a/K_s analysis was conducted by the Pamilo–Bianchi–Li method as implemented in MEGA.

AVIAN INFLUENZA OUTBREAK IN THAILAND: CURRENT POLICIES[14]

Chantanee Buranathai

Bureau of Disease Prevention Control and Veterinary Services
Department of Livestock Development
Thailand

---

[14]This paper was written about the first wave of the avian influenza outbreak—from January to May 2004. Since then, some policies and measures have been changed to correspond with the second wave of the outbreak—from July to the time of publication (December) in 2004.

The current policies and strategies implemented by the Department of Livestock Development (DLD) during the outbreak of highly pathogenic influenza outbreak (HPAI) in 2004 are aimed to (1) contain and eradicate the disease, (2) compensate and restore the loss, (3) improve biosecurity of the poultry system, (4) ensure public safety, and (5) establish a reliable early warning system.

Stamping-Out and Preemptive Culling

Because HPAI is an emerging disease in Thailand, the policy is to contain and eradicate the disease as fast as possible. Therefore, the most stringent measures have been applied. During the initial phase, HPAI-infected premises were stamped-out and disinfected, and preemptive culling was done on premises in the 5-kilometer-radius zone. In the second phase, infected premises and poultry within a 1-kilometer radius were depopulated, followed by disinfection. During the final phase, where sporadic cases were found, infected premises were stamped-out, then samples from the neighboring population were collected for virus isolation. If an HPAI-positive premise was detected, that particular premise was depopulated.

Compensation Scheme

Farmers whose farms are depopulated are compensated by the government in two phases. The initial compensation, right after their farms are stamped-out, is 40 baht ($1) per layer and 20 baht per broiler as well as payment for eggs that had been destroyed. The initial compensation is meant to support farmers when they lose income. The second compensation is arranged when farmers are ready to restock their farms. They can choose between cash or poultry to start the flock. If they prefer cash, the government will pay 100 baht per layer and 20 baht per broiler. The total of 140 baht per layer is equal to or slightly more than average market price, which means 100 percent compensation. HPAI is a special case which the Thai Government agreed to pay 100 percent compensation.

Farm Standard and Biosecurity System

The Department of Livestock Development established the "Farm Standard" for layer, broiler, duck, and other species of poultry. The standard is also divided by nature of the house, size, and type of the farm. The standard is a guideline for poultry farmers to improve the biosecurity system on their farms to prevent avian influenza outbreak. The DLD provides several training courses to educate farmers on disease prevention and control, on the concept of biosecurity, and on how to improve the animal house to meet the biosecurity standard. Only a farm that complies with all requirements will be allowed to restock. Noncompliant farms will not be given permission and infringement of this regulation in unlawful.

Movement Control

From the start of the outbreak until the present, movement control measures have been enforced in every province. Sixty-five checkpoints were set up by the DLD; in addition, more checkpoints can be set by the command of provincial governors, in cooperation with police or military. The DLD is the national authority that issues permits for animal movement. Stringent procedures for movement control have been implemented to prevent spread of the disease. Ten days prior to the movement, cloacal swabs are taken for virus isolation. Only HPAI-negative farms can obtain the movement permit.

Traceability

A database on poultry population is being updated and improved to facilitate planning for disease control, movement control, and epidemiology study in the future.

Vaccination

The Ministry of Agriculture and Cooperatives has a policy of no avian influenza (AI) vaccination. This policy is currently emphasized and implemented.

Surveillance

Three rounds of active and proactive surveillance have been conducted. Collection of samples prior to movement is also considered active surveillance. Passive surveillance from avian cases that come to the DLD laboratory network for diagnosis is ongoing. In addition, DLD staff have been conducting a slaughterhouse surveillance program at the ante-mortem area and checking for virus residue in the finished products. After the final phase of the outbreak, sero-surveillance will be conducted nationwide to evaluate the infection status and identify risk areas. Clinical surveillance will be applied at all times. To support the national surveillance program for AI, the DLD allocated funding to the National Institute of Animal Health, and all Regional Diagnostic Centers were mandated to improve their facilities and increase capacity. Information technology will be developed to ensure the reliability of an early warning system.

Slaughterhouse Standard

Guidelines for standard slaughterhouse and sanitary practice were established and distributed. The DLD is proposing a law to enforce the standard slaughterhouse practice and to regulate the registration of slaughterhouses.

THE 2003–2004 H5N1 AVIAN INFLUENZA OUTBREAK IN VIETNAM

T.D. Nguyen, DVM, PhD[15]

National Institute for Veterinary Research

Introduction

Avian influenza, also known as bird flu, was officially declared to have occurred in Vietnam for the first time on December 23, 2003. The outbreak was first reported in south Vietnam and spread at a galloping speed. Within 6 weeks, 57 of the 64 Vietnamese provinces were affected. However, the outbreak was contained within 2 months. Important lessons can be learned from analyzing the rapid spread of the outbreak and the relatively rapid response to it. This section describes how poultry is raised in Vietnam, how the avian influenza outbreak occurred, and how the country tried to control the disease. It also discusses factors that influenced the effectiveness of AI control measures as applied in Vietnam.

Poultry Production in Vietnam

Vietnam has a population of 260 million domestic birds, including 192 million chickens and 68 million ducks. The population of geese and ratites is very small and that of quails and pigeons and other birds is not known.

Poultry production consists mainly of chickens and ducks raised by individual families, often in their backyards. Chickens are bred in farms that provide chicks both to the poultry industry for broiler stock and to households. Poultry farms are often small and typically contain only 100 to 500 broilers. A few chicken breeding farms supply day-old chicks to nearly all of the country.

Ducks are largely raised in the traditional way, which consists of growing laying ducks throughout the year and meat ducks in the months of May

[15]We would like to thank Kenjiro Inui, DVM, PhD, of the Japanese International Cooperation Agency Project in Vietnam for the initial comments and critique of this manuscript.

and October. Laying ducks are normally unconfined; they scavenge in the rice fields during the day and return home at night. The more numerous meat ducks are kept in the rice fields to collect the fallen rice grains during the harvest seasons. Recently, with the introduction of supermeat ducks and Muscovy ducks from abroad, industrial duck raising has begun in some places.

Many households own both ducks and chickens, housing them together in the backyard. For farmers, keeping chickens and ducks provides one of the most important sources of income. Because of the small scale of poultry production, traders go from house to house buying live birds to sell at the markets. This practice renders the control of animal movement nearly impossible.

Chicken and duck pens are made of local materials such as bamboo, wood, or brick. The pens—even pens used for growing industrial broilers—are sometimes located next to human dwellings. The diversity of chicken-raising settings greatly complicates the practice of biosecurity.

The birds are sold alive because Vietnamese consumers prefer their poultry to be as fresh as possible. Live chickens, especially cockerels, also serve an important ceremonial and spiritual function. They are used as a tribute dedicated to people's ancestors in the New Year or to their deceased parents on their memorial days. As a result, industrial slaughterhouses for birds are almost nonexistent and sanitary meat inspection cannot effectively be implemented.

Vietnam is not a poultry-exporting country; rather, poultry for breeding stock is imported into Vietnam. Poultry imports from neighboring countries are largely unregulated by such practices as animal health inspection.

This is the environment into which AI was introduced in Vietnam.

The Avian Influenza Outbreak

First Signs of the Outbreak

Birds began to die on many farms in the Tien Giang and Long An provinces in December 2003. The local veterinary officials initially reported the cause of death as *Pasteurella*, a common bacterium that is particularly virulent in Southeast Asia; subsequently, the disease was said to be caused by an unknown virus. At the same time, the disease was reported in the Province of Ha Tay in North Vietnam. Avian influenza was eventually diagnosed based on the nonreactivity of the virus toward anti-Newcastle serum and its characteristic behavior in the hemagglutination inhibition test. Thus confirmed, avian influenza was officially declared to have occurred in the country on December 23. Urgent measures, such as circling the outbreak, control of animal and human movement, establishment of checkpoints, disinfection, and culling diseased birds, were recommended. However, these measures cannot, by law, be implemented until a state of emergency (literally the presence of epidemic disease) is declared by the Chairman of the province or by the Minister of Agriculture. The state of emergency was imposed in a timely manner in some provinces, but others were slow to take this step. In some cases, delayed AI confirmation resulted from a lack of diagnostic facilities; in others, government officials failed to recognize the importance of the threat. The outbreak peaked at the beginning of February 2004, when four million birds were destroyed in a single day, on February 6 (Ministry of Agriculture and Rural Development of Vietnam, 2004).

Features of the Outbreak in Vietnam

- Both terrestrial birds (chickens and quails) and aquatic birds (ducks and Muscovy ducks), particularly adult animals, developed clinical disease and suffered high rates of both morbidity and mortality.
- AI infected more birds in industrial operations than in backyard settings.
- The patchy distribution of infected farms and the results of genetic viral analysis suggest that there was a single infection source, and that the disease spread from bird to bird.
- The high virulence of the H5N1 virus was characterized not only by acute and severe infection in humans, but also by the sudden death of chickens without AI typical lesions. Beyond the 15 AI confirmed cases in humans, the flu failed to infect chicken farmers and veterinarians who were in direct contact with diseased birds.
- When human cases of H5N1 influenza were confirmed and publicized in the media, farmers were willing to cull their chickens.

Control Program

Diagnostic testing. The following methods were used: isolation of the virus in embryonated chicken eggs, and hemagglutination (HA), and hemagglutination inhibition (HI) tests; the Directigen Flu A (Becton & Dickinson, Cockeysville, MD), which detects the NP protein; and RT-PCR tests. At the beginning of the outbreak, each infected farm was sampled and tested. Later, as the number of infected farms ballooned, any farm that experienced a massive sudden death of birds (more than 10 percent of the population within 2 days), or at which dead birds had hemorrhagic lesions in the internal organs, was considered to be infected with avian influenza.

Information. A headquarters was established in the main building of the Ministry of Agriculture and Rural Development. Every province reported new AI cases and related issues to the headquarters on a daily basis.

Animal transport restriction. Early in the outbreak, the transport of birds in and out of affected provinces was prohibited. Nevertheless, although checkpoints were set up, birds continued to move in and out of affected areas. Chickens from outbreak regions continued to be sold until the Prime Minister launched a coordinated effort to control AI on February 4.

Disposal. Burial was the main method of bird disposal, but the disposal of culled chickens was difficult to enforce at first because no compensation was offered to farmers. Later, differences in the compensation rates between provinces resulted in birds being moved from provinces that offered relatively low compensation rates to provinces that offered farmers more money for their birds.

Disinfection. The government provided free disinfectants that were widely used in both affected and nonaffected farms. In many breeding farms, disinfection was performed as a preventive measure to preserve the breeding stock.

Despite several requests by poultry companies, the government decided not to vaccinate against AI, and instead relied on disease detection and stamping-out to control the outbreak.

Government Response

The Vietnamese government issued several important and decisive directives and orders in response to the AI outbreak, including the following:

- A Steering Committee led by the Director of the Department of Animal Health was established on January 10, 2004, as a result of the Prime Minister's telegram to the Chairmen of provinces (No. 71/CP-NN dated on January 8), that officially declared the AI outbreak in Vietnam.
- A new National Steering Committee, led by the Minister of Agriculture, was established on January 28 following the Prime Minister's decision (No. 13/2004/QD-TTg) concerning the AI outbreak. This decision was significant because it described AI as a threat to the health of humans as well as animals, and required agencies other than Agriculture to take part in the effort to control the outbreak.
- Following the Prime Minister's telegram to the Chairmen of provinces (No. 159/CP-NN on February 4), members of the government were

sent to every province to provide direct guidance on the control of AI. This decision also led to the implementation of severe control measures, such as prohibiting the circulation and consumption of poultry and poultry products.

• On February 6, Vietnam's most powerful political body, the Politics Bureau, issued a Directive (No. 35) requesting all levels of government and every citizen to participate in the effort to stop the spread of AI.

Containment of the Outbreak

Following the implementation of control measures, the outbreak began to wane from its peak on February 6, 2004. After that date, the number of reported new cases steadily decreased (Figure 2-5).

No new cases of AI were reported in the weeks following February 27, 2004. At the end of March, the government declared that the AI outbreak had been contained. The outbreak resulted in the loss of 40 million chickens and ducks worth an estimated US$120 million (according to the World Bank). This figure does not include the cost of compensating farmers for their losses.

Vietnam's response to AI, and its control of the outbreak within 2 months, was comparable to that of other countries at similar stages of scientific and economic development that were affected by AI.

Key Factors in Controlling the Outbreak

Several positive factors contributed to the control of the AI outbreak in Vietnam. These include:

• The decisive determination of the Vietnamese government to extinguish the outbreak by applying lessons learned from efforts to control Severe Acute Respiratory Syndrome (SARS) in Vietnam in early 2003.

• Vietnam's political structure, which organizes and involves every citizen. Orders and directions from the central government effectively reach every person and can be clearly understood, observed, and fulfilled.

• The decision to ban the movement and consumption of poultry and poultry products. This decision, which was based on advice from scientific experts, limited the spread of disease and allowed officials to detect the appearance of new cases following a 21-day incubation period. This measure was also hoped to reduce the risk of human infection with AI, both within Vietnam and throughout the world.

• Public awareness of the AI outbreak. The media provided news of the development of the outbreak, information regarding the nature of the disease, and descriptions of effective measures against AI. The government's awareness campaign helped people to understand the crisis and enlisted

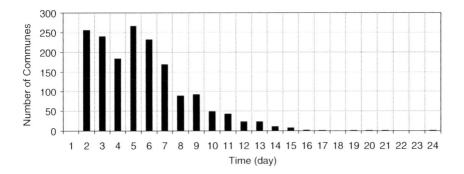

FIGURE 2-5 Number of communes declared as newly affected by the highly pathogenic avian influenza (HPAI) during February 2004 in Vietnam.
SOURCE: Animal Health Department (2004).

public support to stop the transport of birds. This proved far more effective than checkpoints in controlling the spread of disease.
- The virulence of H5N1 and the severity of its avian symptoms (rapid death), which made its presence easy to detect.
- Public fear of becoming infected with AI, which led to increased cooperation with infection control measures.

Lessons Learned

In retrospect, efforts to control infectious diseases can always be improved. The following aspects of the recent response to AI demand critical examination in order to improve the response to future outbreaks:

1. The 1-month delay between official recognition of the outbreak (on January 8) and the decision, following the appearance of human cases of AI, to ban poultry movement and establish the National Steering Committee (February 4). This delay allowed farmers to sell infected chickens and consequently spread the disease. A thorough, consistent, and updated scientific understanding of AI and consensus on the risk it poses to human health is clearly needed. Several scientific workshops have been organized since then to build such a consensus.

2. Vietnam's preparedness for AI. H5N1 AI has been reported repeatedly in neighboring Hong Kong and in the nearby southern provinces of China, a region considered to be the epicenter of influenza. Logically, Vietnam should have been prepared to face influenza in general and AI in particular. The following specific areas require attention to prepare Vietnam against influenza:

- Diagnosis and virus typing. The confirmation of H5N1 AI virus was possible thanks to the generous aid from the Centers for Disease Control and Prevention (CDC) in Atlanta, Georgia. This agency provided NA protein typing and reagent supplies, as well as a team of workers who performed direct diagnosis during the outbreak. However, because this process is time consuming, it would be better to put in place a system of early, on-the-spot detection and virus characterization. This would help Vietnamese authorities react in time to prevent farmers from selling infected birds, thereby limiting disease transmission.

- Disease and virus surveillance and monitoring. Like many other developing countries, Vietnam had no systemic surveillance or program to monitor AI viral circulation. The unprecedented outbreak, therefore, surprised Vietnam.

- Institutional preparedness. Although Vietnam has made general preparations for infectious disease, there is no institutional preparedness for specific diseases; it can thus be argued that the country was insufficiently prepared for AI. Many other countries have detailed plans for AI that include a compensation policy for farmers who cull their flocks; regulations on bird disposal; and guidelines outlining the responsibilities of various governmental authorities in such public health emergencies and the paths of communication among them. Such a plan would help with the timely and efficient control of infectious disease. However, there is an important cultural hurdle that needs to be overcome: In the Vietnamese language, the equivalent in English for "declaration of a state of emergency" is *cong bo dich*, literally "public declaration on the epidemic." Many people would perceive such a declaration as a concern only to animal health officials; instead, there needs to be a way to declare a state of emergency that duly activates other state agencies.

- Technical preparedness. Before 2003, Vietnam had never experienced an AI outbreak. The disease was not included in the curriculum of any of the country's veterinary schools; consequently, many veterinarians incorrectly assumed that its symptomology would resemble influenza in humans and did not suspect that influenza was causing massive mortality in chickens. The country was also ill prepared to deal with the diagnosis and typing of the virus, and had to rely on CDC for help in this effort.

In general terms, Vietnam responded effectively to the AI outbreak; thankfully, no human-to-human transmission occurred. However, if Vietnam had been better prepared for AI, the country would not have lost 15 human lives and as much as 40 million poultry, which has severely affected the rural economy.

Considerations for the Future

It is widely accepted that new influenza viruses will continue to emerge as a result of mutation and genetic reassortment (Guan et al., 1999; Hoffmann et al., 2000; Xu et al., 1999). Research indicates that virus-receptor specificity does not prevent the direct transmission of avian influenza to humans, as was once believed (Matrosovich et al., 2004), and it is now known that any animal, not just the pig (Guan et al., 1999), can serve as the vessel for viral reassortment. The process that allowed H5N1 and H9N2 (Katz, 2003) and H7N7 avian influenza viruses to directly and readily infect humans on other occasions occurred during the 2003–04 AI outbreak in Asia and can be expected to continue (Guan et al., 2004) as the virus becomes increasingly virulent. Consequently, the more we know about this virus, the more we recognize that it is unpredictable and mysterious, and the more we are frightened by it.

One of the issues that arose during the AI outbreak in Vietnam was how to adequately raise government and public awareness of the threat posed by a newly emerged virus, and who should alert decision makers and the public to this danger. The World Health Organization (WHO) Global Influenza Program has foreseen a potential conflict of interest between public health and agriculture/veterinary sectors in relation to surveillance and reporting of animal influenza (Stöhr, 2003). Moreover, evidence indicates that all human influenza viruses are of avian origin. WHO advises that "assessment of the risk to humans needs to be based on a risk assessment of the disease situation in poultry that considers the prevalence of highly pathogenic avian influenza and the adequacy of the surveillance system. A reliable system of review and verification is needed to ascertain that poultry are disease free in an area or country" (WHO, 2004b). Clearly, cooperation between animal and human health institutions should be strengthened. A designated group of experts in both fields in each country could effectively take responsibility for monitoring influenza and notifying government decision makers in the event of an outbreak.

If the next influenza pandemic is imminent, it will probably strike first in poor countries, where public health services are meager and veterinary services are even worse, where vaccine and anti-influenza drugs are not likely to be available, and where disease management is often disorganized and ineffective. Therefore, such countries should be provided with a basic system for AI detection based on cheap and simple techniques. As previously discussed, the highly pathogenic avian influenza (HPAI) virus is readily infecting humans, but there has been no pandemic yet. Most major avian influenza epidemics have been caused by novel HPAI viruses that resulted from reassortment (Sturm-Ramirez et al., 2004). However, the low pathogenic avian influenza (LPAI) viruses that became HPAI after several passages through chickens can also cause epidemic avian influenza. Will the next human influenza pandemic follow the same pattern or will it be caused by a reassorted virus?

To avert an influenza pandemic, it will also be necessary to prioritize the mobilization of public health resources both before and during an influenza outbreak. Three months after the AI outbreak was controlled, attention to AI in Vietnam was already decreasing, as it naturally must. Influenza viruses can change the world, but life must and will go on. The best preparation would be to devise monitoring and reporting mechanisms that guarantee that an outbreak of disease receives appropriate attention from decision makers and the public in time to avert major consequences.

REFERENCES

Animal Health Department. 2004. Number of communes declared as newly affected by the HPAI during February in Vietnam. Animal Health Department of Vietnam.

Claas EC, Osterhaus AD, van Beek R, De Jong JC, Rimmelzwaan GF, Senne DA, Krauss S, Shortridge KF, Webster RG. 1998. Human influenza A H5N1 virus related to a highly pathogenic avian influenza virus. *Lancet* 351:472–477.

Fouchier RA, Schneeberger PM, Rozendaal FW, Broekman JM, Kemink SA, Munster V, Kuiken T, Rimmelzwaan GF, Schutten M, Van Doornum GJ, Koch G, Bosman A, Koopmans M, Osterhaus AD. 2004. Avian influenza A virus (H7N7) associated with conjunctivitis and a fatal case of acute respiratory distress syndrome. *Proc Natl Acad Sci U S A* 101:1356–1361.

Guan Y, Shortridge KF, Krauss S, Webster RG. 1999. Molecular characterization of H9N2 influenza viruses: Were they the donors of the "internal" genes of H5N1 viruses in Hong Kong? *Proc Natl Acad Sci USA* 96:9363–9367.

Guan Y, Shortridge KF, Krauss S, Chin PS, Dyrting KC, Ellis TM, Webster RG, Peiris M. 2000. H9N2 influenza viruses possessing H5N1-like internal genomes continue to circulate in poultry in southeastern China. *J Virol* 74:9372–9380.

Guan Y, Peiris JS, Lipatov AS, Ellis TM, Dyrting KC, Krauss S, Zhang LJ, Webster RG, Shortridge KF. 2002. Emergence of multiple genotypes of H5N1 avian influenza viruses in Hong Kong SAR. *Proc Natl Acad Sci USA* 99:8950–8955.

Guan Y, Poon LL, Cheung CY, Ellis TM, Lim W, Lipatov AS, Chan KH, Sturm-Ramirez KM, Cheung CL, Leung YH, Yuen KY, Webster RG, Peiris JS. 2004. H5N1 influenza: A protean pandemic threat. *Proc Natl Acad Sci USA* 101:8156–8161.

Ha Y, Stevens DJ, Skehel JJ, Wiley DC. 2001. X-ray structures of H5 avian and H9 swine influenza virus hemagglutinins bound to avian and human receptor analogs. *Proc Natl Acad Sci USA* 98:11181–11186.

Hatta M, Gao P, Halfmann P, Kawaoka Y. 2001. Molecular basis for high virulence of Hong Kong H5N1 influenza A viruses. *Science* 293:1773–1775.

Hien TT, Nguyen TL, Nguyen TD, Luong TS, Pham PM, Nguyen VC, Pham TS, Vo CD, Le TQ, Ngo TT, Dao BK, Le PP, Nguyen TT, Hoang TL, Cao VT, Le TG, Nguyen DT, Le HN, Nguyen KT, Le HS, Le VT, Christiane D, Tran TT, Menno de J, Schultsz C, Cheng P, Lim W, Horby P, Farrar J; World Health Organization International Avian Influenza Investigative Team. 2004. Avian influenza A (H5N1) in 10 patients in Vietnam. *N Engl J Med* 350:1179–1188.

Hoffmann E, Stech J, Leneva I, Krauss S, Scholtissek C, Chin PS, Peiris M, Shortridge KF, Webster RG. 2000. Characterization of the influenza A virus gene pool in avian species in southern China: Was H6N1 a derivative or a precursor of H5N1? *J Virol* 74:6309–6315.

Holsinger LJ, Shaughnessy MA, Micko A, Pinto LH, Lamb RA. 1995. Analysis of the post-translational modifications of the influenza virus M2 protein. *J Virol* 69:1219–1225.

Iwatsuki-Horimoto K, Kanazawa R, Sugii S, Kawaoka Y, Horimoto T. 2004. The index influenza A virus subtype H5N1 isolated from a human in 1997 differs in its receptor-binding properties from a virulent avian influenza virus. *J Gen Virol* 85:1001–1005.

Katz JM. 2003. The impact of avian influenza viruses on public health. *Avian Disease* 47: 914–920.

Kaverin NV, Rudneva IA, Ilyushina NA, Varich NL, Lipatov AS, Smirnov YA, Govorkova EA, Gitelman AK, Lvov DK, Webster RG. 2002. Structure of antigenic sites on the haemagglutinin molecule of H5 avian influenza virus and phenotypic variation of escape mutants. *J Gen Virol* 83:2497–2505.

Kumar S, Tamura K, Jakobsen IB, Nei M. 2001. MEGA2: Molecular evolutionary genetics analysis software. *Bioinformatics* 17:1244–1245.

Li KS, Xu KM, Peiris JS, Poon LL, Yu KZ, Yuen KY, Shortridge KF, Webster RG, Guan Y. 2003. Characterization of H9 subtype influenza viruses from the ducks of southern China: A candidate for the next influenza pandemic in humans? *J Virol* 77:6988–6994.

Matrosovich M, Zhou NN, Kawaoka Y, Webster RG. 1999. The surface glycoproteins of H5 influenza viruses isolated from humans, chickens, and wild aquatic birds have distinguishable properties. *J Virol* 73:1146–1155.

Matrosovich MN, Matrosovich TY, Gray T, Roberts NA, Klenk HD. 2004. Human and avian influenza viruses target different cell types in cultures of human airway epithelium. *Proc Natl Acad Sci USA* 101:4620–4624.

Ministry of Agriculture and Rural Development of Vietnam. 2004 (May). *Final Report of Avian Influenza Outbreak in Vietnam*. Ministry of Agriculture and Rural Development of Vietnam.

Peiris JS, Guan Y, Markwell D, Ghose P, Webster RG, Shortridge KF. 2001. Co-circulation of avian H9N2 and contemporary "human" H3N2 influenza viruses in pigs in southeastern China: Potential for genetic reassortment? *J Virol* 75:9679–9686.

Presgraves DC, Balagopalan L, Abmayr SM, Orr HA. 2003. Adaptive evolution drives divergence of a hybrid inviability gene between two species of *Drosophila*. *Nature* 423:715–719.

ProMED-mail. 2004a (August 13). PRO/AH/EDR> Avian influenza, human—East Asia (38). Published date: August 13, 2004. Archive number: 20040813.2249. Available at http://www.promedmail.org. Source: WHO Outbreak News, 13 Aug 2004 [edited]: http://www.who.int/csr/don/2004_08_13/en/print.html. "Human cases of avian influenza: situation in Viet Nam."

ProMED-mail. 2004b (September 29). PRO/AH/EDR> Avian influenza, human—East Asia (49): Viet Nam. Published date: September 29, 2004. Archive number: 20040929.2692. Available at http://www.promedmail.org.

ProMED-mail. 2004c. PRO/AH/EDR> Avian influenza—Eastern Asia (98): Viet Nam, Thailand. Published date: July 27, 2004. Archive number: 20040727.2058. Available at http://www.promedmail.org.

ProMED-mail. 2004d (October 25). PRO/AH/EDR> Avian influenza, human—Thailand (08). Published date: October 25, 2004. Archive number: 20041025.2886. Available at http://www.promedmail.org.

ProMED-mail. 2004e. PRO/AH/EDR> Avian influenza, human—East Asia (46): Thailand, susp. Published date: September 25, 2004. Archive number: 20040925.2647. Available at http://www.promedmail.org.

Scholtissek C, Quack G, Klenk HD, Webster RG. 1998. How to overcome resistance of influenza A viruses against adamantane derivatives. *Antiviral Res* 37:83–95.

Seo SH, Hoffmann E, Webster RG. 2002. Lethal H5N1 influenza viruses escape host antiviral cytokine responses. *Nature Med* 8:950–954.

Shortridge KF, Zhou NN, Guan Y, Gao P, Ito T, Kawaoka Y, Kodihalli S, Krauss S, Markwell D, Murti KG, Norwood M, Senne D, Sims L, Takada A, Webster RG. 1998. Characterization of avian H5N1 influenza viruses from poultry in Hong Kong. *Virology* 252:331–342.

Sims LD, Ellis TM, Liu KK, Dyrting K, Wong H, Peiris M, Guan Y, Shortridge KF. 2003. Avian influenza in Hong Kong 1977–2002. *Avian Diseases* 47:832–838.

Stöhr K. 2003. The WHO Global Influenza Program and its Animal Influenza Network. *Avian Diseases* 47:934–938.

Sturm-Ramirez KM, Ellis T, Bousfield B, Bissett L, Dyrting K, Rehg JE, Poon L, Guan Y, Peiris M, Webster RG. 2004. Reemerging H5N1 influenza viruses in Hong Kong in 2002 are highly pathogenic to ducks. *J Virol* 78(9):4892–4901.

Swofford DL. 2001. *PAUP*: Phylogenetic Analysis Using Parsimony (and Other Methods) 4.0 Beta*. Sunderland, MA: Sinauer Associates.

Thomas JM, Stevens MP, Percy N, Barclay WS. 1998. Phosphorylation of the M2 protein of influenza A virus is not essential for virus viability. *Virology* 252:54–64.

Webster RG, Bean WJ, Gorman OT, Chambers TM, Kawaoka Y. 1992. Evolution and ecology of influenza A viruses. *Microbiol Rev* 56:152–179.

WHO (World Health Organization). 2004a. Avian influenza A (H5N1). *Weekly Epidemiol Rev* 79:65–70.

WHO. 2004b. *Assessment of Risk to Human Health Associated with Outbreaks of Highly Pathogenic H5N1 Avian Influenza in Poultry*. [Online]. Available: http://www.who.int/csr/disease/avian_influenza/assessment2004_05_14/en/.

Xu X, Subbarao K, Cox NJ, Guo Y. 1999. Genetic characterization of the pathogenic influenza A/Goose/Guangdong/1/96 (H5N1) virus: Similarity of its hemagglutinin gene to those of H5N1 viruses from the 1997 outbreaks in Hong Kong. *Virology* 261:15–19.

3

Toward Preparedness:
Opportunities and Obstacles

OVERVIEW

The odds of detecting, controlling, and perhaps preventing the spread of an influenza virus with pandemic potential have improved dramatically since 1918, and they continue to increase with expanding knowledge of influenza viruses and the threat they present to human and animal health. Today, international programs permit the characterization of thousands of viral isolates each year and support worldwide surveillance and communications networks. These efforts are informed by research on viral molecular biology and evolution, and bolstered by simultaneous preparations against the threat of bioterrorism.

Yet major challenges to pandemic preparedness remain to be overcome. The world's growing—and increasingly urbanized—population and the speed and volume of international travel create abundant opportunities for widespread viral transmission. Some countries will respond to a pandemic with abundant resources and expertise, but many others remain essentially defenseless. Even populations wealthy enough to obtain vaccine are unlikely to get enough to prevent significant morbidity and mortality from pandemic influenza unless more rapid vaccine production methods or novel prophylactic vaccines can be introduced before the next pandemic strikes. The circumstances surrounding 2 consecutive years of interpandemic flu vaccine shortages in the United States clearly illustrate this vulnerability. The 2003–2004 shortage, discussed by Glen Nowak in Chapter 6, resulted from increased demand for vaccine during an early and intense flu season, while the 2004–2005 shortage resulted from contamination that rendered half of the U.S. vaccine supply—the product of a single manufacturer, Chiron, Inc.—unusable.

This chapter discusses challenges to pandemic preparedness at international, national, and state levels. It begins with the executive summary of a technical consultation convened by the World Health Organization (WHO) in March 2004 in response to the threat posed by H5N1 avian influenza, and in particular to the evidence that this virus had been transmitted to humans in Vietnam and Thailand, with deadly results. More than 100 experts from 33 countries discussed a broad range of measures that could be introduced by WHO and national authorities to forestall emerging pandemics, slow their spread, and reduce their potential toll of morbidity, mortality, and social disruption. The executive summary presents the recommendations and conclusions of four working groups (surveillance, public health interventions, antivirals, and vaccines) regarding key issues in pandemic preparedness.

In the United States, the Department of Health and Human Services released a draft *Pandemic Preparedness and Response Plan* for a 60-day period of public comment on August 26, 2004. This chapter includes an executive summary and a synopsis of this plan, which describes coordination and decision making at the national level; provides an overview of key issues; and outlines steps that should be taken at the national, state, and local levels before and during a pandemic. It is followed by two contributions that further discuss pandemic planning from the perspective of state and local public health officials, who will be largely responsible for implementing pandemic prevention and control actions in the United States. The first essay discusses pandemic planning as a collaborative process that involves officials at all levels of government and that is guided by federal priorities. The second essay highlights the importance of strengthening influenza surveillance at the state and local levels, both as a means to early detection of an emerging pandemic and to inform the public health response to interpandemic influenza.

The chapter continues with a consideration of pharmaceutical defenses against pandemic influenza. Vaccines significantly reduce morbidity and mortality during annual (interpandemic) flu seasons, but as this chapter demonstrates, considerable obstacles currently hinder the production of a vaccine against a pandemic strain of influenza. The critical role of vaccine manufacturers in addressing a pandemic is described, accompanied by a review of methods and logistics for the development and production of a pandemic vaccine.

Demand for vaccine during a pandemic will likely far exceed supply. These considerations are subsequently explored first in a discussion of the challenges to equitable and effective vaccine distribution, and then in a description of the potential use of antiviral drugs to fill unmet need for vaccine, particularly during the initial phase of a pandemic. David Fedson advises that efforts toward pandemic vaccine development should initially focus on producing the largest possible supply of pandemic vaccine as quickly as possible. Europeans will most likely pursue this goal by developing a low-dose adjuvant pandemic vaccine, which differs from the strategy that will be undertaken by the National Institute of Allergy and Infectious Diseases in the United States. He also describes the potential advantages of engineering viral seed strains with reverse genetics and urges a quick resolution to the ongoing dispute regarding ownership of intellectual property for this technology.

Given these obstacles to the timely production of pandemic vaccine, it is also imperative to develop near-term strategies to address a pandemic threat without recourse to vaccination. Dr. Fedson recounts recent findings suggesting that prophylaxis with statins or other commonly available therapeutic agents, which have recently been found to reduce serum concentrations of several inflammatory mediators, might mitigate the clinical course of human influenza. He suggests next steps in pursuing this idea, but it is not without risk or controversy. For example, a recent case study describes a patient undergoing therapy with two statins (cerivastatin and bezafibrate) who developed acute renal failure due to rhabdomyolysis only after being administered an influenza vaccine; similar cases had occurred in several patients receiving this combined therapy who had contracted influenza (Plotkin et al., 2000). Researchers have also reported that the in-vitro treatment of macrophages with another statin (lovastatin) did not decrease tumor necrotic factor (TNF) production, as would be expected to occur with lovastatin-induced immunosuppression, but instead resulted in increased production of TNF (Monick et al., 2003). The apparent contradiction between this observation and the reports cited by Dr. Fedson may be explained by tolerance induced in vivo subsequent to lovastatin-induced TNF production, or perhaps by differences between the long-term and acute effects of lovastatin.

A second, more widely accepted strategy for coping with pandemic influenza in absence of vaccine is described in the subsequent review by Frederick Hayden, which focuses on the potential role of currently available antiviral drugs in such a pandemic response. However, as this review makes clear, a variety of supply and distribution problems must be solved before this promising strategy could be implemented.

Although the American health care system is overwhelmingly privatized, little attention has yet been paid to private medicine's potential role in preparing for pandemic influenza. This chapter concludes with a description of the status of pandemic planning within the private health care system, and suggestions for ways that private health care organizations could contribute to pandemic preparedness at all levels of government.

WHO CONSULTATION ON PRIORITY PUBLIC HEALTH
INTERVENTIONS BEFORE AND DURING INFLUENZA PANDEMIC
EXECUTIVE SUMMARY

World Health Organization[1]

Reprinted with permission from the World Health Organization,
Copyright World Health Organization, 2004, All Rights Reserved

Background

In January 2004, health authorities in Viet Nam and Thailand reported
their first human cases of infection with avian influenza, caused by an
H5N1 strain. The cases in humans are directly linked to outbreaks of highly
pathogenic H5N1 avian influenza in poultry initially reported in the Re-
public of Korea in mid-December 2003 and subsequently confirmed in an
additional seven Asian countries (Viet Nam, Japan, Thailand, Cambodia,
China, Laos, and Indonesia). As at end-March 2004, no countries other
than Viet Nam and Thailand had reported human cases. The number of
human cases has remained small to date, but treatment has been largely
ineffective and case fatality rates have been high. Moreover, the situation
has several disturbing features, including the historically unprecedented
scale of the outbreak in poultry.

Of foremost concern is the risk that conditions present in parts of Asia
could give rise to an influenza pandemic. Pandemics, which recur at unpredictable intervals, invariably cause high morbidity and mortality and great
social disruption and economic losses. Conservative estimates based on
mathematical modelling suggest that the next pandemic could cause from 2
million to 7.4 million deaths.

Conditions favourable to the start of a pandemic are now much better
understood than in the previous century, which witnessed three pandemics.
Influenza research was greatly stimulated in 1997, when the world's first
known cases of human infection with the H5N1 strain of avian influenza
virus were documented in Hong Kong Special Administrative Region of
China. Investigations launched by that outbreak, including studies in molecular biology and epidemiology, helped elucidate the mechanisms by
which pandemic viruses could emerge and further clarified the conditions
that favour such an event. These studies also demonstrated, for the first

---

[1]Editor's note: During the production of this report, the WHO Executive Board released
additional recommendations. For more information, see the following (1) *Influenza Pandemic
Preparedness and Response*, available at: http://www.who.int/gb/ebwha/pdf_files/EB115/
B115_44-en.pdf and (2) *Strengthening Pandemic Influenza Preparedness and Response*, available at: http://www.who.int/gb/ebwha/pdf_files/EB115/B115_R16-en.pdf.

time, that the H5N1 strain can infect humans directly without prior adaptation in a mammalian host. On that occasion, the culling within three days of Hong Kong's poultry population, estimated at 1.5 million birds, is thought to have possibly averted a pandemic.

Some experts believe that this improved understanding, when combined with efficient surveillance and immediate and aggressive action, might make it possible to detect events with pandemic potential and delay—or even prevent—their escalation and global spread. Research has identified three essential prerequisites for the start of a pandemic. First, a novel influenza subtype must be transmitted to humans. Second, the new virus must be able to replicate in humans and cause disease. Third, the new virus must be efficiently transmitted from one human to another; efficient human-to-human transmission is expressed as sustained chains of transmission causing community-wide outbreaks. Since 1997, the first two prerequisites have been met on four occasions: Hong Kong in 1997 (H5N1), Hong Kong in 2003 (H5N1), the Netherlands in 2003 (H7N7), and Viet Nam and Thailand in 2004 (H5N1). Of these outbreaks, those caused by H5N1 are of particular concern because of their association with severe illness and a high case fatality. Of even greater concern is the uniqueness of the present H5N1 situation in Asia. Never before has an avian influenza virus with a documented ability to infect humans caused such widespread outbreaks in birds in so many countries. This unprecedented situation has significantly increased the risk for the emergence of an influenza pandemic.

A pandemic virus capable of efficient human-to-human transmission could arise via two mechanisms: virus reassortment (the swapping of genetic material between viruses) when humans or pigs are co-infected with H5N1 and a human influenza virus, and adaptive mutation during human infection. The risk that either event will occur remains so long as H5N1 is present in an animal reservoir, thus allowing continuing opportunities for human exposure and infection. The level of risk is determined most directly by the prevalence of the virus in poultry and the frequency of its transmission to humans. The risk also depends on the co-circulation of human and avian influenza viruses and the inherent propensity of these viruses to reassort. Most experts agree that control of the present outbreaks in poultry will take several months or even years; some believe that the virus may have already established endemicity in domestic poultry. The recent detection of highly pathogenic avian influenza in wild birds adds another layer of complexity to control.

The world may therefore remain on the verge of a pandemic for some time to come. At the same time, the unpredictability of influenza viruses and the speed with which transmissibility can improve mean that the time for preparedness planning is right now. Such a task takes on added urgency because of the prospects opened by recent research: good planning and preparedness might mitigate the enormous consequences of a pandemic, and this opportunity must not be missed.

The Consultation

In response to these concerns, WHO convened a technical consultation on preparedness for an influenza pandemic from 16 to 18 March 2004. The consultation, attended by more than 100 experts from 33 countries, considered a wide range of measures that could be introduced, by WHO and national authorities, both before and during a pandemic. Three main objectives were identified: to forestall potential pandemics as they emerge, to slow national and international spread, and to reduce the usually high levels of morbidity, mortality, and social disruption. Participants agreed that the effectiveness of specific interventions would change over time in line with distinct phases, defined by epidemiological criteria, during the progression from an incipient pandemic situation to the declaration of a pandemic. Interventions were therefore discussed in terms of their objectives and likely impact at different phases as well as their feasibility in different resource settings. Epidemiological triggers for shifting objectives and adapting the recommended mix of measures were also identified. The consultation fully recognized that the best opportunity for mitigating the consequences of a pandemic would occur early on, and that planning and preparedness, at both national and global levels, would be needed to take full advantage of this opportunity.

Many key characteristics of a new pandemic virus—its pathogenicity, attack rate in different age groups, susceptibility to antivirals, and response to other treatments—would guide the selection of control measures, but could not be known with certainty in advance. In addition, many characteristics of normal human influenza, such as the role of asymptomatic transmission and the effectiveness of non-medical control measures, are poorly understood. During the chaos of a pandemic, health authorities would almost certainly need to make decisions, often with major social and economic consequences, in an atmosphere of considerable scientific uncertainty. To reduce some of this uncertainty, participants based their recommendations on relevant lessons from the recent SARS outbreak, knowledge about the epidemiology of previous influenza pandemics, and clinical data from outbreaks of H5N1 infection in Hong Kong in 1997 and Viet Nam and Thailand in 2004. Modelling of various scenarios for the emergence of a pandemic strain provided an especially useful planning tool.

Against this background, three main questions were addressed: what reporting and monitoring systems are needed to detect the start of a pandemic at the earliest possible stage and track its evolution, which interventions will be both feasible and effective at different phases and in different resource settings, and what policy options might best cope with the inevitable shortage of vaccines and antivirals. These questions were considered by four working groups focused on surveillance, public health interventions, antivirals, and vaccines. A more complete account of the deliberations and conclusions of each working group is provided in the main body of this report.

Some discussion centered on the question of whether—with better scientific knowledge, better control tools, and the international solidarity shown during the SARS response—something might be done to prevent the present situation from evolving towards a pandemic. In this regard, good surveillance in all countries experiencing outbreaks of highly pathogenic avian influenza in poultry was considered to be a fundamental prerequisite. Guarding against the start of a pandemic would also depend on rapid detection, prompt laboratory confirmation, and accurate reporting of human cases, and the transparent sharing of all relevant information with WHO.

Participants readily agreed that vaccines—the first line of defence for reducing morbidity and mortality—would not be available at the start of a pandemic and would remain in short supply throughout the first wave of international spread. For this reason, efforts to prevent or delay initial spread would have paramount importance. All countries would need to prioritize vaccine distribution and consider difficult ethical and practical questions of eligibility. Developing countries would face the most acute shortages, as manufacturing capacity is concentrated in Europe and North America, and countries can be expected to reserve scarce supplies for their own populations. In the absence of vaccines, antivirals would initially assume greater importance as a prophylactic and treatment tool for reducing morbidity and mortality. In practice, however, this potential role could be undermined by several problems, including high costs, uncertain efficacy, propensity to develop resistance, and extremely limited supplies, further constrained by the absence of any surge capacity for production.

With the first line of defence not a viable option at the start of a pandemic, participants looked at interventions that could forestall or delay national and international spread pending antiviral availability, the augmentation of vaccine supplies, and the implementation of mass vaccination strategies. This strategy of "buying time" was linked to assumptions, partially based on modelling, that the first chains of human-to-human transmission might not reach the efficiency needed to initiate and sustain pandemic spread. In such a scenario, the first evidence of limited human-to-human transmission, most likely expressed as clusters of cases, would be the epidemiological trigger for intense international efforts aimed at interrupting further transmission or at least delaying further national and international spread. For this reason, surveillance systems in countries with outbreaks in animals caused by H5N1 or other influenza viruses of known human pathogenicity should be oriented towards early detection, reporting, and investigation of clusters of human cases, followed by aggressive containment measures, including tracing and management of contacts, targeted prophylactic use of antivirals, and travel-related measures. Participants recommended consideration of whether an international stockpile of antivirals should be established for use exclusively during this critical window of opportunity.

Should early containment fail, the consultation concluded that, once a certain level of efficient transmission was reached, no interventions could halt further spread, and priorities would need to shift to the reduction of morbidity and mortality. It was also recognized that a reassortment event could result in a virus fully equipped for efficient human-to-human transmission, thus immediately curtailing opportunities to "buy time" through measures aimed at preventing geographical spread. Should early surveillance fail, the detection of transmission would likely take place only after efficient transmission was established, again curtailing opportunities to intervene. However, in these cases as well, advance planning had much to offer. As the consequences of a pandemic became apparent, public health authorities would face great public and political pressure to maintain or introduce often drastic, costly, and disruptive protective measures (travel restrictions, screening measures at borders, contacting tracing, isolation and quarantine) which, though useful at earlier stages, might have little or no impact once efficient transmission was established. By including provisions for stopping or adjusting measures in line with clear epidemiological criteria, preparedness plans would help public health authorities withstand this pressure and thus conserve resources for the next objectives: constraining transmission, preventing severe disease, and reducing case fatality.

When objectives shift, clear and frank public information and good communications systems would be essential in helping lower expectations and discouraging the continuation of personal protective measures no longer considered effective. Participants agreed that, once a pandemic begins, its overall management would move outside the public health sector and take on great political and economic significance. Good public information might also protect governments from accusations that extraordinary measures introduced at earlier phases—causing great economic costs and social disruption—failed and were therefore inappropriate. In addition, populations would need to be prepared for the even greater social disruption, linked to high morbidity and mortality that could be expected as the pandemic progressed.

Conclusions

Some General Conclusions

During the deliberations of the working groups and discussions in plenary session, the picture that emerged was one of a world inadequately prepared to respond to an influenza pandemic. Response capacity was considered insufficient at levels ranging from vaccine manufacturing to the sensitivity of surveillance systems, the number of hospital beds, the affordability of diagnostic tests, and the supply of respirators and face masks. A recurring theme was the need to engage government departments beyond the health sector. At the same time, the urgency of the present situation was fully appreciated, and participants made a number of suggestions for improving capacity now. For example, better use of vaccines and antivirals during the inter-pandemic period would improve manufacturing capacity while also helping to reduce the estimated 250,000 to 500,000 deaths caused by seasonal influenza epidemics each year. The burden of influenza in developing countries, including its contribution to overall morbidity and mortality and economic impact, was virtually unknown in most cases. Studies of this burden would give national authorities a better foundation for making influenza a priority and bargaining for a share of resources. Establishment of vaccine manufacturing capacity in developing countries could be expected to improve access while reducing costs.

Moreover, most participants agreed that, under the pressures of an eminent or unfolding pandemic, innovative solutions to some problems would be found. For example, manufacturing capacity for vaccines might be augmented by decreasing the antigen quantity per dose or using adjuvants. Research on antivirals could determine whether reduced drug dose or shortened treatment course might still have a prophylactic or therapeutic effect, and whether administration later in the course of infection might influence transmission dynamics by reducing virus shedding.

As in all public health emergencies caused by an infectious agent, international mechanisms for alert and response can go only a certain way towards mitigating the consequences of an influenza pandemic. In the final analysis, each national health system will bear the burden of protecting populations and managing the emergency. The consultation concluded that international solidarity would have the greatest role to play at the start of human-to-human transmission, when an all-out effort would have the best chance of halting or at least delaying further national and international spread. Should that effort fail, inequities in capacity and the distribution of resources mean that the consequences of a pandemic would almost certainly be most severe in the developing world. Participants stressed the importance of addressing these inequalities now—before a pandemic makes the ethical implications of failing to do so both blatantly apparent and irrevocable.

Conclusions from the Working Groups

Working Group One: Surveillance for pandemic preparedness

1. One of the most important functions of surveillance is to ensure the detection of unusual clusters of cases and of the occurrence of human-to-human transmission at the earliest possible stage, when public health interventions have the greatest chance to prevent or delay further national and international spread. Once a pandemic is fully under way, no interventions are likely to halt further international spread during the first wave of infection.

2. Influenza pandemics are, by their very nature, matters of global concern. Prompt and transparent reporting of early cases and results from the investigation of clusters related to novel influenza viruses is essential for the protection of international public health.

3. The use of limited supplies of vaccines and antivirals will depend on the national situation and should consider the protection of essential community functions and the treatment of groups at highest risk of severe disease. Data from a national risk assessment and internationally coordinated epidemiological investigations will assist in the development of policies for vaccine and antiviral utilization. Data to inform policy decisions need to be produced as quickly and cost-effectively as possible.

4. As the origins of pandemic influenza viruses have historically involved animal species, surveillance activities surrounding the emergence of a potentially pandemic virus require intersectoral collaboration with veterinarians as well as with clinicians, virologists, epidemiologists, and public health professionals.

5. Given resource constraints in many countries, strengthening existing systems to include a capacity to detect and investigate clusters of acute febrile respiratory disease may be the best value for money.

6. The objectives, methods, and attributes of an influenza surveillance system will vary according to different phases in the pre-pandemic and pandemic periods.

7. To assist in preparedness planning, the group set out recommended objectives for influenza surveillance and identified the corresponding methods and activities appropriate at different inter-pandemic, pre-pandemic, and pandemic phases. These recommendations appear as a table in the working group's report.

Working Group Two: Public health interventions

1. An influenza pandemic is a public health emergency that rapidly takes on significant political, social, and economic dimensions. A broad

range of government departments apart from public health should be engaged in pandemic preparedness planning and will need to be involved in decisions regarding interventions having potentially broad impact outside the health sector.

2.   Emergency decisions will need to be made in an atmosphere of scientific uncertainty. Health authorities may need to change recommended measures as data about the causative agent become available and the epidemiological situation evolves, and as interventions either succeed in containing transmission or lose their effectiveness. The basis for all interventions should be carefully explained to the public and professionals, as well as the fact that changes can be expected.

3.   Non-medical interventions will be the principal control measures pending the availability of adequate supplies of an effective vaccine. Many will have their greatest potential impact in pre-pandemic phases while others will have a role after a pandemic has begun. In some resource-poor settings, non-medical interventions will be the only control measures available throughout the course of a pandemic.

4.   Non-medical interventions considered by the consultation include public risk communication, isolation of cases, tracing and appropriate management of contacts, measures to "increase social distance" (such as cancellation of mass gatherings and closure of schools), limiting the spread of infection by domestic and international travel, and the targeted use of antiviral drugs. Certain measures are recommended for consideration based on a public health perspective, although it is recognized that other factors (such as availability of health resources, political, economic and social considerations) and a country's special circumstances will legitimately influence national decisions regarding prioritization and implementation of the various options.

5.   In general, providing information to domestic and international travellers (risks to avoid, symptoms to look for, when to seek care) is a better use of health resources than formal screening. Entry screening of travellers at international borders will incur considerable expense with a disproportionately small impact on international spread, although exit screening should be considered in some situations.

6.   Emerging virus strains with pandemic potential require urgent and aggressive investigation to provide a stronger scientific basis for control recommendations and the strategic use of resources. Confirmation of early episodes of human-to-human transmission is especially important. Biological specimens as well as epidemiological and clinical data must be obtained and shared with extreme urgency, under the leadership of WHO. Advance planning is needed to take advantage of this narrow window of opportunity to contain or slow transmission, which will close quickly once a pandemic begins.

7. Health authorities may need to introduce extraordinary measures under emergency conditions. This is likely to require improvement of public health capacities and modernization of public health laws at national and international levels. The necessary legal authority for implementation of these measures must be in place before a pandemic begins. Respect for public health ethics and fundamental human rights is critical.

8. To assist in preparedness planning, the group assessed more than 30 public health interventions in terms of their feasibility and likely effectiveness at each of four phases in the progression from a pre-pandemic situation to the declaration of a pandemic. Recommended measures, at national and international level, appear as tables in the working group's report.

Working Group Three: Antivirals—their use and availability

1. Antivirals are expected to be effective against human illness caused by avian influenza and human pandemic strains. Pending the availability of vaccines, they will be the only influenza-specific medical intervention for use in a pandemic.

2. Inadequate supplies are a major constraint. Supplies are presently extremely limited and manufacturing capacity could not be augmented during the course of a pandemic. At current capacity, several years would be needed to increase supplies appreciably.

3. Most countries will have no access to antivirals throughout the course of a pandemic and will need to rely on public health measures and supportive care until vaccines become available.

4. Conditions of access will be best in countries that have manufacturing capacity, regularly purchase antivirals for seasonal use, or have stockpiled drugs in advance.

5. Stockpiling of drugs in advance is currently the only way to ensure sufficient supplies at the start of a pandemic. Governments with adequate resources should consider pursuing this option as a precautionary measure.

6. Establishment of an international stockpile of antivirals should be considered for use for specific objectives in the pre-pandemic period, when opportunities for averting a pandemic or delaying its further spread are likely to be greatest. An international stockpile could not be used to meet the needs of individual countries once a pandemic is fully under way.

7. Increased use of antivirals during the inter-pandemic years, based on better understanding of the medical and economic burden of annual influenza epidemics, is one strategy for augmenting production capacity.

8. Price is the second major constraint. Current costs for widespread use of even the shortest duration of treatment place these drugs outside health budgets in the vast majority of countries.

9. Additional obstacles to wide-scale use include side effects of certain agents (especially amantadine), the risk of drug resistance, and limited safety data in key sub-populations.

10. Early treatment is a more efficient use of resources than prophylaxis, which requires a prohibitively large stockpile.

11. Where available, the neuraminidase inhibitors are the preferred drugs for treatment. If the M2 inhibitors must be used for treatment, this should be done with a full awareness of their side effects and propensity to develop resistance.

12. Scarce supplies of an emergency intervention create ethical dilemmas of priority access both within and among countries. Ethical dilemmas regarding fair access and rationing of finite supplies will be difficult to resolve but must be addressed.

Working Group Four: Better vaccines—better access

1. Vaccines are the single most important intervention for preventing influenza associated morbidity and mortality during both seasonal epidemics and pandemics.

2. No country will have adequate supplies of vaccine at the start of a pandemic. At least 4 to 6 months will be needed to produce the first doses of vaccine following isolation of a new pandemic virus. The subsequent augmentation of supplies will be progressive. Stockpiling in advance is not an option.

3. Global manufacturing capacity, which is driven by vaccine demand during the inter-pandemic years, is finite and inadequate. More than 90 percent of current production capacity is concentrated in countries in Europe and North America accounting for less than 10 percent of the world's population.

4. Equitable access will not be possible so long as global manufacturing capacity remains inadequate. Countries without manufacturing capacity will face the most acute vaccine shortages, as countries with manufacturing capacity can be expected to reserve scarce supplies for their own populations.

5. The production of a vaccine for a pandemic virus is a unique process that requires emergency procedures for its development, licensing, production, and delivery.

6. Important constraints to rapid and large-scale production of a pandemic vaccine include intellectual property rights, biosafety requirements for production facilities, and coordination and funding of clinical trials. A global effort to address these constraints is an efficient approach.

7. Country-specific issues to be addressed by national authorities in-

clude procedures for licensing and testing and liability issues surrounding mass use of a new vaccine with an unknown safety profile.

8. Short-term solutions for augmenting supplies include the development of vaccines using a lower antigen content, use of adjuvants to improve immunogenicity, and outsourcing of certain production steps. Another strategy involves advance preparation of pilot lots of vaccine against virus subtypes with pandemic potential. To pursue this strategy, manufacturers may need financial or other incentives to support investments in a product that might never be used.

9. Public funding should give priority to research on cross-subtype vaccines conferring long-lasting protection. Development of vaccines protective against several candidate pandemic viruses is a particularly effective long-term solution, as it opens possibilities for stockpiling. If the vaccine confers long-lasting immunity, preventive vaccination for a future pandemic will be possible as a major step forward.

10. Increased vaccine use during the inter-pandemic years will increase production capacity, but depends upon the burden of influenza within individual countries compared with other health priorities. Regional production strategies and purchasing schemes should be explored as a strategy for increasing vaccine use during the inter-pandemic years.

11. All countries should decide in advance on priority groups for vaccination when supplies are limited and develop strategies for expanding coverage when supplies increase.

12. Vaccine manufacturers in developing countries should participate in the influenza vaccine supply task force of the International Federation of Pharmaceutical Manufacturers.

PANDEMIC INFLUENZA PREPAREDNESS AND RESPONSE PLAN

Department of Health and Human Services[2]

August 2004 Draft Version for Public Comment
Reprinted with permission from
Department of Health and Human Services
Available online: http://www.hhs.gov/nvpo/pandemicplan/

---

[2]Comments on this plan should be forwarded to: National Vaccine Program Office, Office of the Assistant Secretary for Health, Department of Health and Human Services, Hubert H. Humphrey Building, 200 Independence Ave, SW—Room 725H, Washington, DC 20201-0004, e-mail: pandemicinfluenza@osophs.dhhs.gov.

Executive Summary

An influenza pandemic has a greater potential to cause rapid increases in death and illness than virtually any other natural health threat. Planning and preparedness before the next pandemic strikes—the interpandemic period—is critical for an effective response. This Draft Pandemic Influenza Preparedness and Response Plan describes a coordinated strategy to prepare for and respond to an influenza pandemic. It also provides guidance to state and local health departments and the health care system to enhance planning and preparedness at the levels where the primary response activities in the United States will be implemented.

Influenza causes seasonal epidemics of disease resulting in an average of 36,000 deaths each year. A pandemic—or global epidemic—occurs when there is a major change in the influenza virus so that most or all of the world's population has never been exposed previously and is thus vulnerable to the virus. Three pandemics occurred during the twentieth century, the most severe of which, in 1918, caused over 500,000 U.S. deaths and more than 20 million deaths worldwide. Recent outbreaks of human disease caused by avian influenza strains in Asia and Europe highlight the potential of new strains to be introduced into the population. Recent studies suggest that avian strains are becoming more capable of causing severe disease in humans and that these strains have become endemic in some wild birds. If these strains reassort with human influenza viruses such that they can be effectively transmitted between people, a pandemic can occur.

Characteristics of an influenza pandemic that must be considered in preparedness and response planning include: (1) simultaneous impacts in communities across the United States, limiting the ability of any jurisdiction to provide support and assistance to other areas; (2) an overwhelming burden of ill persons requiring hospitalization or outpatient medical care; (3) likely shortages and delays in the availability of vaccines and antiviral drugs; (4) disruption of national and community infrastructures including transportation, commerce, utilities and public safety; and (5) global spread of infection with outbreaks throughout the world.

The Department of Health and Human Services (HHS) continues to make progress in preparing to effectively respond to an influenza pandemic. This has been done through programs specific for influenza and those focused more generally on increasing preparedness for bioterrorism and other emerging infectious disease health threats. Substantial resources have been allocated to assure and expand influenza vaccine production capacity; increase influenza vaccination use; stockpile influenza antiviral drugs in the Strategic National Stockpile (SNS); enhance U.S. and global disease detection and surveillance infrastructures; expand influenza-related research; support public health planning and laboratory; and improve health care system readiness at the community level.

Additional preparation is also ongoing in several critical areas. Vaccination is the primary strategy to reduce the impact of a pandemic but the time required currently to develop a vaccine and the limited U.S. influenza vaccine production capacity represent barriers to optimal prevention. Enhancing existing U.S. and global influenza surveillance networks can lead to earlier detection of a pandemic virus or one with pandemic potential. Virus identification and the generation of seed viruses for vaccine production is a critical first step for influenza vaccine development.

In addition to expanding the number of global surveillance sites and extending existing sentinel surveillance sites to perform surveillance throughout the year, there has been a concomitant enhancement of laboratory capacity to identify and subtype influenza strains. Vaccine research and development can be accelerated during the inter-pandemic period by preparing and testing candidate vaccines for influenza strains that have pandemic potential, conducting research that will guide optimal vaccine formulation and schedule, and assessing techniques that can enhance manufacturing yields using current and prospective production methods. Plans are in place to increase U.S. influenza vaccine manufacturing capacity through a partnership with industry to assure that vaccine can be produced at any time throughout the year. This includes increasing the demand for annual influenza vaccine by the Centers for Medicaid and Medicare Services (CMS) and the Centers for Disease Control and Prevention (CDC), which will have the dual benefits of improving annual influenza prevention and control by strengthening the vaccine delivery system, and expanding manufacturing capacity to meet this increased demand—and also promoting the diversification of existing vaccine production with technology that is amenable to rapid expansion to meet vaccine needs in a pandemic. Enhanced planning by the public and private health care sectors to assure the ability to distribute vaccine, targeting available supply to priority groups, and monitoring vaccine effectiveness and adverse events also are critical to meet pandemic response goals.

Early in a pandemic, especially before vaccine is available or during a period of limited supply, use of other interventions may have a significant effect. For example, antiviral drugs are effective as therapy against susceptible influenza virus strains when used early in infection and can also prevent infection (prophylaxis). In 2003, the antiviral drug oseltamivir was added to the SNS. Analysis is ongoing to define optimal antiviral use strategies, potential health impacts, and cost-effectiveness of antiviral drugs in the setting of a pandemic. Results of these analyses will contribute to decisions regarding the appropriate type and quantity of antiviral drugs to maintain in the SNS. Planning by public and private health care organizations is needed to assure effective use of available drugs, whether from a national stockpile, state stockpiles or in private sector inventories.

Implementing infection control strategies to decrease the global and community spread of infection, while not changing the overall magnitude of a pandemic, may reduce the number of people infected early in the course of the outbreak, before vaccines are available for prevention. Travel advisories and precautions, screening persons arriving from affected areas, closing schools and restricting public gatherings, and quarantine of exposed persons may be important strategies for reducing transmission. The application of these interventions will be guided by the evolving epidemiologic pattern of the pandemic.

Planning by state and local health departments and by the health care system and coordination between the two is critical to assure effective implementation of response activities and delivery of quality medical care in the context of increased demand for services. Guidance included in this plan and from other organizations, as well as technical assistance and funding are available to facilitate planning. Coordination in planning and consistency in implementation with other emergency response plans, such as those for bioterrorist threats and SARS can improve efficiency and effectiveness. In addition, other public health emergency programs such as the Health Resources and Services Administration (HRSA) Hospital Preparedness Program and the CDC Public Health Preparedness and Response Cooperative Agreements are providing states with resources to strengthen their ability to respond to bioterror attacks, infectious diseases and natural disaster. For example, initiatives and funding being provided by HRSA will help states improve coordination of health care services and emergency response capacity and facilitate preparedness for influenza, smallpox, SARS, as well as other public health emergencies. In FY 04, HHS introduced a cross-cutting critical benchmark for state pandemic influenza preparedness planning as part of the Department's awards to states to improve hospitals' response to bioterrorism and other diseases. The goal of this planning activity is to assure implementation of an effective response including the delivery of quality medical care in the context of the anticipated increased demand for services in a pandemic (www.hhs.gov/asphep/FY04benchmarks.html). Completing pandemic preparedness and response plans and testing them in tabletop and field exercises are key next steps. All totaled since September 11, 2001, HHS has invested more than $3.7 billion in strengthening the Nation's public health infrastructure.

Preparedness for an influenza pandemic is coordinated in the office of the Assistant Secretary for Health, HHS. Response activities will be coordinated by the Assistant Secretary for Public Health Emergency Preparedness, on behalf of the Secretary in close coordination with the Department of Homeland Security as stipulated in HSPD#5. Other federal agencies will play critical roles as well.

Pandemic influenza response activities are outlined by pandemic phase, a classification system developed by the World Health Organization (WHO) in 1999. Phase 0, the inter-pandemic phase, is divided into 4 levels: Phase 0, Level 0 (0.0; with no recognized human infections caused by a novel influenza strain; Phase 0, Level 1 (0.1; ("new virus alert") with a case of human infection caused by a novel strain; Phase 0, Level 2 (0.2; with two or more human cases but no documented person-to-person transmission and unclear ability to cause outbreaks; and phase 0, Level 3 (0.3; ("pandemic alert") with person-to-person spread in the community and an outbreak in one country lasting for more than two weeks. Progression from a new virus alert to a pandemic alert will be accompanied by response activities that include intensified U.S. and global surveillance; investigation of the virology and epidemiology of the novel influenza strain including collaboration with international partners on containment; vaccine development and clinical testing leading toward licensure of a pandemic vaccine; coordination with health departments and activation of local plans, and implementation of the communications plan which includes education of health care providers and the public.

Pandemic Phase 1 occurs with confirmation that the novel influenza virus is causing outbreaks in one country, has spread to others, and disease patterns indicate that serious morbidity and mortality are likely to occur. In Phase 2, outbreaks and epidemics occur in multiple countries with global disease spread. Response activities during these phases depend, in part, on the extent of disease internationally and in the U.S. community-level interventions and travel restrictions may decrease disease spread. Once vaccine becomes available, immunization programs will begin. At this phase, antiviral prophylaxis and therapy targeted to maximize impact, local coordination of hospital and outpatient medical care and triage, and activation of emergency response plans to preserve community services also will occur. Federal agencies and personnel will support response activities, monitor vaccine effectiveness and adverse events following vaccination and antiviral drug use, conduct surveillance to track disease burden, and disseminate information.

Widespread pandemic disease, as with annual influenza outbreaks, is likely to be seasonal. Thus, Phase 3 signals the end of the first pandemic wave and may be followed by a second seasonal wave in Phase 4. A pandemic will end, Phase 5, as population immunity to the pandemic strain becomes high due to disease or vaccination, the virus changes, and/or another influenza strain becomes predominant. Phase 3 activities include recovery, assessment and refinement of response strategies, ongoing vaccine production and vaccination and restocking supplies such as antiviral drugs. Greater vaccine availability, experience with and improved strategies for a pandemic response, and increased immunity to the pandemic strain should decrease the impact of the second pandemic wave.

Synopsis

Purposes of the Pandemic Influenza Preparedness and Response Plan

• To define and recommend preparedness activities that should be undertaken before a pandemic that will enhance the effectiveness of a pandemic response.

• To describe federal coordination of a pandemic response and collaboration with state and local levels including definition of roles, responsibilities, and actions.

• To describe interventions that should be implemented as components of an effective influenza pandemic response.

• To guide health departments and the health care system in the development of state and local pandemic influenza preparedness and response plans.

• To provide technical information on which recommendations for preparedness and response are based.

Components of the Pandemic Influenza Preparedness and Response Plan

• The plan includes this core section and twelve annexes.

• The core plan describes coordination and decision making at the national level; provides an overview of key issues for preparedness and response; and outlines action steps to be taken at the national, state, and local levels before and during a pandemic.

• Annexes 1 and 2 provide information to health departments and private sector organizations to assist them in developing state and local pandemic influenza preparedness and response plans.

• Annexes 3–12 contain technical information about specific preparedness and response components. They include a description of influenza disease and pandemics; surveillance; vaccine development and production; vaccine use strategies; antiviral medication use strategies; strategies to decrease transmission of influenza; communications; research; observations and lessons learned from the 1976 swine influenza program; and comparisons between planning for an influenza pandemic and Severe Acute Respiratory Syndrome (SARS) outbreaks.

Pandemic Plan Development Process

• The first national pandemic influenza plan was developed in 1978, shortly after the swine influenza cases and vaccination campaign in 1976.

• In 1993, a U.S. Working Group on Influenza Pandemic Preparedness and Emergency Response was formed to draft an updated national plan. This group included representatives from the HHS agencies (CDC, FDA, NIH, HRSA and others) and coordinated by the National Vaccine Program Office (NVPO).

• Comments and input on specific issues included in the plan has been obtained from a wide range of groups in the public and private sectors; and from other pandemic influenza preparedness plans (see weblinks) or planning guides (such as the Association of State and Territorial Health Officials [ASTHO]).

• Recent developments that have influenced the influenza pandemic planning process include experience gained through planning for bioterrorist events and other health emergencies such as the international response to SARS and the national responses to anthrax cases and the implementation of a the US smallpox vaccination program.

• Ongoing enhancements in public health and communications infrastructure and development of new technologies, for example in vaccine development and production, are likely to influence portions of the plan. Therefore, it is envisioned that the Plan will be an evergreen document, which will be modified as new developments warrant. Supporting materials (such as educational materials, fact sheets, question and answer documents, etc.) will be added to the Plan or modified as needed.

Goals of a Pandemic Response

• Limit morbidity and mortality of influenza and its complications during a pandemic.
• Decrease social disruption and economic loss.

Key Pandemic Preparedness and Response Principles

• Detect novel influenza strains through clinical and virologic surveillance of human and animal influenza disease.
  ♦ Global surveillance networks identify circulating influenza strains informing recommendations for annual influenza vaccines in the U.S. and around the world.
  ♦ Surveillance also has identified novel strains that have caused outbreaks among domestic animals and persons in several countries.
  ♦ Given the speed with which infection may spread globally via international travel, effective international surveillance to identify persons who have influenza illness coupled with laboratory testing to determine the infecting strain is a critical early warning system for potential pandemics.

   ◆   Effective U.S. surveillance systems also are fundamental in the
       detection of influenza disease and the causative strains, and to
       monitor the burden of morbidity and mortality.

•   Rapidly develop, evaluate, and license vaccines against the pandemic
strain and produce them in sufficient quantity to protect the population.
   ◆   The production timeline of the annual influenza vaccine. The
       time from identification of a new influenza strain to produc-
       tion, licensure, and distribution- is approximately six to eight
       months. In contrast to the protracted timelines in the develop-
       ment, licensure and use of other vaccines, the accelerated
       timeline for the annual influenza vaccine reflects active col-
       laboration and coordination of the World Health Organiza-
       tion, HHS agencies and influenza vaccine manufacturers.
   ◆   Use of new molecular techniques to develop high-yield vaccine
       reference strains (the "seed" viruses that will be prepared by
       public sector labs and provided to vaccine manufacturers) and
       production of monovalent vaccine containing only the pan-
       demic strain could shorten the timeline to initial availability of
       a pandemic vaccine.
   ◆   Currently, three manufacturers produce influenza vaccine that
       is licensed for the U.S. market, two with all or part of the
       production process located in the United States. The amount of
       pandemic influenza vaccine produced depends on the physical
       capacity of the manufacturing facilities, the growth character-
       istics of the pandemic virus in embryonated chicken eggs used
       for vaccine production, and the amount of influenza virus pro-
       tein that is included in each dose to achieve optimal protection.
       The number of available doses also is limited by manufacturing
       capacity for filling and labeling vials or syringes. In 2004, HHS
       worked with industry to assure year-round supply of eggs for
       vaccine production. In addition HHS is supporting the expan-
       sion of production capacity and diversification of influenza
       manufacturing technology, particularly the development of in-
       fluenza vaccines made in cell culture.

•   Implement a vaccination program that rapidly administers vaccine
to priority groups and monitors vaccine effectiveness and safety.
   ◆   In contrast to the childhood immunization program, the dis-
       tribution and administration of influenza vaccine during the
       annual seasonal epidemic occurs largely through the private
       sector.

♦ In a pandemic, vaccine supply levels will change over time.

(1)   When a pandemic first strikes vaccine will likely not be ready for distribution. Because of this, antiviral drug therapy and preventive use in those not infected (prophylaxis), quality medical care, and interventions to decrease exposure and/or transmission of infection will be important approaches to decrease the disease burden and potentially the spread of the pandemic until vaccine becomes available.

(2)   Vaccine will require six to eight months to produce. Once the first lots of vaccine are available, there is likely to be much greater demand than supply. Vaccine will need to be first be targeted to priority groups that will be defined on the basis of several factors. These may include the risk of occupational infections/transmission (e.g., health care workers); the responsibilities of certain occupations in providing essential public health safety services; impact of the circulating pandemic virus on various age groups; and heightened risks for persons with specific conditions. Although the priority groups for annual influenza vaccination will provide some guidance for vaccine priority-setting for a pandemic, the risk profile for a pandemic strain and the priorities for vaccination may differ substantially and therefore will need to be guided by the epidemiologic pattern of the pandemic as it unfolds.

(3)   Later in the pandemic, vaccine supply will approximate demand, and vaccination of the full at-risk population can occur.

♦ Given the time required for vaccine development and vaccine production capacity, shortages may exist throughout the first pandemic wave.

♦ In recent years when influenza vaccine was delayed or in short supply for annual influenza epidemics, many persons were vaccinated who were not in recommended priority groups, vaccine distribution was inequitable, and a gray market developed in response to increased demand, with high prices being paid for some vaccine doses. During a pandemic, increased demand for vaccine could exacerbate these problems.

♦ Several options exist for purchase and distribution of influenza vaccine during a pandemic. The Federal government could purchase all available pandemic influenza vaccine with pro rata distribution to state and local health departments; there could be a mixed system of Federal and private sector purchase; or the current, primarily private system could be utilized. It should be noted that the Federal government already finances a substantial portion of influenza vaccine, including that purchased for eligible children under the Vaccines for Children (VFC) program and reimbursement for doses administered to persons 65 years old or older under the Medicare Modernization Act. In a mixed system with public and private vaccine supply, the proportion in each sector may change as target groups and available vaccine supply change during the course of a pandemic response. The range of options is currently being considered by HHS.

• Determine the susceptibility of the pandemic strain to existing influenza antiviral drugs and target use of available supplies; avoid inappropriate use to limit the development of antiviral resistance and ensure that this limited resource is used effectively.

♦ The objective of antiviral prophylaxis is to prevent influenza illness. Prophylaxis would need to continue throughout the period of exposure in a community. The objective of treatment is to decrease the consequences of infection. For optimal impact, treatment needs to be started as soon as possible and within 48 hours of the onset of illness.

♦ Two classes of drugs are used to prevent and treat influenza infections.

o *Adamantines* (amantadine and rimantadine) are effective as prophylaxis and have been shown to decrease the duration of illness when used for treatment of susceptible viruses. However, resistance often develops during therapy. The adamantines are available from proprietary and generic manufacturers.

o *Neuraminidase inhibitors* (NI; oseltamivir and zanamivir) also are effective for prophylaxis and treatment of susceptible strains. New data suggests that NI treatment can decrease complications such as pneumonia and bronchitis, and decrease hospitalizations. The development of antiviral resistance, to date, has been uncommon. The NIs are produced by European manufacturers. The U.S. supply of NIs is limited as demand for these drugs during annual influenza outbreaks is low. Zanamivir supply is limited in the United States.

♦ The available supply of influenza antiviral medications is limited and production cannot be rapidly expanded: there are few manufacturers and these drugs have a long production process. In 2003, oseltamivir was added to the SNS. Analysis is ongoing to define optimal antiviral use strategies, potential health impacts, and cost-effectiveness of antiviral drugs in the setting of a pandemic. Results of these analyses will contribute to decisions regarding the appropriate antiviral drugs to maintain in the SNS. Planning by public and private health care organizations is needed to assure effective use of available drugs, whether from a national stockpile, state stockpiles or the private sector.

♦ Developing guidelines and educating physicians, nurses, and other health care workers before and during the pandemic will be important to promote effective use of these agents in the private sector.

• Implement measures to decrease the spread of disease internationally and within the United States guided by the epidemiology of the pandemic.

♦ Infection control in hospitals and long-term care facilities prevents the spread of infection among high-risk populations and health care workers.

♦ Because influenza strains that cause annual outbreaks are effectively transmitted between people and can be transmitted by people who are infected but appear well, efforts to prevent their introduction into the United States or decrease transmission in the community have limited effectiveness.

♦ If a novel influenza strain that is not as efficiently spread between people causes outbreaks in other countries or the United States, measures such as screening travelers from affected areas, limiting public gatherings, closing schools, and/or quarantine of exposed persons could slow the spread of disease. Decisions regarding use of these measures will need to be based on their effectiveness and the epidemiology of the pandemic.

• Assist state and local governments and the health care system with preparedness planning in order to provide optimal medical care and maintain essential community services.

♦ An influenza pandemic will place a substantial burden on inpatient and outpatient health care services. Because of the increased risk of exposure to pandemic virus in health care settings, illness and absenteeism among health care workers in the context of increased demand will further strain the ability to provide quality care.

♦ In addition to a limited number of hospital beds and staff shortages, equipment and supplies may be in short supply. The disruptions in the health care system that result from a pandemic may also have an impact on blood donation and supply.

- ♦ Planning by local health departments and the health care system is important to address potential shortages. Strategies to increase hospital bed availability include deferring elective procedures, more stringent triage for admission, and earlier discharge with follow-up by home health care personnel. Local coordination can help direct patients to hospitals with available beds and distribute resources to sites where they are needed.
- ♦ Health care facilities may need to be established in nontraditional sites to help address temporary surge needs. Specific challenges in these settings such as infection control must be addressed.
- ♦ Not all ill persons will require hospital care but many may need other support services. These include home health care, delivery of prescription drugs, and meals. Local planning is needed to address the delivery of these and essential community functions such as police, fire, and utility service.

- • Communicate effectively with the public, health care providers, community leaders, and the media.
  - ♦ Informing health care providers and the public about influenza disease and the course of the pandemic, the ability to treat mild illness at home, the availability of vaccine, and priority groups for earlier vaccination will be important to ensure appropriate use of medical resources and avoid possible panic or overwhelming of vaccine delivery sites. Effective communication with community leaders and the media also is important to maintain public awareness, avoid social disruption, and provide information on evolving pandemic response activities.

Coordination of a Pandemic Response

An influenza pandemic will represent a national health emergency requiring coordination of response activities. As outlined in Homeland Security Presidential Directive 5 (http://www.fema.gov/pdf/reg-ii/hspd_5.pdf), the Department of Homeland Security (DHS) has primary responsibility for coordinating domestic incident management and will coordinate all non-medical support and response actions across all federal departments and agencies. HHS will coordinate the overall public health and medical emergency response efforts across all federal departments and agencies. Authorities exist under the Public Health Service Act for the HHS Secretary to declare a public health emergency and to coordinate response functions. In addition, the President can declare an emergency activating the Federal

Response Plan, in accordance with the Stafford Act, under which HHS has lead authority for Emergency Support Function #8 (ESF8)

- HHS response activities will be coordinated in the Office of the Assistant Secretary for Public Health Emergency Preparedness in collaboration with the Office of the Assistant Secretary for Public Health and Science and will be directed through the Secretary's Command Center. The Command Center will maintain communication with HHS agency emergency operations centers and with other Departments.
- HHS agencies will coordinate activities in their areas of expertise. Chartered advisory committees will provide recommendations and advice. Expert reviews and guidance also may be obtained from committees established by the National Academy of Sciences, Institute of Medicine or in other forms.

Preparedness Activities

- During the inter-pandemic period many activities can be pursued to assure that the government is as prepared as possible for a pandemic. These include:
  - ◆ Expand manufacturing capacity for influenza vaccine, develop surge capacity for a pandemic vaccine production, and assess potential approaches to optimize vaccine dose, and diversify manufacturing.
  - ◆ Strengthen global surveillance—human and veterinary—leading to earlier detection of novel influenza strains that infect humans, cause severe disease and are capable of person-to-person transmission such that they have a high probability of international spread and assess the susceptibility of the pandemic virus to antiviral drugs. Enhanced surveillance infrastructure also will strengthen detection of other respiratory pathogens—as occurred with SARS. In addition to coordination between HHS and USDA, building and strengthening a global veterinary surveillance network will complement the existing clinical laboratory network organized by WHO.
  - ◆ Strengthen U.S. surveillance by expanding to year-round surveillance for influenza disease and the viral strains that cause it. Develop hospital-based surveillance for severe respiratory illness (e.g., influenza and other infectious agents) and identify methods to rapidly expand the current sentinel physician surveillance system during an influenza pandemic or other health emergency.
  - ◆ Conduct research to better understand the pathogenic and

transmission potential of novel influenza viruses in order to improve predictions about the strains that could trigger an outbreak that could lead to a pandemic.

♦ To shorten the timeline to vaccine availability in a pandemic, develop collections (libraries) of novel influenza strains that may cause a pandemic; prepare reagents to diagnose infection and evaluate candidate vaccines; and develop high-growth reference strains that can be used for vaccine production.

♦ For selected novel influenza strains, develop investigational vaccine lots and perform clinical studies to evaluate immunogenicity, safety, and whether one or two doses are needed for protection. In the determination of the optimal vaccine dose, studies should also be performed to assess whether adding an adjuvant—a substance to enhance the immune response to vaccination—or alternative vaccine administration approaches will lead to improved protection and/or the ability to protect more people with the available amount of vaccine virus and effectively expand the vaccine supply.

♦ Conduct research to develop new influenza vaccines that are highly efficacious, are easier to administer, or that are directed against a constant portion of the influenza virus and thus sidestepping the need to develop a new vaccine every year to match the predominant viral strains that are most likely to cause disease. With this approach it may be possible to create an influenza vaccine stockpile in the future.

♦ Continue efforts to expand annual influenza vaccine use and provide appropriate incentives to strengthen the vaccine delivery system, increase vaccine use and acceptance by the public, and to manufacturers to increase overall capacity.

♦ Improve capacity to monitor influenza vaccine effectiveness and to track vaccine distribution and coverage.

♦ Periodically assess the appropriateness of the types and quantities of antiviral drugs included in the SNS.

♦ Promote planning and provide guidance to groups that will have the lead role in a pandemic response such as state and local health departments, the public and private health care organizations, and emergency response groups; and review, test and revise the plans, as needed.

♦ Evaluate the potential impacts of interventions to decrease transmission of infection such as travel advisories, school closings, limiting public gatherings, and quarantine and isolation.

♦ Develop materials for various audiences that will inform and educate them about influenza and pandemic influenza.

CONSIDERATIONS FOR PANDEMIC INFLUENZA PLANNING:
A STATE PERSPECTIVE

Kathleen F. Gensheimer, MD, MPH

Maine Department of Health and Human Services

Need for a National Plan

Planning for pandemic influenza is a critical process that needs to take place at the local, state, and national levels. Planning at any of these government levels is interdependent on the process taking place at any of these levels, and cannot be viewed as an isolated or independent process. State and local planning is especially dependent on decisions, guidance, and priorities established by the federal government. Not only do state and local government agencies lack the specific expertise in pandemic influenza that could best guide the planning process, but independent and potentially disparate decisions made at the state and local levels will ultimately result in public confusion and mistrust. For example, if one state established a response to issues posed by a pandemic that differed dramatically from a neighboring state, such as totally dissimilar priority groups for influenza vaccine, chaos would ensue. Therefore, the national plan needs to address many of the decision-making aspects unique to pandemic influenza in order to avoid such confusion, versus leaving "100 flowers to bloom" at the state and local levels. Furthermore, given the influenza clock whereby we truly do not "know what time it is," it is critical to have the national plan completed, approved, and distributed as soon as possible, allowing states to be better informed as they move forward with their own planning process.

Public Health Preparedness: A Never-Ending Process

Public health preparedness for an act of bioterrorism has only begun to raise the importance of pandemic influenza planning. It is critical to emphasize the "dual use" concept and to avoid a categorical "stovepipe" approach that has been so characteristic of federally funded projects in the past. An integrated planning approach is not only more efficient and effective, but can allow lessons learned from previous crises—whether they are of a natural, environmental, or infectious disease etiology—to be incorporated into revising what should be a dynamic and continuous process.

Lack of Human Resources

Planning requires professional human resources to adequately initiate and complete the process. Qualified and experienced public health professionals represent a limited resource. This core group is becoming increasingly burned out responding around the clock to one perceived crisis after the next, whether it is smallpox, SARS, monkeypox, or West Nile virus. Thus the planning process needs to be efficient to conserve these limited human resources. However, such limitations also argue in favor of the dual use concept and of finalizing and distributing a national plan, enabling states to have access to a rich resource afforded by a carefully written and fully documented national plan.

Public Health Powers

Public health authorities may need to revert to nontraditional means of disease control in the event of a pandemic. Although public health holds broad powers, such authority has not been tested within the United States in the twenty-first century. SARS introduced the concept of quarantine into everyday vocabulary in the spring of 2003. Although the public may not question the legality of such broad public health powers, the societal acceptance of such authority may be questioned. Even though the Toronto experience suggested that the Canadians were compliant with quarantine, and that future public health measures may be informed by the Toronto experience, serious doubt remains that the rural Mainer is going to passively sit home in a state of quarantine when an imminent plague is present. Northern New England Yankees have demonstrated a fierce independence when confronted with various crises in the past, and tout "Live Free or Die" on their license plates.

Risk Communication

Clearly a risk communication nightmare will be on our hands if discussions regarding specific controversial aspects of the pandemic plan are not communicated to the public prior to the crisis. Such discussions need to address controversial public health control measures, such as imposition of quarantine, as well as decisions regarding priority groups targeted to receive limited amounts of vaccines or antivirals. Preferably, the general public will be a player in the decision-making and planning process, thus enhancing the public's acceptance of such deliberations as a workable public health tool. By addressing the public's concerns now, in the prepandemic planning stages, the ultimate outcome will be a more realistic approach to dealing effectively with the crisis at hand and to soliciting the cooperation of the public in accepting protective courses of action. In addition, public health needs to advocate for research into the effectiveness of nonmedical interventions, such as masks and banning of mass gatherings, creating a sound scientific base that can lend further support to such recommendations.

Sustainability of Preparedness Funding

In recent years, local and state public health agencies have received substantial funding resources for bioterrorism/catastrophic planning. Such funding has been critical in addressing the languishing infrastructure that has characterized public health in this country for too long. Considerable strides have been made, including engaging most states in pandemic influenza planning. Such funding support needs to be sustained into the future to reap the benefits of recent efforts, recognizing that the payoff is enhanced capacity to monitor, respond, investigate, and ultimately, prevent the next public health crisis. Reducing funding support at this point will only repeat the age-old truism in public health, which sadly has been to eliminate the program before the disease is eliminated. In this instance, it would be a disaster to reduce funding support for planning efforts prior to the inescapable fact that there will be another pandemic. Investing in public health is an investment in securing the public's health and well-being.

Narrowing the Gap Between Public Health and the Health Care/Hospital Community

The age-old gap between funding support for public health, which targets control and prevention, and the traditional health care community, which emphasizes diagnosis and treatment, could potentially be narrowed if the two components work together to address the core need to promote influenza vaccination of health care workers. By promoting health care worker acceptance of influenza vaccine, we would also protect the patients those health care workers serve, representing a boost for this cost-effective prevention strategy. Furthermore, improving on the current 34 percent acceptance rate of influenza vaccine among health care workers will also boost demand for the vaccine during the interpandemic years, which will result in an increased number of doses of influenza vaccine produced by manufacturers annually. Enhanced demand and production will ultimately represent a key component to pandemic influenza preparedness.

Integrated, Coordinated Surveillance Systems Monitoring the Impact of the Population Affected

Influenza-like illness (ILI) is a hallmark of not only influenza, but of other viral syndromes and other potential bioterrorist events. For this reason, ILI should be at the top of the list of syndromes that receive priority for surveillance purposes. Such surveillance systems need to be expanded from seasonal to year round. As evidenced from this past influenza season, during an influenza outbreak the media and the public demand accurate, timely, and local surveillance data to respond to the questions that will be posed to public health authorities: Who is affected? When is the peak of the out-break and over what time period do we expect to see disease reports? Where is influenza activity currently most active? Not only are such questions posed during the interpandemic years, but accurate responses to such inquiries will be critical during a pandemic.

Uniform criteria for influenza surveillance need to be strengthened across the nation to encompass not only outpatient visits as ascertained through the current sentinel physician surveillance system, but to expand to a surveillance system that can encompass significant morbidity such as patients hospitalized with pneumonia or other ILI complications. Strategies to obtain prompt and timely reporting of pneumonia and influenza deaths need to be extended beyond the current 122-city death reporting system to address surveillance gaps in those states not represented in this system. Finally, as was demonstrated in 1999 with the arrival of West Nile virus in the Western Hemisphere, surveillance for emerging and remerging infectious diseases needs to involve our wildlife and veterinarian partners. The current H5N1 scenario in southeast Asia is one more example of where animal and human health surveillance data need to be exchanged on a regular and ongoing basis if we are to effectively monitor for pandemic influenza and other zoonoses.

Don't Repeat Swine Flu

The response to disease crises from yesterday should assist us in planning for the crises of tomorrow. We need to take seriously lessons learned from recent events such as SARS and smallpox vaccine initiatives and to incorporate those lessons in our pandemic planning efforts. We need to be proactive in our planning, not reactive; establish priorities for scarce resources; and invest in a wide range of activities that will enhance our collective response. We can't just "turn on the faucet" when the next crisis hits, but utilize limited resources strategically, allowing an effective collective response.

Invest in the Future

The influenza virus obeys or recognizes no rules. Ultimately, we need a collective change in mindset regarding influenza—in that it is not an entity that we just "have to tolerate" every winter, but rather a serious vaccine-preventable disease that results in 38,000 deaths annually in the United States. A recent call from a Maine nursing home nursing supervisor sums up the current mentality regarding influenza. She called to report an outbreak of influenza-like illness in a 60-bed nursing home. The supervisor realized she was obligated by law to report such outbreaks and provided the off-handed comment that 12 residents had died of ILI complications within the past several days. However, she was quick to note the deceased were all elderly and "would have died anyway." Why is it that the public and medical communities have chosen to ignore what could be a preventable disease entity?

Conclusion

In summary, the challenges are many, but the issues are real. We cannot afford to lose the momentum afforded by public interest in influenza as generated during the 2003–04 season, to squander the financial resources currently dedicated to bioterrorism/catastrophic public health planning, or to turn our backs on a significant vaccine-preventable disease. Instead, we need to collaboratively accept the challenges posed by the virus that follows no rules, and to embark on a coordinated planning effort at the national, state, and local levels.

PREPARING FOR PANDEMIC INFLUENZA: THE NEED FOR ENHANCED SURVEILLANCE

Kathleen F. Gensheimer,[3] Keiji Fukuda,[4]
Lynette Brammer,[3] Nancy Cox,[4] Peter A. Patriarca,[3]
Raymond A. Strikes[3]

Reprinted from *Vaccine*, vol. 20, Gensheimer et al.,
Preparing for pandemic influenza:
The need for enhanced surveillance, pp. 63–65,
Copyright 2002, with permission from Elsevier

Abstract

In the United States, planning for the next influenza pandemic is occurring in parallel at the national, state and local levels. Certain issues, such as conducting surveillance and purchasing pandemic vaccine, require coordination at the national level. However, most prevention and control actions will be implemented at the state and local levels, which vary widely in terms of population demographics, culture (e.g., rural versus urban) and available resources. In 1995, a survey by the Council of State and Territorial Epide-

[3]Division of Disease Control, Augusta, ME, 04333.
[4]Centers for Disease Control and Prevention, Atlanta, GA.

miologists (CSTE) found that only 29 (59%) states perceived a need to develop a specific influenza pandemic plan for their jurisdiction. Since then, the process of developing slate and local plans has gained considerable momentum. Integration of these efforts with the national planning process has been facilitated by: (1) the mutual involvement of state and federal staff in both processes; (2) the sharing of draft documents; (3) the ongoing occurrence of local and national coordinating meetings; (4) the provision of financial resources by the federal government. So far, approximately 12 states either have drafted or begun drafting a state and local influenza pandemic plan. One of the benefits of the collaborative planning process has been the development of new working relationships and partnerships among several agencies at the state, local and national levels. Such efforts will improve our collective ability to rapidly investigate and control other emerging or re-emerging public health threats in the twenty-first century, be it a bioterrorist event, pandemic influenza, or any other catastrophic health event.

Introduction

In the United States, public health services, including surveillance, are provided most directly by municipal, county and state health departments, or a combination of all three. The scope and extent of these services depend upon the resources and interests of each particular state. However, all states recognize the importance of sharing their surveillance data. This is accomplished through the close working relationship established between the states and the national centers for disease control and prevention.

Although a surveillance system for influenza has historically been in place in the United States, the system is in jeopardy due to the misperception that influenza is not an important public health problem and the continued erosion of resources supporting the public health infrastructure at the state and local levels over the years. Critical health department services, including disease and virologic surveillance activities, have been dismantled in many states. As a result, a piecemeal type of surveillance for influenza exists within the United States with 50 states each having their own surveillance system, some being extensive, and others practically non-existent.

National Influenza Pandemic Preparedness

In 1993, the National Working Group on influenza pandemic preparedness and emergency response (GrIPPE), began to develop an updated, comprehensive blueprint for an action influenza pandemic plan for the United States. The GrIPPE identified influenza surveillance as a key component of the pandemic plan. This national group includes experts from the public and private sectors, including. those listed as contributors to this paper because of their support for influenza surveillance at the state and local levels. The group has also recognized that to effectively address the threat of an influenza pandemic, measures to reduce the impact of influenza must be in place and operational at the state and local levels now, during the pre-pandemic period. Because more influenza-related illness and death occur in the aggregate during regularly recurring influenza epidemics than during the pandemics themselves, the GrIPPE has attempted to link its plan to other relevant public health initiatives such as those related to emerging infections and adult immunization.

Process

In 1994, the Council of State and Territorial Epidemiologists (CSTE) was formally asked by the GrIPPE to participate in the national pandemic influenza planning process. The CSTE is a professional association of 400 epidemiologists in the United States and territories working together to detect, prevent and control conditions of public health significance through actively promoting disease surveillance activities. As part of this effort, the CSTE conducted a survey of state epidemiologists in 1995 to assess influenza surveillance systems currently in place. All 50 states and the DC responded to the survey.

All 51 respondents reported at least one source of influenza surveillance information, and 39 (77%) identified sentinel physicians as the primary source of disease reports. However, in 1995, the sentinel physicians were not a definable entity as they are now. Forty-eight (94%) states had the capacity, either through some private or public health laboratory, to identify influenza viruses isolated in tissue culture. Of 47 laboratories that indicated to what degree they could characterize influenza viruses, 37 (79%) could subtype the viruses, while 10 (21%) could identify viruses only as influenza A or B. Another 1995 survey by the Association of State and Public Health Laboratory Directors (ASTHPHL) of its membership was more specific in defining influenza virologic resources available at each state's public health laboratory, with 10 (20%) states indicating no state public health laboratory capacity to isolate viruses and 13 (25%) state public laboratories reporting no ability to subtype influenza isolates.

In the CSTE survey, 34 (67%) states responded that their laboratory surveillance system would be adequate to detect a new pandemic virus, with 29 (57 percent) states indicating that their disease surveillance system would be adequate. Among the reasons given for the difficulty in detecting a new pandemic strain: 20 (83%) respondents indicated inadequate financial resources; 19 (79%) reported inadequate personnel; and 10 (42%) responded that influenza was not considered a high priority.

However, if targeted resources were made available, 44 (86%) respondents indicated that they would increase laboratory surveillance for influenza, and 39 (76%) indicated they would increase disease surveillance activities. The estimates provided for surveillance activities were modest ranging from US$ 2000-100,000 (mean of US$ 37,602) for laboratory surveillance and US$ 2000-100,000 (mean US$ 40,914) for disease surveillance.

In summary, the 1995 CSTE survey found that many states lacked surveillance activities dedicated to influenza, but that many states would expand virologic and disease-based surveillance systems if nominal resources were made available.

Pandemic Planning at State and Local Levels

Several efforts have been undertaken at the national level to respond to states needs and to promote enhanced preparedness for pandemic influenza. A "Pandemic Influenza Planning Guide for State and Local Health" officials was developed as a result of these efforts.

The surveillance component of the planning guide calls for enhancements in virologic and disease-based surveillance, and improvements in surveillance information systems. The planning guide makes the following recommendations during the pre-pandemic period:

- Virologic surveillance capability must be improved by ensuring that at least one laboratory in each state and/or major metropolitan area has the capacity of to isolate and subtype influenza viruses.
- Disease-based surveillance capacity must also be improved by defining the existing sentinel physician network, with the aim of establishing a population based system of approximately one sentinel physician per 250,000 population.
- Contingency plans for enhancing state and local virologic and disease-based surveillance systems in the event of a novel virus or pandemic alert must be developed.
- Electronic and telecommunications capability with neighboring jurisdictions and with CDC needs to be enhanced

One component of the existing influenza surveillance system is weekly reports to CDC's national notifiable disease system from each state epidemiologist designating the level of influenza activity during the preceding week. Levels of estimated activity were reported as widespread, regional, sporadic, or non-existent. The validity of these estimates has long been questioned, since they may primarily reflect local interest or availability of resources. The means of collecting the information does not appear to be consistent across geographic regions. As a result, it is difficult to determine the extent of influenza-related morbidity on a regional or national level on the basis of reports from state epidemiologists.

Many states lack the financial resources to conduct influenza virologic surveillance. State public health laboratories are under attack by state legislatures and many are being dismantled or privatized, which has led to the loss of core public health activities. State public health laboratories need consistent financial support to culture and characterize isolates on a timely basis. However, one concern is that specimen submissions will diminish as health maintenance organizations implement cost-cutting measures. In addition, submissions of specimens for virus isolation are expected to decrease as rapid antigen test kits are improved and become more widely available. Having fewer isolates available for characterization is a potential public health problem.

The demands of pandemic planning have prompted CDC and CSTE to begin to change influenza surveillance. Disease and laboratory-based surveillance are being reinforced as a result of these pandemic planning efforts and other databases are explored as potential sources of additional qualitative or quantitative data. Efforts are under way to:

- upgrade the sentinel physician network by enlisting and retraining more participants;
- use uniform definitions and outcomes, integrating influenza reporting with other state-based systems;
- standardize reporting procedures by adopting uniform methods of data transmission;
- develop a semi-automated data management system to provide rapid feedback.

One benefit of such efforts may be to increase the public's, medical providers' and public health practitioners' understanding of influenza as a potentially preventable disease.

Conclusion

National efforts to prepare for the next influenza pandemic require the support and interaction from partners at the state, local and federal levels. A solid influenza surveillance system in place at the state and local levels will assist in proactively planning for the regularly recurring epidemics as well as for the inevitable pandemic. We will need initiatives such as the national pandemic planning effort to direct financial resources dedicated to influenza surveillance activities. I too would like to commend Dr. Alan Kendal for his comments yesterday urging that we share our limited resources with the developing countries around the world throughout the pandemic planning process and into the pandemic itself. I would also like to congratulate the organizers of this conference for bringing together the world community to discuss surveillance, so that we may all benefit from the lessons learned in recent.

PREPAREDNESS OPPORTUNITIES AND OBSTACLES

Philip H. Hosbach

Aventis Pasteur

Pandemic Planning: Vaccine Development and Production Issues

Aventis Pasteur is one of the world's leading vaccine manufacturers. Today, the company accounts for approximately 40 percent of the world's influenza vaccine supply. It manufactures influenza vaccine in the France and the United States, and has the only U.S. manufacturing site for inactivated influenza vaccine. In the 2003–2004 season, Aventis Pasteur shipped more than 43 million influenza doses in the United States. This year we intend to ship between 48 and 50 million doses.

In addition to its vaccines to protect against influenza and a host of other diseases, including meningitis, pertussis, tetanus, and polio, the company has entered into agreements with the National Institute of Allergy and Infectious Diseases (NIAID) to conduct research and development on an inactivated SARS vaccine and an avian influenza vaccine.

Experts believe that an influenza pandemic originating from natural origins will inevitably occur (Patriarca and Cox, 1997) and will likely cause substantial illness, death, social disruption, and widespread panic. In the United States alone, the next pandemic could cause an estimated 89,000 to 207,000 deaths, 314,000 to 734,000 hospitalizations, 18 to 42 million outpatient visits, and 20 to 47 million additional illnesses (Meltzer et al., 1999).

Among the necessary preparations for any catastrophic infectious disease event, such as pandemic influenza, planning appropriately for the supply and delivery of vaccines is essential. The expertise of vaccine manufacturers, particularly those with a track record of influenza vaccine production and distribution, should be utilized at the earliest stage of planning and vaccine development. Manufacturers have access to vaccine production information regarding the timeframes needed to implement specific policy changes. They are also in direct contact with health care providers and are in a strong position to understand how policies will be accepted (or not accepted) and applied (or not)—particularly in the private sector. Also critical is their unequaled experience and resources in the efficient distribution of large amounts of vaccine to numerous distribution and provider locations in short periods of time. Manufacturers' knowledge and experience with the complex processes, logistics, and all the associated moving parts make industry an essential partner in pandemic planning and policy formulation.

Possibly the most practical and cost-effective strategy for ensuring pandemic readiness involves maximizing immunization rates during interpandemic years in order to build demand and supply. The company believes that the work of the influenza immunization enterprise to increase the availability and use of influenza vaccine over the past 10 years has provided a solid foundation for a pandemic immunization program.

Aventis Pasteur's preparations for an influenza pandemic are well underway. The company has entered into an agreement with NIAID to produce influenza vaccine based on a potential pandemic strain. Previously, the company responded to an NIAID challenge grant to develop a variety of potential pandemic strains to see if they could be produced in egg or cell cultures.

We have started production of two pilot H5N1 lots of 8,000 doses. Also, the company plans to continue to expand its operations and will complete a new formulation and filling plant, which is expected to be online in 2006 or 2007.

In addition, Aventis Pasteur entered into a strategic agreement with Crucell N.V. that gives it an exclusive license to research, develop, manufacture, and market cell-based influenza vaccines based on Crucell's proprietary PER.C6™ cell line technology.

While the industry continues to explore newer methods for producing influenza vaccines, manufacturers must recognize that egg-based production is the only proven and rigorously tested large-scale production method and it will remain so for the near- to mid-term future. Companies must work off this assumption and ensure flock protection and egg reserves. Also, manufacturers should consider the use of alternative methods to enhance the supply and performance of the vaccine, including the consideration of appropriate adjuvants and delivery devices.

As the government and industry work together toward pandemic preparedness, manufacturers have requested that the government issue Requests for Proposals (RFP) that realistically reflect pandemic requirements and that there is clear and effective coordination throughout the U.S. government of various RFPs. Furthermore, the U.S. government must supply the proper liability protection for full industry participation in pandemic influenza planning and preparedness. This is a key lesson we learned from past experiences and it is crucial to avoiding potentially life-threatening delays.

Manufacturing of Influenza Vaccine

The production of influenza vaccine is based on a multitiered process with extensive quality assurance and quality control. A number of internal and external factors affect production, including guidance and requirements from government agencies, how quickly vaccine strains grow, manufacturing capacity, forecasts, and the timing of orders. Therefore, it is essential to have realistic vaccine production timelines.

To prepare for a pandemic, production capacity and capabilities will need to be significantly increased. This is feasible, but supply and demand factors must be considered. When it comes to influenza vaccine, these two elements are inextricably connected.

On the "supply" side are three principal elements. First is the length of time required to produce vaccine. Then there is the need for a system to get those doses to immunization providers as quickly as we can make the vaccine. This is something we do regularly with influenza as we are producing an essentially new vaccine every year. Third, we need manufacturing capacity—including physical facilities, validated equipment and processes, and trained personnel—dedicated to producing this one vaccine in a short period of time.

Three main variables govern the amount of traditional trivalent influenza vaccine that Aventis Pasteur can produce in any season. The first is the timing of the selection of the three strains of the virus. Manufacturers receive word of the strains to be used as soon as the World Health Organization has the information from its worldwide monitoring operation. If the announcement of the third strain runs late—that is, past mid-March—and that third strain proves difficult to grow, it makes for a more challenging production schedule. If *any* of the strains produces lower yields than expected, there can be delays in getting vaccine to market. During the time period of January through May, industry is consumed with the virus-growing process. We do not actually begin to fill even the first vials with finished vaccine until early summer. Subsequently, each and every lot needs to be tested separately by the FDA before release to health care providers.

When looking at the manufacturing process, the single most important element is capacity. The doses of trivalent vaccine that the company currently produces translate to up to 150 million doses of monovalent vaccine for pandemic use. For an influenza pandemic, it is estimated that as many as 600 million pandemic doses need to be produced, which means that capacity to routinely produce between 150 and 200 million trivalent doses is required annually. Clearly, we must work to increase immunization rates (demand) and bring the nation closer to the immunization goal of 185 million Americans, who the CDC considers at "high risk" for complications associated with influenza. Manufacturers will invest (supply) to meet rising demand, expanding capacity to meet our nation's pandemic needs.

In addition to the need for significantly expanded capacity, the other challenges facing the industry as it prepares for pandemic influenza include the limited advance notice between production waves and the requirement for additional materials (e.g., syringes, vials) to expand industry surge capacity. At the same time, the FDA's Center for Biologics Evaluation and Research (CBER) will need to significantly increase its own capacity in order to test more quickly and expedite the release process. In recognition of the importance of CBER and the challenges it faces in the twenty-first century, Aventis Pasteur continues to call for additional agency funding.

Today, distribution of influenza vaccine rests primarily in the private sector, which has expertise in order processing, storage, distribution, and shipment. In the United States, 85 percent of influenza vaccine is sold, distributed, and administered in the private market. This approach is working well and should serve as the basis in preparing for a pandemic vaccine. Although the system is not perfect, we should build on the existing private–public system rather than trying to replace the system during a pandemic event.

Other planning assumptions include the need for enhanced worldwide surveillance and detection; the ability to relay information quickly to private industry; rapid strain identification and seed preparation; maximization of internal and external industry communications; and government policies regarding exports of vaccine during a pandemic. There must also be flexibility in sending influenza vaccine overseas to stem small, virulent outbreaks. We recognize that the threat from influenza does not have borders and that preventing the spread of the disease may greatly reduce mortality rates in all countries. If more influenza vaccine were manufactured in the United States, we would be in a better position to consider global needs.

Increasing Interpandemic Influenza Vaccine Demand

Increasing interpandemic influenza vaccine demand is essential for improving public health today, enabling predictable and steady vaccine supply, and preparing for pandemic influenza.

In 2003, the late season spike in influenza vaccine demand dramatically reinforced the need to develop a national consensus in the United States about how to predictably increase the annual demand for influenza vaccine immunization. Manufacturers will respond to increased demand by producing as much product as they can sell and will continue to invest to expand current capabilities.

Increased demand will drive increases in the annual vaccine supply. Government health planners have recognized the importance of influenza immunization. As part of the Healthy People 2010 program, they have set ambitious but imminently achievable goals for influenza. The year 2010 is not many influenza seasons away. The focus on influenza immunization demand is essential to achieve Healthy People 2010 goals and to effectively plan for a pandemic event. Although the Healthy People 2010 goal is to immunize 185 million Americans, currently only 75 to 85 million Americans are immunized annually and only 38 percent of health care workers receive influenza vaccination. Increased immunization rates in this group are especially critical.

As a charter member of the National Influenza Summit's private–public partnership and the global leader in influenza vaccine development and production, Aventis Pasteur has recommended a number of steps, described below, to increase influenza immunization. These principles were proposed by the company to the National Vaccine Advisory Committee in Washington, D.C., in February 2004, and reiterated at the Influenza Summit in Atlanta, Ga., in April 2004.

Best practices. Encourage practitioners, managed care organizations, insurers, health care institutions, and community-based immunizers to develop, share, and implement best practices to run seasonal surge adult/ pediatric immunization campaigns. This begins with timely prebooking and may include flexible scheduling of patients, periodic reminders from physicians, and implementation of standing orders to offer immunization to meet patient care quality objectives.

Annual national awareness and educational campaigns. Support public health authorities, the National Influenza Summit, and advocacy organizations and coalitions in managing sustained, annual public awareness/education programs. These programs should convey consistent information about high-risk groups (e.g., health care workers, first responders, and police), articulate key influenza recommendations to the public, and communicate information regarding the timing and length of the influenza immunization season. Programs should also be tailored to "at risk" target groups, including minorities.

Support the U.S. Department of Health and Human Services' agencies in meeting their annual influenza immunization goals as a unified Department, including:

• National Vaccine Program Office: Gain consensus among public and private partners about national immunization goals, and convene annual reviews of progress toward objectives for supply and demand goals.
• Centers for Disease Control and Prevention: Support annual widespread practitioner and public education and awareness campaigns and advocacy coalitions. Add routine publication of adult/pediatric influenza

immunization rates by risk group and states to help target and measure specific improvements.

• Centers for Medicare & Medicaid Services: Annually inform all Medicare and Medicaid providers and other parties about influenza recommendations, coverage and reimbursement, and the importance of early prebooking to implement successful seasonal campaigns. Publish adequate and timely reimbursement notices for providers and make available Medicare immunization rate information to public health to measure further improvement.

• Food and Drug Administration: Support FDA efforts to provide up-to-date technical expertise and oversight in order to ensure vaccine safety, the timely availability of vaccine, and increased public confidence in vaccines.

Extend immunization season. Consider expanding the immunization season into December and possibly beyond.

Emphasize exemplary health care worker immunization efforts. Identify and resolve barriers to health care worker immunization by emphasizing the responsibilities to protect oneself, one's patients, and one's family. Provide workers with information designed to educate patients year round concerning influenza and immunization.

Mobilize insurers/managed care providers. Secure agreement among managed care/insurance companies about the importance of covering influenza immunization and administration; ensure that managed care system, health care professionals, relevant institutions, and all immunizers understand the need to preorder vaccine; remind at-risk patients why immunization is so important; and implement standing orders.

Establish strategic influenza vaccine reserves. Immediately establish shared risk reserves for influenza vaccine to ensure protection for unforeseen outbreaks and/or in the event of a pandemic. Influenza vaccine cannot be stockpiled from year to year, but government negotiations with the private sector of an annual strategic vaccine shared-risk reserve could offer the public and health care providers additional confidence that supply will meet ever-increasing demand.

Looking beyond influenza vaccines, stockpiles for all other routine pediatric vaccines must be in place before a pandemic due to the need for manufacturers to focus their efforts on the manufacture, formulation, and filling of 300 to 600 million monovalent doses for a pandemic. During a pandemic, which can last more than 2 years, Aventis Pasteur would need the flexibility to shift resources and facilities to the production and filling of influenza vaccine, which could postpone or delay the filling and release of the other routinely used vaccines.

A 6-month stockpile should be sufficient to enable manufacturers to make their way through the rescheduling process. In support of stockpiles, government funding has been allocated and the CDC has developed a strategic plan. Still, certain accounting rules of the Securities and Exchange Commission are severely hindering the establishment of stockpiles.

Looking ahead to the 2004–2005 influenza season and beyond, it is imperative for planning to begin as early as possible. Planning early assists all stakeholders and allows manufacturers to more precisely forecast demand. Manufacturers recommend that providers prebook vaccines every year because prebookings drive annual supply and ensure a more stable process. Prebookings for the 2004–2005 influenza season began in December 2003. The estimated capacity in the United States for this upcoming season is 90 to 100 million doses of trivalent vaccine. Production will, as always, depend on strain yields.

In summary, there are a number of key lessons and principles that the industry, government, and medical community must consider for pandemic influenza planning:

- Demand drives supply; industry can optimize and expand influenza production if demand is stable and predictable
  - ♦ Sustainable initiatives are needed to drive demand
- Manufacturers' expertise should be utilized at the earliest stage of the policy process
  - ♦ Companies with a track record of influenza vaccine production should be involved in policy development; pandemic plans conceived without manufacturer involvement run the risk of not being executable
- RFP deliverables should realistically reflect pandemic requirements and include appropriate liability protection
- The current private–public distribution system provides a strong foundation on which to build
- Identify high-risk groups and establish priorities for phased immunization
- Extend the immunization season
- Send influenza vaccine overseas to stem small, virulent outbreaks
- Develop shared-risk reserves for unanticipated demand/outbreaks on an annual basis and establish stockpiles of routinely used vaccines

PANDEMIC INFLUENZA VACCINES:
OBSTACLES AND OPPORTUNITIES

David Fedson

Sergy Haut, France

This section highlights opportunities and obstacles presented by two key issues in pandemic preparedness: the development and registration of a "pandemic-like" vaccine, and the use of reverse genetics to prepare seed strains for vaccine development. These issues are introduced with an overview of global vaccine production and distribution and followed by an exploration of the idea that prophylaxis and/or treatment with certain commonly available therapeutic agents such as statins could possibly have beneficial effects on the clinical course of human influenza. If these effects could be confirmed, they could potentially mitigate the morbidity and mortality of pandemic influenza when there are limited supplies of vaccines and antiviral drugs.

Global Distribution of Influenza Vaccine, 2000–2003

According to a recent report by the Influenza Vaccine Supply (IVS) Task Force, 230 million doses of influenza vaccine were distributed worldwide in 2000, of which 162 million (70 percent) were distributed in Canada, the United States, Western Europe, Australasia, and Japan (Table 3-1). In 2003, vaccine distribution increased to 292 million doses, of which 207 million (71 percent) were distributed in the same countries. During this 4-year period, vaccine distribution increased 20 percent in Canada and the United States, 18 percent in Western Europe, 25 percent in Australasia, and 134 percent in Japan. For the rest of the world, vaccine distribution increased from 69 million doses to 85 million doses, a 23 percent increase. For these other countries, the use of influenza vaccine was largely limited to four countries in South America (Argentina, Brazil, Chile, and Uruguay), several countries in Central Europe (especially Hungary and Poland), Russia, and South Korea. When individual countries were compared according to per capita vaccine distribution levels in 2003, the leading countries (doses distributed/1,000 total population) were Canada (344), South Korea (311), the United States (286), and Japan (230) (Macroepidemiology of Influenza Vaccination Study Group, unpublished observations).

Nearly all of the world's influenza vaccine is produced in nine countries: Australia, Canada, France, Germany, Italy, Japan, Netherlands, United Kingdom, and United States. In 2003, these countries had only 12 percent of the world's population, yet they produced 95 percent of the world's influenza vaccine. Almost none of the doses produced in Canada, Japan,

TABLE 3-1 Global Distribution of Influenza Vaccine, 2000–2003

WHO Region	Total Doses Distributed (000s)			
	2000	2001	2002	2003
Europe	93,004	99,094	103,824	102,891
Western Europe	65,130	67,864	72,812	76,523
Central and Eastern Europe	27,874	31,230	31,012	26,368
Americas	104,593	114,389	122,348	123,578
Canada	11,900	10,600	9,700	11,100
United States	68,000	78,345	82,705	84,913*
Mexico, Central and South America	24,693	25,444	29,943	27,565
Western Pacific	29,916	39,424	41,795	61,189
Australia	3,415	3,632	4,087	4,357
Japan	12,491	17,440	20,802	29,253
New Zealand	646	627	668	715
Other countries	13,364	17,725	16,238	26,864
Southeast Asia	82	95	134	253
Eastern Mediterranean	1,043	1,201	1,163	1,540
Africa	2,291	2,530	1,298	1,230
GLOBAL TOTAL	230,929	256,733	270,562	291,979*

*The data for the United States do not include doses of cold-adapted, live-attenuated trivalent influenza vaccine distributed by MedImmune. In 2003, MedImmune produced ~4–5 million doses of CAIV-T and distributed ~830,000 doses, but only ~250,000 doses were actually sold.

and the United States were exported to other countries. Companies located in five Western European countries produced 190 million doses, 65 percent of the world's supply. Excluding the 13.8 million doses produced in Hungary, Romania, and Russia (all of which were distributed domestically), these companies produced 99.3 percent of the 79 million doses of influenza vaccine used in countries outside Western Europe, Canada, the United States, Australasia, and Japan.

These results demonstrate that in the event of a new pandemic, most countries in the world will be critically dependent on vaccines produced in five Western European countries. Although the United States is unlikely to contribute any supplies of influenza vaccine to other countries, it can and should contribute in other ways to help prepare the global community for the next pandemic.

Pandemic Vaccine Development and Registration

Recent outbreaks of avian influenza in Asia and other parts of the world suggest it is unwise to assume that the next pandemic will delay its appearance for another 5 years. Thus the strategy for pandemic vaccine development should initially focus on what needs to be done to ensure that the largest possible supply of pandemic vaccine can be made available as quickly as possible in order to respond to the needs of populations in all countries. It should be based on the existing global capacity to produce trivalent influenza vaccines in egg-based production systems. Its goal should be to determine the lowest amount of HA antigen that can be included in an adjuvanted vaccine that will be acceptably immunogenic when given in a two-dose schedule to a population.

The low-dose adjuvanted pandemic vaccine development strategy is one that will most likely be pursued by European vaccine companies in collaboration with the European Medicines Evaluation Agency (EMEA). It differs from the strategy that will be undertaken by NIAID in the United States. Both strategies are described in detail below.

Pandemic Vaccine Development and Registration in Europe

European vaccine companies have a unique responsibility to the 25 countries that are now part of the European Union (EU) and to the many non-EU countries that will be entirely dependent on European companies for supplies of pandemic vaccine. For this reason, in September 2002, representatives of the member companies of the IVS Task Force met with staff of WHO and its Collaborating Centers and with a representative of the EMEA. The purpose of the meeting was to review steps needed to develop and register pandemic vaccines in Europe.

In the EU, the annual updating of marketing authorizations for interpandemic influenza vaccines is handled by a "fast track" variation of a decentralized registration procedure (Official Journal of the European Community, 1995; Wood and Lewandowski, 2003). Unlike registration of influenza vaccines in the United States, EU registration requires demonstration of safety and satisfactory serum anti-HA antibody responses for each company's vaccine (CPMP, 1997; Wood and Lewandowski, 2003). The process can take as long as 73 days. Registration of a pandemic vaccine will be handled differently for several reasons. The vaccine will likely not be a variation of a current vaccine, but an entirely new vaccine. The EU centralized procedure will be used, and this will be especially important if the vaccine is produced using a reverse genetics-engineered seed strain and is thus considered a biotechnology product. The pressure of time will be severe. Fortunately, in the event of a pandemic threat, an EU regulation allows national authorities to "exceptionally and temporarily consider the variation to be accepted after a complete application has been lodged and *before* the end of the procedure . . ." (Official Journal of the European Community, 2003). This regulation provides the legal basis for the European approach to developing and registering pandemic vaccines.

In September 2002, the EMEA began a process of discussion and collaboration with the Regulatory Working Group of the European Vaccine Manufacturers (EVM) to discuss basic principles for the development and the regulatory strategy for pandemic vaccines. (All European vaccine manufacturers are members of the EVM.) In April 2004, the results of this process were published by the EMEA in the form of two "Notes for Guidance" documents (CPMP, 2004a; CPMP, 2004b), which set forth requirements for demonstrating the quality, safety, and immunogenicity of a "mock-up" (i.e., candidate) pandemic vaccine that will be developed during the interpandemic period.

The core pandemic dossier will document the production process for the "mock-up" vaccine and its final formulation (CPMP, 2004a). With these data, a company can submit its dossier and receive a marketing authorization via the EMEA centralized procedure. When a pandemic threat is declared and a true pandemic vaccine is produced, only quality data related to the pandemic variation need to be submitted. Each pandemic vaccine variation will receive a fast-track assessment (within 3 days) and approval by the Committee for Proprietary Medicinal Products (CPMP) and a final European Community decision within another 24 hours (Official Journal of the European Community, 2003; CPMP, 2004b). Approval will be given with the understanding that companies will gather safety, immunogenicity, and effectiveness data on the pandemic vaccine during clinical use (CPMP, 2004b). Precise details on how this will be done have yet to be worked out.

The EMEA scientific guidance for a "mock-up" vaccine recognizes that clinical data on interpandemic vaccines cannot be extrapolated to a pandemic situation because the pandemic vaccine will be different (CPMP, 2004a). It will be monovalent, have a different antigen content, probably be adjuvanted, contain preservatives, and probably require a different vaccination schedule, especially for immunologically naive subjects. Consequently, companies have been asked to develop prototype pandemic vaccines during the interpandemic period. They must include viral antigens to which humans have had no previous exposure (e.g., H5N1). Companies will be required to conduct clinical trials for safety and to establish the dosage and schedule for their "mock-up" vaccines in order to obtain marketing authorization for their pandemic vaccines.

The EMEA has not published its own clinical development plan for a "mock-up" pandemic vaccine. However, the EVM Clinical Working Group, which represents all major European vaccine companies, has proposed a step-wise clinical development plan of its own. The plan calls for an initial set of safety and immunogenicity studies in healthy adults 18 to 40 years of age. Each study group will include at least 30 immunologically naive subjects. Three hemagglutinin antigen (HA) dosages will probably be tested, each with and without an adjuvant. Two doses will be given 3 weeks apart. The goal of the initial studies will be to determine the formulation that best balances acceptable immunogenicity with an antigen-sparing dosage level that will maximize pandemic vaccine supply. Following initial studies, larger (>300 subjects) safety and immunogenicity studies will be conduced in immunologically naive, healthy younger (18 to 59 years of age) and older (>60) adults. Two doses of the chosen formulation will be given, vaccine safety will be evaluated over 6 months, and a booster dose will be given at 6 (and perhaps also 12) months. Primary immunogenicity will be assessed on day 42, and secondary immunogenicity on day 21 and at 6 ± 12 months. According to the EMEA, immunogenicity will be judged as satisfactory only if all three CPMP criteria (seroconversion, seroprotection, and geometric mean titers (GMT)) are met (Official Journal of the European Community, 1995). These criteria are stricter than those for interpandemic vaccines and may be modified later.

The EMEA procedural guidance sets up several task force groups (CPMP, 2004b). The Joint EMEA-Industry Task Force will meet yearly and have a general advisory role. During the interpandemic period, it will monitor the availability of reference strains and reagents, the status of core dossier authorizations, and manufacturing issues. The EMEA Task Force will provide advice to regulatory authorities, work with companies before they submit their pandemic variation applications, and review safety and effectiveness data obtained during the pandemic. Because of the global implications of European vaccine production, WHO will probably be represented on the EMEA Task Force. The EMEA Evaluation Project Team will evaluate the pandemic variation applications for each product.

Over a period of 18 months, EMEA staff vaccine experts and European vaccine companies put together an integrated "roadmap" that outlines most of the steps for developing and registering a "mock-up" pandemic vaccine. Once a company obtains a marketing authorization for its core dossier, regulatory approval for a true pandemic vaccine can be quickly obtained. Australian regulatory authorities will likely follow the European approach, but it is unclear what will be done in Canada, Japan, Russia, and other vaccine-producing countries.

In spite of having a strategy for developing "mock-up" pandemic vaccines, it is uncertain whether European companies will actually follow through on the strategy. The companies may be reluctant to pay for developing vaccines that will never be marketed (unless the "mock-up" vaccine and pandemic viruses are closely matched). Expectations that the sunk costs of "mock-up" vaccine development will be quickly recovered when a pandemic arrives will be tempered by uncertainty over vaccine prices, liability issues, purchasing guarantees, and political takeover of pandemic vaccination programs. Although all companies are interested in developing "mock-up" vaccines, they know that the early costs will be modest compared with the much larger costs of full-scale clinical development later on. EC officials and vaccine companies have yet to discuss EC funding for the more expensive stages of clinical development. If the emergence of the next pandemic virus is delayed for several years, Europeans may have enough time to solve these difficult problems. However, if the pandemic virus emerges within the next year or two, Europeans, like their colleagues in the United States and elsewhere, will need to make their decision on how to formulate a pandemic vaccine based on existing clinical data. In all likelihood, they will choose a low-dose, alum-adjuvanted vaccine because it appears to be the only vaccine formulation that will meet the population needs of Europeans and those of other countries that will depend on Europe for supplies of pandemic vaccines (Fedson, 2003a,b; Wood, 2001; Hehme et al., 2002; Hehme et al., 2004).

Pandemic Vaccine Clinical Trials in the United States

In May 2004, the U.S. government awarded contracts to Aventis Pasteur and Chiron[5] to produce pilot lots of monovalent H5N1 "pandemic-like" vaccines. These vaccines will be formulated at two dosage strengths:

---

[5]Editor's note: This vaccine is being manufactured at a different facility from the one making the interpandemic, seasonal influenza vaccine that was recently cited for "good manufacturing practice violations" by the FDA (Chiron Corporation, 2004; NIAID, 2004).

15 µg and 45 µg of HA antigen (standard and high dose, respectively). These two dosages comply with FDA requirements for currently licensed influenza vaccines. The vaccines will be tested in the National Institutes of Health Vaccine Trial and Evaluation Units.

If a pandemic virus emerges within the next year or two, the national governments of vaccine-producing countries will probably not allow their companies to export pandemic vaccine to other countries until their own domestic needs have been met (Fedson, 2003a,b). Any doses left over will likely be exported to countries that have no vaccine-producing capacity. As a result, the United States will be forced to depend on its sole domestic producer for supplies of pandemic vaccine. Moreover, in the event of a pandemic, it will probably be necessary to administer two doses of vaccine to a largely if not entirely immunologically naive population (Fedson, 2003a,b; Wood, 2001). How will the United States be able to adequately meet its needs for pandemic vaccine?

In 2004, domestic vaccine production in the United States will be approximately 50 million doses of trivalent vaccine. Assuming a comparable 6-month production cycle, this will be equivalent to 150 million doses of standard-dose (15 µg HA) monovalent pandemic vaccine and 50 million doses of high-dose (45 µg HA) vaccine. This would be enough to vaccinate (with two doses) 75 million people with a standard-dose pandemic vaccine and only 25 million people with a high-dose vaccine, fewer people than are now being vaccinated each year with the trivalent vaccine. For the United States to be able to offer two doses of standard-dose or high-dose pandemic vaccine to each person (assume 300 million people), domestic production of trivalent vaccine would have to increase to either 200 million or 600 million doses per year. Even with greatly expanded domestic vaccine production, it is clear that the number of doses of pandemic vaccine formulated according to the NIH strategy will fall far short of meeting the needs of the American people. Furthermore, the United States will have no pandemic vaccine to offer people in other countries.

European investigators have shown that two doses of a pandemic vaccine (perhaps whole virus), formulated with a low amount of HA antigen per dose (perhaps as low as 1.875 µg HA) and combined with an alum adjuvant, could realistically offer significant clinical protection to large populations of immunologically naive individuals (Wood, 2001; Hehme et al., 2002; Hehme et al., 2004). For example, if all of the world's vaccine companies were instructed to produce a 1.875 µg HA alum-adjuvanted monovalent subunit pandemic vaccine, they could hypothetically produce (over 6 months) 7.2 billion doses of pandemic vaccine (300 million × 3 × 8). This would be enough to vaccinate 3.6 billion people, more than half the world's population. This amount of vaccine would probably exceed the combined capacities of the world's health care systems to deliver it. For the

United States, with its vaccine production capacity limited to 50 million doses of trivalent vaccine, the low-dose strategy would allow the United States to produce enough vaccine to vaccinate 600 million people: 300 million Americans and 300 million people in other countries. Even more important, in the early weeks of the pandemic, this strategy would increase by 8-fold the number of doses available for use each week compared with the standard-dose strategy and by 24-fold the number of doses compared with the high-dose strategy.

The low-dose, adjuvanted pandemic vaccine strategy is central to the thinking of major influenza vaccine companies located outside the United States. The EMEA Vaccine Expert Group considers it the most promising approach for producing adequate supplies of pandemic vaccines. Experts who work with WHO regard it as essential. It figures prominently among the recommendations on priorities for pandemic preparedness recently published by WHO. How low the HA content of an "antigen-sparing" adjuvanted pandemic vaccine can be set is uncertain. This can best be determined in large multinational, publicly funded clinical trials of one or more pandemic-like vaccines produced by all companies that intend to produce true pandemic vaccines (Fedson, 2003a,b). In the United States, however, the strategy for developing an H5N1 vaccine appears to be based on determining a dosage that is optimally immunogenic and safe for an individual rather than one that is acceptably immunogenic for a population. The U.S. strategy also seems to assume that the pandemic will not emerge for 5 or more years.

During this 5-year period, the U.S. government hopes to accelerate the introduction of cell culture vaccine production and expand the supply of embryonated eggs. These efforts could increase domestic capacity to produce trivalent and pandemic vaccines. Given enough time, U.S. investigators might also settle on a low-dose, adjuvanted formulation for a pandemic vaccine. However, if the pandemic arrives within the next few years, current efforts will not lead to a greatly expanded capacity for vaccine production and will not provide information on the pandemic vaccine formulation and vaccination schedule that will meet the needs of public health.

Conclusion

The United States can learn an important lesson from the rapid progress Europeans have made in conceptualizing a process for pandemic vaccine development and registration. Likewise, Europeans can learn from Americans that public funding will play an essential role in accelerating the clinical development process. Given the common needs of nations on both sides of the Atlantic, Americans and Europeans should develop a common process for publicly funding clinical trials of low-dose, adjuvanted candidate ("mock-up") pandemic vaccines.

Reverse Genetics, Intellectual Property, and Influenza Vaccination

Each year, the production of influenza vaccines begins when reference strains are provided to vaccine companies by WHO. Since the early 1970s, the reference strains have been prepared using the technique of genetic reassortment. With this technique, embryonated eggs are co-infected with an influenza virus considered most likely to cause epidemic disease and a high-growth strain of influenza A/PR8 virus. Following subsequent cloning, a progeny genetic reassortant virus is isolated that has two genes coding for the surface (HA and neuraminidase [NA]) antigens of the epidemic virus and six PR8 genes that are associated with high growth.

Genetic reassortants have been essential to the success of influenza vaccine production for more than 30 years, but they have disadvantages. The time needed to isolate a genetic reassortant suitable for commercial vaccine production can take many weeks. The reassortants do not always grow efficiently in egg-based production systems. Importantly, the avian H5N1 viruses associated with human disease are lethal for embryonated eggs. Largely for this reason, no commercially viable H5N1 seed strain for human vaccine production has yet been prepared using genetic reassortment.

In the past few years, reference strains suitable for producing human H5N1 influenza vaccines have been prepared in several laboratories using the techniques of reverse genetics (RG) (Fodor et al., 1999; Subbarao et al., 2003; Webby et al., 2004). With these techniques, the polybasic amino acids associated with H5N1 virulence are removed from the HA cleavage site. Plasmids containing the genes for the avian virus HA and NA antigens are then cloned and transfected into Vero cells along with plasmids containing the six PR8 genes. The progeny virus is rescued from cell culture, purified, propagated in embryonated eggs, and tested for stability and pathogenicity. The methods for preparing RG-engineered viruses are straightforward, the results are predictable, and the process can take as little as 15 to 20 days. Moreover, it can be used with avian viruses that cannot be propagated in eggs.

The techniques of reverse genetics differ from genetic reassortment in one important respect; they are associated with patents. The intellectual property (IP) rights for RG are held by at least two academic institutions (Mt. Sinai Medical Center and the University of Wisconsin) and one pharmaceutical company (MedImmune, Inc.). At least one patent holder has agreed to allow RG to be used to prepare reference strains for research purposes. However, all patent holders expect to be paid royalties if RG-engineered seed strains are used for commercial vaccine production.

If we were now facing a true pandemic threat from an H5N1 virus, most vaccine companies would be uncertain about the precise ownership of the IP rights for the RG-engineered seed strains they would be called on to use. Some companies have already undertaken their own analyses of RG patent rights, but they should not be expected to disclose their findings. DHHS has conducted a patent search of its own and formulated its policy options, but they are not publicly known. Even if they were, the patent rights would apply only to the United States; patent rights in Europe and Japan are independent of those in the United States. In the absence of knowing who owns the intellectual property for RG, it would be difficult for a vaccine company to enter into negotiations on royalty payments for pandemic vaccine production. If negotiations with only one patent holder were attempted, litigation by the others could follow. Given these uncertainties, if presented with a pandemic threat, the United States and other national governments would probably exercise government use or similar rights for RG. Royalty payments would not be negotiated between patent holders and patent users; they would be determined by courts or governments.

A strong argument can be made for resolving RG-IP ownership *before* the next pandemic threat appears. This would allow companies to determine whether using RG-engineered seed strains would offer advantages over genetic reassortants for interpandemic as well as pandemic vaccine production. Companies would have time to respond to regulatory requirements to upgrade their production facilities. Because European countries regard RG-engineered viruses as genetically modified organisms (GMOs), there would be time for European-based companies to resolve uncertainties over GMO issues with regulators and with the public. Royalty payments could be negotiated with the RG patent holders, avoiding litigation. However, several obstacles still stand in the way. In interpandemic years, companies have enough time to produce their vaccines using genetic reassortants, which are provided free of charge. They have no compelling commercial reasons to use RG-engineered seed strains. If they did, their vaccines could not command higher prices and consequently paying royalties would erode their profit margins. The RG patent holders could facilitate negotiations with the companies by forming a patent pool, but thus far they have shown no interest in doing so.

One way to accelerate the introduction of RG-engineered seed strains during the interpandemic period would be to conduct multinational, publicly funded clinical trials of candidate pandemic-like vaccines (Fedson, 2003a,b). This "dress rehearsal" strategy would challenge companies and their production facilities, national regulatory agencies, and European public opinion on GMO issues. All would gain the practical experience needed to prepare them for pandemic vaccine production. However, most vaccine companies won't fund expensive clinical trials of vaccines that won't be marketed. The U.S. clinical development program for H5N1 vaccine responds only to U.S., not global, needs, and only two companies will participate. Although the EMEA has developed a thoughtful process that will lead to licensure of a true pandemic vaccine, it has yet to identify public funding for the clinical trials that will make it a reality. More disturbing are recent decisions by three of the four major European vaccine companies not to produce pilot lots of a European H5N1 "mock-up" vaccine. Although these vaccines would be used only for research purposes, the companies are unwilling to participate largely because of restrictions and uncertainties related to intellectual property rights for reverse genetics.

Experts in intellectual property describe the RG-IP issue as a classic example of market failure. Unless the public sector provides a framework for negotiations for RG-IP during interpandemic years, companies will not be prepared to produce pandemic vaccines using RG-engineered seed strains. Moreover, because IP issues are governed by national patent laws, the negotiating framework must be international. The need for an international solution has been acknowledged by WHO (WHO, 2004), but WHO has authority and capability to address the technical but not the IP issues related to RG.

Because of its importance to the global supply of pandemic vaccine, efforts must be undertaken immediately to solve the intellectual property issues related to reverse genetics. An international solution is not readily apparent. The national governments of vaccine-producing countries must take an interest in solving this problem (Hollis, 2002). The intellectual property rules of the World Trade Organization and the needs of international public health must be reconciled (Novak, 2003). Political and technical support might be sought from organizations such as the Organization for Economic Cooperation and Development (OECD); nearly all countries with vaccine companies are OECD Member States. The technical assistance of the World Intellectual Property Organization (WIPO) and the WIPO Arbitration and Mediation Center could be especially important (see http://www.wipo.int/). It may be adequate to bring together the various patent holders, assuming they see the possibility of a substantial market. Whatever process is chosen, achieving a solution to the problem of intellectual property for reverse genetics represents an important criterion for judging the ability of countries to work together to achieve good governance for global public health (Fidler, 2004).

**Please see the statement immediately following this paper for MedImmune, Inc.'s comments on the above section.

Clinical and Experimental Studies of the Molecular Pathophysiology of Influenza

Recent studies suggest that the biological basis for severe disease associated with influenza virus infections is virus-induced cytokine dysregulation

(Julkunen et al., 2001). Avian H5N1 influenza viruses are potent inducers of proinflammatory cytokines (TNF-alpha and interferon beta) (Cheung et al., 2002). High serum concentrations of the chemokine interferon induced protein-10 (IP-10) and the monokine induced by interferon gamma (MIG) have been reported in patients with H5N1 disease (Peiris et al., 2004). In addition to these laboratory findings, epidemiologists have long recognized that influenza is associated with an increased risk of hospitalization and death due to cardiovascular and cerebrovascular diseases (Madjid et al., 2003; Reichert et al., 2004). Observational studies have documented a reduction in hospitalizations for congestive heart failure, recurrent myocardial infarction, and stroke following influenza vaccination (Nichol et al., 2003; Majid et al., 2003). Given these findings, recent advances in cardiovascular treatment could have important implications for the prophylaxis and treatment of interpandemic and pandemic influenza.

Much attention has been given recently to the effects of high-intensity statin treatment for coronary heart disease (Sacks, 2004; Cannon et al., 2004; Topol, 2004). The protection afforded by these agents seems to be above and beyond their effects in lowering serum levels of low-density lipoprotein cholesterol. The "cholesterol-centric" explanation for the clinical benefits of statins appears to be giving way to their "pleiotropic" effects. One recent study showed that patients with nonischemic dilated cardiomyopathy who were treated with low-dose simvastatin resulted in clinical improvement that was associated with a substantial lowering of serum concentrations of several inflammatory mediators, including TNF-alpha and IL-6 (Node et al., 2003). Similar effects have been seen on levels of C-reactive protein and the results have been dose related (Sacks, 2004). Finally, experimental (Merx et al., 2004) and clinical (Almog et al., 2004) studies have shown that statins have a dramatic effect in protecting against mortality caused by bacterial sepsis. These findings suggest that prophylaxis with statins or perhaps other commonly available therapeutic agents could possibly have beneficial effects on the clinical course of human influenza. Although this is only an idea, given the need for effective interventions in an emergent pandemic, it is one worth pursuing.

Several avenues of study could be considered. First, during the next influenza season (or for past influenza seasons for which appropriate administrative databases exist), case-control studies could be undertaken to determine whether common treatments for cardiovascular and cerebrovascular diseases are associated with reductions in all influenza-related hospitalizations and deaths, not just those associated with underlying cardiovascular or cerebrovascular diseases. Second, the existing databases for large-scale prospective trials of cardiovascular therapies could be reanalyzed to determine whether treatment is associated with reductions in influenza-related events that are independent of the effects of influenza vaccination. Third, studies of influenza in experimental animals could be undertaken to determine whether any of these treatments has an effect on clinical illness and/or virus shedding. Special attention could be given to the effects of treatment on the development of secondary bacterial pneumonia (McCullers and Rehg, 2002). Finally, in vitro studies could be undertaken to determine whether treatment of cell cultures with statins and other agents before or shortly after infection with influenza viruses has any effect on their subsequent production of proinflammatory cytokines.

If the studies outlined above should prove to be positive, their benefits for the next pandemic could be overwhelmingly important because, unlike antiviral agents and vaccines, supplies of these agents will be abundant and their availability widespread.

STATEMENT FROM MEDIMMUNE, INC., REGARDING REVERSE GENETICS TECHNOLOGY

MedImmune, Inc.

Mountain View, California

There are generally regarded to be four patent portfolios associated with the reverse genetics technology. An earlier filed portfolio developed by Palese et al. (WO 91/03552) at Mt. Sinai School of Medicine is owned by MedImmune, Inc. Later filed portfolios developed by Kawaoka et al. (WO 00/60050) at University of Wisconsin and Hoffmann (WO 01/83794) at St. Jude Children's Research Hospital are exclusively licensed by MedImmune, Inc. Finally, another later filed portfolio, also developed by Palese et al. (U.S. Patent No. 6,544,785), is owned by Mt. Sinai. Thus, these four patent portfolios are currently controlled by two parties.

For its part, MedImmune, Inc., has taken steps to ensure that its patent rights do not inhibit the development and commercialization of a pandemic influenza vaccine. Specifically, MedImmune, Inc., proactively notified the World Health Organization in December 2003 that it would grant free access to its intellectual property to government organizations and companies developing pandemic influenza vaccines *gratis* for public health purposes. In addition, MedImmune, Inc., has given similar notification to NIH and NVPO in the United States, and the National Institute for Biological Standards and Control (NIBSC) in the United Kingdom. For corporate manufacturers considering the *commercial* sale of pandemic influenza vaccines produced by reverse genetics, MedImmune, Inc., has sent out letters to all such manufacturers offering licenses to its intellectual property under reasonable terms. MedImmune, Inc., has made it clear to its commercial peers that it will waive royalties on its intellectual property for any and all pandemic influenza vaccines that are offered free of charge in the interest of public health. MedImmune, Inc., expects to apply this same pandemic licensing policy to any additional intellectual property rights for reverse genetics it should control in the future.

This intellectual property landscape is relatively simple compared to the typically complex field of biotechnology, where experienced companies like the influenza vaccine manufacturers are used to securing multiple licenses for a single product. Thus, influenza vaccine manufacturers should face little difficulty in obtaining licenses to the relevant intellectual property, and may direct their resources instead toward obtaining regulatory approval for pandemic vaccines.

PERSPECTIVES ON ANTIVIRAL USE DURING PANDEMIC INFLUENZA

Frederick G. Hayden[6,7,8]

Reprinted, with permission, from Hayden (2001), Copyright 2001 by The Royal Society

Antiviral agents could potentially play a major role in the initial response to pandemic influenza, particularly with the likelihood that an effective vaccine is unavailable, by reducing morbidity and mortality. The M2 inhibitors are partially effective for chemoprophylaxis of pandemic influenza and evidence from studies of interpandemic influenza indicate that the neuraminidase inhibitors would be effective in prevention. In addition to the symptom benefit observed with M2 inhibitor treatment, early therapeutic use of neuraminidase inhibitors has been shown to reduce the risk of lower respiratory complications. Clinical pharmacology and adverse drug effect profiles indicate that the neuraminidase inhibitors and rimantadine are preferable to amantadine with regard to the need for individual prescribing and tolerance monitoring. Transmission of drug-resistant virus could substantially limit the effectiveness of M2 inhibitors and the possibility exists for primary M2 inhibitor resistance in a pandemic strain. The frequency of resistance emergence is lower with neuraminidase inhibitors and mathematical modelling studies indicate that the reduced transmissibil-

[6]Department of Internal Medicine, PO Box 800473, University of Virginia Health Sciences Center, Charlottesville, VA 22908; fgh@virginia.edu.

[7]Keywords: amantadine; rimantadine; oseltamivir; zanamivir; antivirals; resistance.

[8]I would like to thank Dr. Fred Aoki and Dr. Martin Meltzer for their ideas and constructive comments and Diane Ramm for help with manuscript preparation.

ity of drug-resistant virus observed with neuraminidase inhibitor-resistant variants would lead to negligible community spread of such variants. Thus, there are antiviral drugs currently available that hold considerable promise for response to pandemic influenza before a vaccine is available, although considerable work remains in realizing this potential. Markedly increasing the quantity of available antiviral agents through mechanisms such as stockpiling, educating health care providers and the public and developing effective means of rapid distribution to those in need are essential in developing an effective response, but remain currently unresolved problems.

Introduction

This article provides personal perspectives on selected issues that are relevant to the use of antiviral drugs during the next influenza pandemic. It expands on previously published comments (Hayden, 1997) that were made before the availability of the novel class of anti-influenza agents, the neuraminidase inhibitors, and focuses on three areas: antiviral agent selection, antiviral resistance and the application of mathematical models. This discussion does not consider other important public health issues such as costs and their reimbursement, the stability of raw materials or formulated drug and their potential for stockpiling and rationing or distribution of limited drug supplies. However, it is obvious that adequate supplies and rapid access to antiviral drugs are essential if they are to be useful. In this regard, increasing appropriate use and fostering both health care provider and public familiarity with the available agents during the interpandemic period are essential for their effective use during the next pandemic.

Improvements in medical care since the last pandemic, including the introduction of new antiviral drugs that are specific for influenza A and B viruses, offer potential for reducing the impact of the next one. However, the health care systems of the USA and many other countries are sometimes unable to cope with the relatively modest increases in demand that occur with interpandemic disease. Mathematical models based on assumptions derived largely from the 1957 and 1968 pandemic experiences and the recent interpandemic period have estimated that 89,000–207,000 deaths, 314,000–734,000 hospitalizations, 18–42 million out-patient visits and 20–47 million additional illnesses will occur during the next pandemic (Meltzer et al., 1999). A pandemic like that occurring in 1918 would probably increase the impact by another order of magnitude. Most of these illnesses and deaths will occur over a short period of weeks to several months in a given region and overwhelm health care services. The mass casualties, which will include health care workers and providers of the essential community services, will not only rapidly fill hospital beds and exhaust available supplies of antivirals, antibiotics and other essential medications, but could also lead to substantial disruption of societal services, industrial production and infrastructure such as transportation, food supply and communications (Schoch-Spana, 2000). The 1918 pandemic incapacitated the health care system as well as other basic functions of many cities.

Antiviral agents could potentially play a major role in the initial response to pandemic influenza, particularly with the likelihood that an effective vaccine is unavailable, and might substantially reduce morbidity, hospitalizations, other demands on the health care system and mortality. However, a number of limitations regarding antiviral use during a pandemic warrant consideration.

The major current impediment to effective use in a pandemic would be limited availability coupled with high demand during a short period. In particular, restricted availability, drug costs, the risks of adverse effects and the potential for the emergence of drug resistance are constraints on prolonged prophylactic administration during the initial wave or waves of a pandemic. Fair allocation of available resources would be extremely difficult in the context of an ongoing pandemic or even major epidemic. As summarized below, antivirals have proven efficacy in treatment and prevention, but an inadequate supply and limited surge capacity in production would result in lack of use. Markedly increasing the quantity of available antiviral agents through mechanisms such as stockpiling and developing effective means of rapid distribution to those in need are essential in developing an effective response, but remain currently unresolved problems.

Selection of Antivirals

A fundamental question is which agent or agents should be selected for potential stockpiling and widespread use in the population. Most countries currently have one M2 inhibitor (amantadine) and one or two neuraminidase inhibitors (zanamivir and oseltamivir) approved for use in influenza treatment and/or prophylaxis and in the USA four agents including rimantadine are currently available (Table 3-2). Although other neuraminidase inhibitors are in various stages of development, these four agents are the ones that require scrutiny at present with regard to their use in response to a pandemic. Efficacy, tolerability, ease of administration and the potential for clinically important drug resistance are all factors that warrant consideration in selecting among the available agents. Data regarding use in pandemic influenza are only available with the M2 inhibitors, but extensive clinical testing of the neuraminidase inhibitors in interpandemic influenza permits reasonable conclusions regarding their efficacy.

TABLE 3-2 Currently Available Antiviral Agents for Influenza

Class and Agent	Brand Name	Route	Dose Adjustments	Adverse Drug Interactions	Paediatric/ Liquid Formula
M2 Inhibitors Amantadine	Symmetrel	Oral	CC ≤ 50–70 Age ≥ 65 Years	CNS Stimulants, Anticholinergics, Antihistamines, and Certain Diuretics	Yes
Rimantadine	Flumadine	Oral	CC ≤ 10 Age ≥ 65 Years Hepatic Disease	Not Reported	Yes
NA Inhibitors Oseltamivir (GS4104)	Tamiflu	Oral	CC ≤ 30	Not Reported	Yes
Zanamivir (GGl67)	Relenza	Inhalation	No	Not Reported	Not Applicable

NOTE: CC, creatinine clearance (ml min^{-1}). Probenicid inhibits renal excretion as potential drug interaction in the case of oseltamivir.

Efficacy for Prophylaxis

The comparative efficacies of these agents have received limited study. In general, amantadine and rimantadine have comparable antiviral and clinical activities when used in chemoprophylaxis or in the treatment of influenza A virus illness (reviewed in Hayden & Aoki, 1999). The evidence from placebo-controlled, blinded studies of amantadine and rimantadine during the 1968 H3N2 pandemic and 1977 H1N1 reappearance establish that these agents are effective for chemoprophylaxis in immunologically naive adult populations (Table 3-3), although the observed levels of protection against influenza illness varied considerably across studies and were generally lower than the 80–90% protective efficacies against illness observed in studies of interpandemic influenza. Lower protection rates are observed for laboratory documented infection (Table 3-3), an observation that, in part, reflects the occurrence of subclinical and likely immunizing infections during chemoprophylaxis. The neuraminidase inhibitors are highly effective in chemoprophylaxis against epidemic influenza in studies assessing both seasonal prophylaxis in non-immunized adults (Hayden et al., 1989; Monto el al., 1999a) or immunized nursing home residents (Peters et al., 2001) and post exposure prophylaxis in families (Hayden et al., 2000; Welliver et al., 2001). The single study comparing the prophylactic efficacy of an M2 with a neuraminidase inhibitor found that inhaled zanamivir was superior to oral rimantadine in short-term influenza prophylaxis in nursing home outbreaks, largely because of frequent rimantadine prophylaxis failures secondary to resistant virus (Gravenstein et al., 2000). Such results would predict that the neuraminidase inhibitors would also be effective for prophylaxis of pandemic influenza.

TABLE 3-3 Amantadine Prophylaxis During Pandemic Influenza

	Protective Efficacy	
Pandemic/Subtype	Influenza A Illness	Seroconversion
1968 H3N2	59-100	28-52
1977 H1N1	31-71	18-39

NOTE: The values are the percentage ranges of reported efficacies in studies of oral amantadine.
SOURCE: The data are taken from Nafta et al. (1970), Oker-Blom et al. (1970), Smorodintsev et al. (1970), Monto et al. (1979), Pettersson et al. (1980) and Quarles et al. (1981).

Efficacy for Treatment

One clinical feature of previous pandemic influenza, particularly the 1918 disease, was that convalescence was protracted, with fatigue and functional impairment lasting for weeks. Early antiviral treatment has been shown to reduce the time to functional recovery by up to several days in adults and children with acute influenza. Placebo-controlled, blinded studies during the 1968 H3N2 pandemic and 1977 H1N1 reappearance showed that amantadine and rimantadine provided therapeutic benefit in uncomplicated illness in previously healthy adults, with reductions in fever, symptom severity and the time to resuming normal activities (Knight et al., 1970; Galbraith et al., 1971; Van Voris et al., 1981). However, most controlled treatment studies of the M2 inhibitors have enrolled relatively few patients and none to date have documented reductions in complications or antibiotic use.

The antiviral and clinical benefits of early antiviral treatment have not been directly compared between an M2 and a neuraminidase inhibitor. Several large placebo-controlled, blinded studies have shown that treatment with either inhaled zanamivir or oral oseltamivir reduces illness duration, the time to resuming normal activities and the likelihood of physician-diagnosed lower respiratory complications leading to antibiotic use in adults (Monto et al., 1999b; Kaiser et al., 2000; Treanor et al., 2000). Such benefits have also been observed in zanamivir treatment studies involving patients with asthma or chronic obstructive airways disease (Murphy et al., 2000) and in oseltamivir treatment studies involving children aged 1–12 years, in whom new otitis media diagnoses were reduced by over 40% (Whitley et al., 2001). In contrast, one earlier pediatric study of rimantadine found no beneficial effects on earache or presumed otitis media risk following influenza (Hall et al., 1987). Both intranasal zanamivir and oral oseltamivir reduce otologic abnormalities in experimental human influenza (Hayden et al., 1999; Walker et al., 1997), whereas oral rimantadine does not (Doyle et al., 1998). Furthermore, preliminary analysis of the aggregated clinical trials experience with oseltamivir indicates that early treatment is also associated with reductions in hospitalizations. Until a direct comparison of the relative therapeutic effects of an M2 and a neuraminidase inhibitor is performed, the available data indicate that a neuraminidase inhibitor would be the preferred antiviral agent for treatment during pandemic influenza from the perspective of therapeutic benefit.

Ease of Administration

The selection of an antiviral agent for wide-scale use also depends heavily on its pharmacological properties, which in turn influence the complexity of its dose regimens, the route and frequency of administration, the need for therapeutic monitoring and dose adjustments and the potential for clinically important drug-drug or drug-disease interactions. Clinically important differences exist among the M2 inhibitors (reviewed in Hayden & Aoki, 1999) and the neuraminidase inhibitors (reviewed in Gubareva et al., 2000) with regard to their human pharmacology. Each of the available agents can be dosed infrequently, with once daily for prevention and once (rimantadine and amantadine) or twice daily for treatment. Dose adjustments are rarely needed for rimantadine and the neuraminidase inhibitors (Table 3-2). No age related adjustments are required for the neuraminidase inhibitors.

In contrast, amantadine depends directly on renal excretion for elimination and has a narrow therapeutic index (*ca.* 2:1 ratio of the one associated with frequent adverse effects to the therapeutic dose), such that amantadine dose adjustments are required for relatively modest decrements in renal function, including those usually observed with ageing. Furthermore, amantadine has several recognized drug interactions that increase the likelihood of side-effects (Table 3-2) and the need for close clinical monitoring in certain patient groups. The need for individual prescribing of amantadine based on knowledge of renal function is a significant limitation to its wide-scale use. The inhaler device used for zanamivir dosing is also an obstacle with respect to the ease of administration. The current delivery system requires a cooperative, informed patient who is able to make an adequate inspiratory effort. Elderly hospitalized patients often have problems using the delivery system effectively (Diggory et al., 2001) and the current device is not appropriate for use in young children (below 5 years of age) or those with cognitive impairment or marked frailty. While the need for device training is an important concern in treating acutely ill patients, most studies to date have shown good compliance and the inhaled route may offer certain advantages in the chemoprophylaxis of influenza.

Tolerability and Safety

Similarly, the type, frequency, severity and management of adverse drug effects and their relationships to drug dose are all considerations in agent selection (Table 3-4). The duration of drug exposure, short-term treatment versus longer periods for prophylaxis and the timing of onset with regard to initiation of dosing are, again, all considerations in this regard.

Amantadine has the narrowest toxic:therapeutic ratio among the available agents and is commonly associated with dose-related minor central nervous system (CNS) side-effects, that are probably related to its amphetamine like CNS stimulatory properties and, less often, severe CNS toxicities

TABLE 3-4 Adverse Drug Reaction Profiles of Currently Available Anti-Influenza Agents

Agent	Adverse Reaction	Severity	Frequency During Treatment	Dose Related	Reversible
Amantadine	CNS	Mild-moderate	10–30%	Yes	Yes
		Severe	Uncommon	Yes	Yes
	Gastrointestinal	Mild	Common	Yes	Yes
Rimantadine	CNS	Mild-moderate	< 10%	Yes	Yes
	Gastrointestinal	Mild	Common	Yes	Yes
Zanamivir	Bronchospasm	Mild-severe	Very Uncommon	No	Yes
Oseltamivir	Gastrointestinal	Mild	Common (5–15%)	Yes	Yes

(Table 3-4). The latter occur most often in those with high plasma concentrations due to impaired renal excretion. Rimantadine has a significantly lower potential for causing CNS adverse effects, in part related to differences in its pharmacokinetics (Hayden & Aoki, 1999), although dose reductions are recommended in the elderly. For example, one recent crossover study in an elderly nursing home resident population compared prolonged amantadine chemoprophylaxis, at the currently recommended reduced dose of 100 mg day^{-1} further adjusted for renal function, with rimantadine chemoprophylaxis at the same dose and found *ca.* 10-fold higher frequencies of overall adverse events, including confusion and hallucinosis and drop-out during amantadine administration (Keyser et al., 2000).

Inhaled zanamivir treatment has been very infrequently described as causing bronchospasm, sometimes severe or associated with fatal outcome, in acute influenza sufferers with pre-existing airways disease. Influenza itself often causes severe exacerbations in such patients so that the possible causal relationship to zanamivir administration is uncertain, as is the actual frequency of such events. One large placebo-controlled study of influenza-infected patients with underlying mild-moderate asthma or, less often, chronic obstructive airways disease found no excess of serious respiratory adverse events and more rapid clinical recovery including peak expiratory flow rates in zanamivir recipients (Murphy et al., 2000). However, until further data are available, zanamivir use in patients with underlying airways disease requires close clinical monitoring. Like the M2 inhibitors, oseltamivir is associated with mild-moderate gastrointestinal (GI) upset in a minority of patients, but no other serious end-organ toxicity has been recognized to date.

In most instances, the adverse effects associated with these drugs are readily reversible after the cessation of administration. Severe CNS adverse reactions related to excess amantadine accumulation in the blood can be an exception, because such toxicity is usually due to a failure to reduce the dose in the setting of renal impairment with its attendant prolonged elimination half-life. Another concern with regard to extensive community use of antivirals during pandemic influenza is their potential for adverse effects during pregnancy. Amantadine and rimantadine are recognized teratogens in animals and, consequently, are relatively contraindicated in pregnancy. The clinical pharmacology and adverse drug effect profiles of the antivirals for influenza indicate that the neuraminidase inhibitors and rimantadine are preferable to amantadine with regard to the need for individual prescribing, tolerance monitoring and the seriousness of side-effects. When these findings are considered in the context of the available information about efficacy and antiviral resistance (discussed below), it is clear that the neuraminidase inhibitors would be the preferred agent for treatment and, in some instances, prophylaxis during pandemic influenza.

Antiviral Resistance

An important issue in pandemic influenza is the potential for the emergence and spread of drug-resistant influenza A viruses that cause the loss of the clinical effectiveness of antiviral drugs. The M2 and neuraminidase inhibitors have important differences with respect to the frequency and biological properties of resistant variants (Table 3-5). In addition to the selection of drug resistant variants during antiviral use, the possibility of primary or *de novo* drug resistance in a pandemic strain warrants consideration. Primary resistance to the neuraminidase inhibitors has not been described at the enzyme level and these agents are active against all of the nine neuraminidase subtypes recognized in avian influenza viruses (reviewed in Gubareva et al., 2000; Tisdale, 2000). In contrast, primary resistance to the M2 inhibitors has been described in swine influenza viruses of the H1N1 subtype in the 1930s in the absence of selective drug pressure. More recently, swine viruses in Europe and North America and isolates from several zoonotically infected humans of H1N1 and H3N2 subtypes have shown primary resistance (A. Hay, personal communication). Amantadine resistance has also been described in a small portion (<1%) of field isolates (Ziegler et al., 1999) and in those receiving the drug for the treatment of Parkinsonian symptoms (Iwahashi et al., 2001). Such observations raise the concern that amantadine-resistant isolates circulate naturally under certain conditions. In addition, the use of amantadine for influenza management in China also increases the potential that a pandemic strain might show primary resistance to amantadine and rimantadine.

Another generic issue regarding resistance emergence is the proposed tactic for extending the availability of limited antiviral drug supplies during pandemic influenza by reductions in either the dose level or, in the case of treatment, the duration of therapy. Theoretically, a short course therapy of 1–3 days might reduce viral loads sufficiently to provide clinical benefit. Obvious concerns related to this approach would include the potential loss of therapeutic or prophylactic efficacy, rebound in viral replication and symptoms after the cessation of administration and fostering emergence of drug resistance, in part due to continued viral replication in the setting of subinhibitory drug concentrations. The risks of these events would probably be higher in pandemic influenza than in interpandemic disease because of the lack of specific immunity to an antigenic ally novel strain and the potential for higher or more protracted levels of viral replication in affected persons. Indeed, higher drug doses might be required for exerting comparable antiviral effects and clinical benefits in pandemic as compared with interpandemic infections. Consequently, the minimally effective doses and durations of therapy need careful study in epidemic influenza before recommendations might be considered for the pandemic situation. Conducting such studies in unprimed populations such as young children or in immunocompromised hosts might provide useful insights.

TABLE 3-5 Epidemiological and Biological Features of Drug-Resistant Influenza Viruses Recovered During Clinical Use

	Locus of Resistance	Frequency During Therapy	Infectivity in Animals	Virulence in Animals	Person to Person Transmissibility
Amantadine/Rimantadine	M2	High (ca. 30%)	Wild-type	Wild-type	Yes
Zanamivir	NA	Low (?)	Reduced	Reduced	Unstudied
Oseltamivir	NA	Low (ca. 0.4% in adults and 4% in children)	Reduced	Reduced	Unstudied

NOTE: The reported frequency of recovering M2 inhibitor-resistant variants ranges from ca. 10% in elderly adults to over 75% of immunocompromised patients shedding virus 3 days or longer (Hayden, 1996; Englund et al., 1998).
SOURCE: Based on ferret studies by Carr et al. (2001), the person to person transmissibility of one oseltamivir-resistant variant is reduced in animals.

Amantadine and Rimantadine

The M2 inhibitors have been associated with the rapid emergence of high-level resistant variants during therapeutic use and failures of chemo-prophylaxis due to the transmission of such strains under close contact conditions, as in households and nursing homes (reviewed in Hayden, 1996). These variants are due to point mutations in the M gene and corresponding single amino acid substitutions in the target M2 protein (reviewed in Hay, 1996). They show no obvious loss of virulence or transmissibility in animal models or humans (Table 3-5) and have been shown to compete effectively with wild-type, susceptible virus for multiple-cycle transmission in the absence of selective drug pressure in an avian model (Bean et al., 1989). The frequency of observing such resistant variants has averaged *ca.* 30% in treated adults and children, but ranges to over 50% of immuno-compromised hosts (Englund et al., 1998).

A key aspect of the clinical and public health implications of resistance emergence is the transmissibility of resistant variants. For example, one older study employing rimantadine for index case treatment and post-exposure prophylaxis in families observed negligible prophylactic efficacy due to high rates of resistance emergence and probable transmission leading to failures of drug prophylaxis (Hayden et al., 1989). A similar study with amantadine during the 1968 pandemic also found low prophylactic effi-cacy, although the reasons were not elucidated (Galbraith et al., 1969). In contrast, inhaled zanamivir used for both treatment and post-exposure prophylaxis in families was highly effective and not associated with resis-tance emergence (Hayden et al., 2000). A recent nursing home-based study comparing 2 weeks' prophylaxis with oral rimantadine or inhaled zanamivir after recognized outbreaks found over 60% higher protection in zanamivir recipients as compared with rimantadine, in part due to high frequencies of prophylaxis failures due to rimantadine-resistant viruses (Gravenstein et al., 2000). The extensive use of rimantadine for prophylaxis and treatment of non-study participants on the same wards may have contributed to the observed prophylaxis failures. Such experiences highlight the potential for the emergence of amantadine-resistant influenza A viruses and spread under close contact conditions.

Oseltamivir and Zanamivir

The neuraminidase inhibitors appear to be associated with a lower frequency of resistance emergence due to neuraminidase mutations (re-viewed in McKimm-Breschkin, 2000; Tisdale, 2000) and a lower risk of transmission (Table 3-5). To date, only one instance of zanamivir resistance in an immunocompromised host has been documented (Gubareva et al.,

1998) and no resistance has been found in immunocompetent persons receiving treatment (Barnett et al., 2000; Boivin et al., 2000; Hayden et al., 2000). The frequency of recovering resistant variants may be higher with oseltamivir therapy in that variants exhibiting neuraminidase resistance have been recovered from *ca.* 0.4% of treated adults and 4% of treated children (N. Roberts, personal communication; Treanor et al., 2000; Whitley et al., 2001). However, the oseltamivir resistant variants show reduced infectivity and virulence in animal models and the commonest variant with amino acid substitution at position 292 shows reduced transmissibility in a ferret model (Carr et al., 2001). These observations indicate that antiviral resistance due to neuraminidase resistance appears to alter the fitness of influenza viruses and suggests that resistance will be much less likely to be a threat during drug use in epidemic or pandemic influenza.

Modelling Studies

Mathematical models can be used for assessing the potential for the spread of drug-resistant influenza viruses under both epidemic and pandemic circumstances (Stilianakis et al., 1998). Such models can be used for assessing the effectiveness and potential impact of antiviral resistance transmission during different strategies of antiviral intervention, such as chemoprophylaxis alone, the treatment of ill persons alone or combined treatment and prophylaxis. For example, one such study examined the effect of these different approaches using amantadine or rimantadine in a closed population during a theoretical pandemic outbreak in which all residents were assumed to be susceptible and become infected (Stilianakis et al., 1998). The model, which is based on studies with amantadine and rimantadine, predicted that treatment alone would affect the epidemic curve minimally, whereas chemoprophylaxis alone or a combination of treatment and chemoprophylaxis both reduce the number of symptomatic cases (Table 3-6). However, the observed outcomes depended heavily on the transmissibility of drug-resistant virus relative to wild-type, susceptible virus (Table 3-6). When transmissibility of the resistant variant was comparable to the wild-type, prophylaxis failures due to resistant virus were common, particularly with the combined approach for which one-half of illnesses were due to resistant virus. A relatively modest fivefold reduction in transmissibility was associated with substantial reductions in the impact of resistant virus and improved effectiveness for both the prophylaxis alone or combined intervention approaches (Table 3-6). Another recently described model examining the effects of resistance emergence also predicts that decreases in biological fitness and associated transmissibility of drug-resistant virus, as observed with neuraminidase inhibitor-resistant variants, will lead to negligible community spread of such variants (Ferguson and Mallett, 2001).

TABLE 3-6 Effect of the Transmissibility of Drug-Resistant Virus on Outcomes in a Theoretical Closed Population Pandemic Influenza Outbreak

		Percentage of Residents Affected	
Strategy for Drug Intervention	Outcome	Resistant Virus Fully Transmissible	Resistant Virus 20% Transmissible
Treatment only	Infected	100	100
	Ill	56	55
	Ill, Resistant Virus	8	7
Prophylaxis only	Infected	98	90
	Ill	30	23
	Ill, Resistant Virus	11	3
Combined treatment and prophylaxis	Infected	99	87
	Ill	34	23
	Ill, Resistant Virus	17	5

NOTE: The values for the percentage of residents affected were adapted from Stilianakis et al. (1998). They are based on the assumption of a fully susceptible population (n = 578), an overall infection frequency of 100% and an illness frequency of 56% in the absence of drug intervention. The third and fourth columns are the transmission probabilities of resistant virus relative to wild-type, susceptible virus. The assumption regarding drug efficacy and the likelihood of resistance emergence are based on studies with amantadine and rimantadine and are detailed in Stilianakis et al. (1998).

The Economic Impact

In the absence of a mass immunization programme, the costs, excluding disruptions to commerce and society, of the next pandemic are projected to range from US$71.3 billion to US$166.5 billion for hospitalizations, outpatient care, self-treatment and lost work days and wages in the United States alone (Meltzer et al., 1999). Formal pharmacoeconomic analyses of antiviral interventions have not been reported to date for pandemic influenza, but could be helpful in selecting the appropriate strategies and target populations for antiviral use. Through use of the economic model developed by Meltzer et al. (1999) and assumptions regarding drug effectiveness derived from recent therapeutic trials with oseltamivir, preliminary assessment of the economic impact of using antivirals for treatment during an influenza pandemic are possible (Table 3-7). Extensive therapeutic use would be projected to save many days off work, out-patients visits for presumed complications and, particularly in older adults, hospitalizations (M.I. Meltzer and F.G. Hayden, unpublished observations). These preliminary analyses suggest that treatment in high-risk older adults would reduce hospitalizations, whereas treatment in non-high-risk younger adults and

TABLE 3-7 Projected Economic Impact of Neuraminidase Inhibitor Treatment on Selected Outcomes During Pandemic Influenza

	Out-patient Visits Saved per 1000 Ill		Hospitalizations Saved per 1000 Ill		Out-patient-related Days Off Work Saved per 1000 Ill	
	Mean	95% CI	Mean	95% CI	Mean	95% CI
0-19 Years	162	152-171	2.2	0.8-3.5	800	754-847
20-64 Years	296	284-307	4.0	1.8-6.0	585	320-844
65+ Years	227	223-229	14.4	11.3-17.6	745	735-755

NOTE: The days off work saved only refer to out-patient illnesses and do not consider the effect of hospitalization. Paediatric illnesses were assumed to cause days off work for care givers (Meltzer et al. 1999). These outcomes are derived from the use of a previously described mathematical model (Meltzer et al. 1999) and the following assumptions regarding the effects of early antiviral treatment derived from studies with oseltamivir: neuraminidase inhibitor treatment reduces the days of illness by 1.5 days, the number of out-patient visits by 20% (0-19 years), 50% (20-64 years) and 30% (> 65 years) and hospitalizations by 50% compared with no treatment. CI, confidence interval.)
SOURCE: M. I. Meltzer and F. G. Hayden, unpublished observations, et al.

children would reduce out-patient visits and work/school days lost. By assigning direct and indirect dollar valuations to the health outcomes averted, it was estimated that the treatment of high-risk persons aged 65 years and older and non-high-risk persons aged 20–64 years would generate the largest and comparable savings per 1000 ill.

If it were possible to extend early treatment to those who would not seek medical care, considerable savings in indirect costs due to days off work/school could be achieved across all age groups. However, the actual implementation of that strategy would require the development and validation of new treatment paradigms, such as telephone triage by non-physician health care providers or self-diagnosis through symptom checklists and then rapid access to antiviral drugs for patient-initiated therapy. Such assessments need to be undertaken during the interpandemic influenza period so that they might be acceptable for use during the next pandemic. In general, the results of such economic analyses depend on the nature of the pandemic and its associated age-related morbidity and mortality rates, the projected costs of outcomes and the assumed effectiveness of the intervention. Future research will need to include estimates of the cost of delivering treatments to various age and risk groups and examine other drug treatments and strategies including prophylaxis. However, such economic models can help guide decisions about the potential benefits of antiviral treatment or prophylaxis in different populations groups.

PARTNERING WITH THE PRIVATE MEDICAL SYSTEM

Gordon W. Grundy, MD, MBA

Aetna, Inc.

Health plans and managed care organizations (MCOs) operate at the center of the private medical system. Over 200 million American citizens are privately insured by more than 1,300 health care organizations. Aetna is among the largest with more than 13 million members. By virtue of financing, facilitating, and coordinating the delivery of health services, health plans have fiduciary and contractual relationships with a variety of constituents. These include individual citizens (health plan members), employers (payers of private health insurance), physicians, hospitals, and other ancillary providers (e.g., home health care agencies, skilled nursing facilities, and urgent care centers).

In planning for pandemic influenza, the role of the private medical system as mediated through health plans and MCOs can be framed by addressing four key questions:

1. What capabilities can private health plans bring to influenza pandemic planning?

2. How and why should health plans and MCOs interface with the planning process?

3. How can health plans and MCOs facilitate the delivery of medical services during an influenza pandemic?

4. How might a public–private partnership to address pandemic influenza be achieved?

Capabilities of Private Health Plans

Health plans and MCOs can contribute a broad range of resources to the pandemic planning process. They are experienced at increasing health awareness through educational initiatives and promoting preventive care with timely reminders to insured members. In addition, health plans often provide performance feedback to the physicians and hospitals with which they have contractual relationships. These activities reach significant numbers of constituents. For example, a single large health plan such as Aetna can communicate nationwide with more than 13 million individuals, 350,000 physicians, and 3,500 hospitals. Because MCO databases contain information on members, physicians' practice locations, and hospital contacts, they are well positioned to conduct outreach in the event of a public health crisis.

Education

Most health plans have developed educational components within their wellness programs as well as in case and disease management functional areas. With some modification, these resources could be adapted to inform the public during an influenza pandemic. Health plans generally find that individual members attend to the topics that are discussed in mailings and in telephone campaigns. Given the proven capability of health plans and MCOs in outreach and education activities, public health agencies should consider them as potential partners in communicating with citizens during an influenza pandemic threat.

Immunization Campaigns

Aetna is one of many health plans that have experience in conducting preventive immunization campaigns and our ability to do so has been measured and accredited. In support of these efforts, we have established alternative sites for providing immunizations, such as retail establishments and pharmacies, and we have developed a variety of ways to get people to sites where they can be appropriately immunized. Aetna's extensive data-base enables us to target high-risk individuals and to build predictive mod-eling tools, including risk stratification. This allows us to identify those individuals within our health plan who would be at high risk for complica-tions from influenza, whether due to age or a chronic condition.

In December 2003, for example, when the influenza season got off to an early and severe start and the potential for a vaccine shortage became apparent, Aetna conducted an outreach campaign within its southeast re-gion to urge health plan members at high risk for flu complications due to a chronic medical condition to be immunized. Over a period of 4 days, Aetna placed more than 134,000 telephone calls to insured members and ultimately contacted more than 100,000 people—many of whom received as many as 4 calls. Information was disseminated rapidly and thoroughly, reaching about 80 percent of our at-risk regional members. This success at sending public health messages quickly and broadly is an asset, and one that we and other health care plans can contribute in addressing pandemic influenza.

Incentives for Physicians and Insured Members

Through contractual relationships with physicians, health plans and MCOs can encourage them to improve annual influenza immunization rates. Physicians can receive feedback on their vaccination rates for mem-bers, especially those at high risk for flu complications. In addition, finan-cial incentives might be established for outstanding performance in this area. Members can also be rewarded for taking appropriate preventive health measures by enhancing their plan benefits.

Research and Demonstration Projects

An Institute of Medicine workshop in 1998 noted a potential role for MCOs in research and demonstration projects related to emerging infec-tions. In the past, however, there has been little incentive for health plans to participate in these projects. With the looming threat of an influenza pan-demic, this worthwhile concept might well be revisited and meaningful incentives considered.

The Planning Process

How then should health plans and MCOs interface effectively with the planning process for pandemic influenza? First and foremost, they need to be part of the planning process. In addition to offering the previously described capabilities, health plan representatives need to be at the table because they understand how specific medical systems in individual communities actually work. Their unique viewpoint can complement the knowledge of local public health departments.

Health plan managers are familiar with each hospital's issues, capacities, referral patterns, and nearby lower level care providers. In the course of health plan work, every effort is made to ensure that members who are hospitalized in acute care facilities are transitioned into lower levels of care as appropriate. Based on that experience, health plans may be able to assist in addressing the expected strain on hospital surge capacity resulting from pandemic influenza, particularly in intensive care units. For example, MCOs may be able to help transition or move hospitalized individuals into alternative sites of care in order to make optimal use of acute care resources.

Health plans also need clear policies, directives, and recommendations from the CDC and other governmental agencies in order to ensure our effective participation in the response to pandemic influenza. In this, as in all medical circumstances, we rely on authoritative sources in the public health field and evidence-based literature to frame and craft our policies. Although health plans recognize the considerable uncertainties inherent in predicting the pandemic course and outcome, the clearer the statements we (and the public) receive, the more support we can provide. For example, if health plans are to encourage and incentivize immunization during a pandemic, we will need to know which populations to target. Will the focus be on people with chronic conditions in order to reduce morbidity and mortality? Alternatively, will the priority be working adults and children in order to reduce the economic impact of lost productivity by ensuring the health of caregivers? Or will we have a universal immunization program to decrease the overall burden of illness? Health plans can most effectively assist in implementing the strategy when it is clearly stated and understood.

Finally, the planning process should recognize the full financial ramifications of an influenza pandemic. This goes beyond calculating the percentage increase in utilization of services and estimates of the aggregate dollar amounts that will be spent as a result. Cost estimates need to reach a more granular level, one that acknowledges that health care is delivered by individuals who get paid for their services. A considerable portion of the health services delivered in a pandemic will be provided by private practitioners who will expect reimbursement. Although certain expenses may be waived, the basic financial support system for the private medical system is carried by employers and needs to stay afloat. This issue requires further study and understanding before positing any recommendations.

Facilitating Delivery of Medical Services

In many circumstances, health plans can most effectively facilitate the delivery of medical services during an influenza pandemic by removing obstacles. More specifically, in the event of a pandemic, health plans will need to temporarily remove or waive many of the policies and procedures that have been established to manage costs but could hinder the response to a public health crisis.

This is exactly what many health plans did following the events of September 11, 2001, as well as after several recent natural disasters and the blackout that affected much of the northeastern United States during the summer of 2003. Most plans in the affected areas issued time-limited waivers of prior approval, referral, and formulary requirements, enabling their members to access care wherever they found it. Aetna even went a step further in September 2001 by bringing counseling teams to worksites in the metropolitan New York area to provide ready access to behavioral health services for plan members.

This precedent to respond quickly and productively in emergency situations will no doubt be replicated during an influenza pandemic. Whether educating their members, promoting immunization, waiving procedures, enhancing surge capacity, or ensuring access to antiviral medications, health plans will play an important role in the day-to-day management of the pandemic. The challenge and responsibility for the private medical system will be to develop a coordinated response that can be launched at the direction of public health officials.

Achieving Public–Private Partnership

To comprehensively address the threat of pandemic influenza, a public–private partnership would most effectively leverage the strengths of health plans and MCOs. Many health plans—potentially every plan—would need to be involved in such an effort. A leading organization that could establish such broad representation is the trade association known as America's Health Insurance Plans (AHIP). Composed of 1,300 health plans that insure more than 200 million citizens, AHIP is engaged in several activities that have public health dimensions. It has had a Disease Prevention and Public Health Work Group in place since 1996 and currently partners with the CDC to work on vaccine surveillance and safety assessment research. In addition, AHIP focuses on emergency preparedness related to bioterrorism and periodically issues public health updates for its member plans.

Another possible partner is the Council for Affordable Quality Health Care (CAQH). Including 22 of the largest national and regional health plans, its member organizations insure more than 100 million Americans. Although less than 5 years old, CAQH is establishing a track record of public awareness initiatives, the most notable of which is a joint effort with the CDC to promote the appropriate use of antibiotics.

The strengths of these national organizations could also be complemented by a series of partnerships with state-based health plan associations that are closer to local public health agencies and often emphasize preventive care and quality.

Should a public–private partnership in pandemic planning be pursued? The advantages are persuasive. Collaboration between public and private entities will bring different techniques and skill sets to bear on public health challenges while fostering innovation. Such partnerships seem likely to increase the chance for success in planning for and managing a future influenza pandemic.

REFERENCES

Almog Y, Shefer A, Novack V, Maimon N, Barski L, Eizinger M, Friger M, Zeller L, Danon A. 2004. Prior statin therapy is associated with a decreased rate of severe sepsis. *Circulation* 110:880–885.

Barnett JM, Cadman A, Gor D, Dempsey M, Walters M, Candlin A, Tisdale M, Morley PJ, Owens IJ, Fenton RJ, Lewis AP, Claas EC, Rimmelzwaan GF, De Groot R, Osterhaus AD. 2000. Zanamivir susceptibility monitoring and characterization of influenza virus clinical isolates obtained during phase II clinical efficacy studies. *Antimicrob Agents Chemother* 44:78–87.

Bean WJ, Thelkeld SC, Webster RG. 1989. Biologic potential of amantadine-resistant influenza A virus in an avian model. *J Infect Dis* 159:1050–1056.

Boivin G, Goyette N, Hardy I, Aoki FY, Wagner A, Trottier S. 2000. Rapid antiviral effect of inhaled zanamivir in the treatment of naturally occurring influenza in otherwise healthy adults. *J Infect Dis* 181:1471–1474.

Cannon CP, Braunwald E, McCabe CH, Rader DJ, Rouleau JL, Belder R, Joyal SV, Hill KA, Pfeffer MA, Skene AM; Pravastatin or Atorvastatin Evaluation and Infection Therapy-Thrombolysis in Myocardial Infarction 22 Investigators. 2004. Intensive versus moderate lipid lowering with statins after acute coronary syndromes. *N Engl J Med* 350:1495–1504.

Carr J, Herlocher L, Elias S, Harrison S, Gibson V, Clark L, Roberts N, Ives J, Monto AS. 2001. Influenza virus carrying an R292K mutation in the neuraminidase gene is not transmitted in ferrets. *Antiviral Res* 50:A85.

Cheung CY, Poon LL, Lau AS, Luk W, Lau YL, Shortridge KF, Gordon S, Guan Y, Peiris JS. 2002. Induction of proinflammatory cytokines in human macrophages by influenza A (H5N1) viruses: A mechanism for the unusual severity of human disease? *Lancet* 360:1831–1837.

Chiron Corporation. 2004. *Chiron to Produce Further Pandemic-Like Influenza Vaccines for National Institutes of Health Clinical Studies.* [Online]. Available: http://phx.corporate-ir.net/phoenix.zhtml?c=105850&p=irol-newsArticle&ID=604514&highlight= [accessed November 10, 2004].

CPMP (Committee for Proprietary Medicinal Products). 1997. *Note for Guidance on Harmonization of Requirements for Influenza Vaccines.* CPMP/BWP/214/96 Circular No. 96-0666, pp. 1–2. [Online]. Available: http://www.emea.eu.int/pdfs/human/bwp/021496en.pdf [accessed December 17, 2004].

CPMP. 2004a. *Guideline on Dossier Structure and Content for Pandemic Influenza Vaccine Marketing Authorisation Applications.* [Online]. Available: http://www.emea.eu.int/pdfs/human/veg/4710703en.pdf [accessed December 17, 2004].

CPMP. 2004b. *Guideline on Submission of Marketing Authorisation Applications for Pandemic Influenza Vaccine Through the Centralized Procedure*. [Online]. Available: http://www.emea.eu.int/pdfs/human/veg/498603en.pdf [accessed December 17, 2004].

Diggory P, Fernandez C, Humphrey A, Jones V, Murphy M. 2001. Comparison of elderly people's technique in using two dry powder inhalers to deliver zanamivir: Randomised controlled trial. *BMJ* 322:1–4.

Doyle WJ, Skoner D, Alper CM, Allen G, Moody SA, Seroky J, Hayden FG. 1998. Effect of rimantadine treatment on clinical manifestations and otologic complications in adults experimentally infected with influenza A (H1N1) virus. *J Infect Dis* 177:1260–1265.

Englund JA, Champlin RE, Wyde PR, Kantarjian H, Atmar RL, Tarrand J, Yousuf H, Regnery H, Klimov AI, Cox NJ, Whimbey E. 1998. Common emergence of amantadine and rimantadine resistant influenza A viruses in symptomatic immunocompromised adults. *Clin Infect Dis* 26:1418–1424.

Fedson DS. 2003a. Pandemic influenza and the global vaccine supply. *Clin Infec Dis* 36: 1552–1561.

Fedson DS. 2003b. Pandemic flu vaccine trials and reverse genetics: Foundation for effective response to next pandemic. Ensuring an adequate global supply of influenza vaccine. *Infect Dis News* 4:13.

Ferguson NM, Mallett S. 2001. An epidemiological model of influenza to investigate the potential transmission of drug resistant virus during community use of antiviral treatment of influenza. *Antiviral Res* 50:A85.

Fidler DP. 2004. Germs, governance, and global health in the wake of SARS. *J Clin Invest* 113:799–804.

Fodor E, Devenish L, Engelhardt OG, Palese P, Brownlee GG, Garcia-Sastre A. 1999. Rescue of influenza A virus from recombinant DNA. *J Virol* 73:9679–9682.

Galbraith AW, Oxford JS, Schild GC, Watson GI. 1969. Study of L-adamantanamine hydrochloride used prophylactically during the Hong Kong influenza epidemic in the family environment. *Bull WHO* 41:677–682.

Galbraith AW, Oxford JS, Schild GC, Potter CW, Watson GI. 1971. Therapeutic effect of L-adamantanamine hydrochloride in naturally occurring influenza A 2-Hong Kong infection. A controlled double-blind study. *Lancet* 2:113–115.

Gravenstein S, Drinka P, Osterweil D, Schilling M, McElhaney JE, Elliott M, Hammond J, Keene O, Krause P, Flack N. 2000. A multicenter prospective double-blind randomized controlled trial comparing the relative safety and efficacy of zanamivir to rimantadine for nursing home influenza outbreak control. In: *Abstracts of the 40th Interscience Conference on Antimicrobial Agents and Chemotherapy*. Washington, DC: American Society for Microbiology. P. 270.

Gubareva LV, Matrosovich MN, Brenner MK, Bethell R, Webster RG. 1998. Evidence for zanamivir resistance in an immunocompromised child infected with influenza B virus. *J Infect Dis* 178:1257–1262.

Gubareva LV, Kaiser L, Hayden FG. 2000. Influenza virus neuraminidase inhibitors. *Lancet* 355:827–835.

Hall CB, Dolin R, Gala CL, Markovitz DM, Zhang YQ, Madore PH, Disney FA, Talpey WB, Green JL, Francis AB, et al. 1987. Children with influenza A infection: Treatment with rimantadine. *Pediatrics* 80:275–282.

Hay AJ. 1996. Amantadine and rimantadine-mechanisms. In: Richman DD, ed. *Antiviral Drug Resistance*. Chichester, United Kingdom: John Wiley & Sons Ltd. Pp. 43–58.

Hayden FG. 1996. Amantadine and rimantadine-clinical aspects. In: Richman DD, ed. *Antiviral Drug Resistance*. Chichester, United Kingdom: John Wiley & Sons Ltd. Pp. 59–77.

Hayden FG. 1997. Antivirals for pandemic influenza. *J Infect Dis* 176(Suppl I):S56–S61.

Hayden FG. 2001. Perspectives on antiviral use during pandemic influenza. *Philos Trans R Soc Lond B Biol Sci.* 356(1416):1877–1884.

Hayden FG, Aoki FY. 1999. Amantadine, rimantadine, and related agents. In: Yu VL, Merigan TC, Barriere SL, eds. *Antimicrobial Therapy and Vaccines*. Baltimore, MD: Williams and Wilkins. Pp. 1344–1365.

Hayden FG, Belshe RB, Clover RD, Hay AJ, Oakes MG, Soo W. 1989. Emergence and apparent transmission of rimantadine-resistant influenza A virus in families. *N Engl J Med* 321:1696–1702.

Hayden FG, Treanor JJ, Fritz RS, Lobo M, Betts RF, Miller M, Kinnersley N, Mills RG, Ward P, Straus SE. 1999. Use of the oral neuraminidase inhibitor oseltamivir in experimental influenza: Randomized controlled trials for prevention and treatment. *JAMA* 282:1240–1246.

Hayden FG, Gubareva LV, Monto AS, Klein TC, Elliot MJ, Hammond JM, Sharp SJ, Ossi MJ. 2000. Inhaled zanamivir for prevention of influenza in families. Zanamivir Family Study Group. *N Eng J Med* 343:1282–1289.

Hehme N, Engelmann H, Kunzel W, Neumeier E, Sanger R. 2002. Pandemic preparedness: Lessons learnt from H2N2 and H9N2 candidate vaccines. *Med Microbiol Immunol* (Berl) 191:203–208.

Hehme N, Engelmann H, Kuenzel W, Neumeier E, Saenger R. 2004. Immunogenicity of a monovalent, aluminum-adjuvanted influenza whole virus vaccine for pandemic use. *Virus Res* 103:163–171.

Hollis A. 2002. The link between publicly funded health care and compulsory licensing. *CMAJ* 167:765–766.

Iwahashi J, Tsuji K, Ishibashi T, Kajiwara J, Imamura Y, Mori R, Hara K, Kashiwagi T, Ohtsu Y, Hamada N, Maeda H, Toyoda M, Toyoda T. 2001. Isolation of amantadine resistant influenza A viruses (H3N2) from patients following administration of amantadine in Japan. *J Clin Microbiol* 39:1652–1653.

Julkunen I, Sareneva T, Pirohonen J, Ronni T, Melen K, Matikainen S. 2001. Molecular pathogenesis of influenza A virus infection and virus-induced regulation of cytokine gene expression. *Cytokine Growth Factor Rev* 12:171–180.

Kaiser L, Keene ON, Hammond J, Elliott M, Hayden FG. 2000. Impact of zanamivir on antibiotics use for respiratory events following acute influenza in adolescents and adults. *Arch Intern Med* 160:3234–3240.

Keyser LA, Karl M, Nafziger AN, Bertino JS Jr. 2000. Comparison of central nervous system adverse effects of amantadine and rimantadine used as sequential prophylaxis of influenza A in elderly nursing home patients. *Arch Intern Med* 160:1485–1488.

Knight V, Fedson D, Baldini J, Douglas RG, Couch RB. 1970. Amantadine therapy of epidemic influenza A2-Hong Kong. *Infect Immun* 1:200–204.

Madjid M, Naghavi M, Litovsky S, Casscells SW. 2003. Influenza and cardiovascular disease. A new opportunity for prevention and the need for further studies. *Circulation* 108:2730–2736.

McCullers JA, Rehg JE. 2002. Lethal synergism between influenza virus and Streptococcus pneumoniae: Characterizations of a mouse model and the role of platelet-activating factor receptor. *J Infect Dis* 186:341–350.

McKimm-Breschkin JL. 2000. Resistance of influenza viruses to neuraminidase inhibitors—a review. *Antiviral Res* 47:1–17.

Meltzer MI, Cox NJ, Fukuda K. 1999. The economic impact of pandemic influenza in the United States: Priorities for intervention. *EID* 5:659–671.

Merx MW, Liehn EA, Janssens U, Lutticken R, Schrader J, Hanrath P, Weber C. 2004. HMG-CoA reductase inhibitor simvastatin profoundly improves survival in a murine model of sepsis. *Circulation* 109:2560–2565.

Monick M, Powers L, Butler S, Hunninghake GW. 2003. Inhibition of Rho family GTPases results in increased TNF-alpha production after lipopolysaccharide exposure. *J Immunol* 171:2625–2630.

Monto AS, Gunn RA, Bandyk MG, King CL. 1979. Prevention of Russian influenza by amantadine. *JAMA* 241:1003–1007.

Monto AS, Robinson DP, Herlocher ML, Hinson JM Jr, Elliott MJ, Crisp A. 1999a. Zanamivir in the prevention of influenza among healthy adults: A randomized controlled trial. *JAMA* 282:31–35.

Monto AS, Webster A, Keene O. 1999b. Randomized, placebo-controlled studies of inhaled zanamivir in the treatment of influenza A and B: Pooled efficacy analysis. *J Antimicrob Chemother* 44(Suppl B):23–29.

Murphy K, Eivindson A, Pauksens K, Stein WJ, Tellier G, Watts R, Leophonte P, Sharp SJ, Loeschel E. 2000. Efficacy and safety of inhaled zanamivir for the treatment of influenza in patients with asthma or chronic obstructive pulmonary disease. *Clin Drug Invest* 20:337–349.

Nafta I, Turcanu AG, Braun I, Companetz W, Simionescu A, Birt E, Florea V. 1970. Administration of amantadine for the prevention of Hong Kong influenza. *Bull WHO* 42:423–427.

NIAID (National Institute of Allergy and Infectious Diseases). 2004. *NIAID Taps Chiron to Develop Vaccine Against H9N2 Avian Influenza.* Award Part of NIAID Pandemic Influenza Preparedness Program. [Online]. Available: http://www2.niaid.nih.gov/newsroom/releases/h9n2.htm [accessed November 10, 2004].

Nichol KL, Nordin J, Mullooly J, Lask R, Fillbrandt K, Iwane M. 2003. Influenza vaccination and reduction in hospitalizations for cardiac disease and stroke among the elderly. *N Engl J Med* 348:1322–1332.

Node K, Fujita M, Kitakaze M, Hori M, Liao JK. 2003. Short-term statin therapy improves cardiac function and symptoms in patients with idiopathic dilated cardiomyopathy. *Circulation* 108:839–843.

Novak K. 2003. The WTO's balancing act. *J Clin Invest* 112:1269–1273.

Official Journal of the European Community. 1995. Article 7b, Regulation 541/95. European Union: Publications Office of the European Union.

Official Journal of the European Community. 2003. Article 8, Regulation 1085/2003. European Union: Publications Office of the European Union.

Oker-Blom N, Hovi T, Leinikki P, Palosuo T, Pettersson R, Suni J. 1970. Protection of man from natural infection with influenza A2 Hong Kong virus by amantadine: A controlled field trial. *BMJ* 3:676–678.

Patriarca PA, Cox NJ. 1997. Influenza pandemic preparedness plan for the United States. *J Infect Dis* 176(Suppl 1):S4–S7.

Peiris JS, Yu WC, Leung CW, Cheung CY, Ng WF, Nicholls JM, Ng TK, Chan KH, Lai ST, Lim WL, Yuen KY, Guan Y. 2004. Re-emergence of fatal human influenza A subtype H5N1 disease. *Lancet* 363:617–619.

Peters PH, Gravenstein S, Norwood P, DeBock V, Van Cauter A, Gibbens M, van Planta T-A, Ward P. 2001. Long term use of oseltamivir for the prophylaxis of influenza in a vaccinated frail older population. *J Am Geriatric Soc* 49:1–7.

Pettersson RF, Hellstrom PE, Penttinen K, Pyhala R, Tokola O, Vartio T, Visakorpi R. 1980. Evaluation of amantadine in the prophylaxis of influenza A (H1N1) virus infection: A controlled field trial among young adults and high-risk patients. *J Infect Dis* 142:377–383.

Plotkin E, Bernheim J, Ben-Chetrit S, Mor A, Korzets Z. 2000. Influenza vaccine—a possible trigger of rhabdomyolysis induced acute renal failure due to the combined use of cerivastatin and bezafibrate. *Nephrol Dial Transplant* 15:740–741.

Quarles JM, Couch RB, Cate TR, Goswick CB. 1981. Comparison of amantadine and rimantadine for prevention of type A (Russian) influenza. *Antiviral Res* 1:149–155.

Reichert TA, Simonsen L, Sharma A, Pardo SA, Fedson DS, Miller MA. 2004. Influenza and the winter increase in mortality in the United States, 1959–1999. *Am J Epidemiol* 160:492–502.

Sacks FM. 2004. High-intensity statin treatment for coronary heart disease. *JAMA* 291:1132–1134.

Schoch-Spana M. 2000. Implications of pandemic influenza for bioterrorism response. *Clinical Infectious Diseases* 31:1409–1413. [Online]. Available: http://www.wipo.int.

Smorodintsev AA, Karpuhin GI, Zlydnikov DM, Malyseva AM, Svecova EG, Burov SA, Hramcova LM, Romanov JA, Taros LJ, Ivannikov JG, Novoselov SD. 1970. The prophylactic effectiveness of amantadine hydrochloride in an epidemic of Hong Kong influenza in Leningrad in 1969. *Bull WHO* 42:865–872.

Stilianakis NI, Perelson AS, Hayden FG. 1998. Emergence of drug resistance during an influenza epidemic: Insights from a mathematical model. *J Infect Dis* 177:863–873.

Subbarao K, Chen H, Swayne D, Mingay L, Fodor E, Brownlee G, Xu X, Lu X, Katz J, Cox N, Matsuoka Y. 2003. Evaluation of a genetically modified reassortant H5N1 influenza A virus vaccine candidate generated by plasmid-based reverse genetics. *Virology* 305:192–200.

Tisdale M. 2000. Monitoring of viral susceptibility: New challenges with the development of influenza NA inhibitors. *Rev Med Virol* 10:45–55.

Topol EJ. 2004. Intensive statin therapy—a sea change in cardiovascular prevention. *N Engl J Med* 350:1562–1564.

Treanor JJ, Hayden FG, Vrooman PS, Barbarash R, Bettis R, Riff D, Singh S, Kinnersley N, Ward P, Mills RG. 2000. Efficacy and safety of the oral neuraminidase inhibitor oseltamivir in treating acute influenza: A randomized controlled trial. U.S. Oral Neuraminidase Study Group. *JAMA* 283:1016–1024.

VanVoris LP, Betts RF, Hayden FG, Christmas WA, Douglas RGJ. 1981. Successful treatment of naturally occurring influenza A/USSR/77 H1N1. *JAMA* 245:1128–1131.

Walker JB, Hussey EK, Treanor JJ, Montalvo A, Hayden FG. 1997. Effects of the neuraminidase inhibitor zanamivir on otologic manifestations of experimental human influenza. *J Infect Dis* 176:1417–1422.

Webby RJ, Perez DR, Coleman JS, Guan Y, Knight JH, Govorkova EA, McClain-Moss LR, Peiris JS, Rehg JE, Tuomanen EI, Webster RG. 2004. Responsiveness to a pandemic alert: Use of reverse genetics for rapid development of influenza vaccines. *Lancet* 363:1099–1103.

Welliver R, Manto AS, Carewicz O, Schatteman E, Hassman M, Hedrick J, Huson L, Ward P, Oxford JS. 2001. Effectiveness of oseltamivir in preventing influenza in household contacts. *JAMA* 285:748–754.

Whitley RJ, Hayden FG, Reisinger K, Young N, Dutkowski R, Ipe D, Mills RG, Ward P. 2001. Oral oseltamivir treatment of influenza in children. *Pediatr Infect Dis J* 20:127–133.

WHO (World Health Organization). 2004 (April 27). *WHO Consultation on Priority Public Health Interventions Before and During an Influenza Pandemic.* [Online]. Available: http://www.who.int/csr/disease/avian_influenza/guidelines/pandemicconsultation/en/ [accessed December 17, 2004].

Wood JM. 2001. Developing vaccines against pandemic influenza. *Philos Trans R Soc Lond B Biol Sci* 356:1953–1960.

Wood JM, Lewandowski RA. 2003. The influenza vaccine licensing process. *Vaccine* 21:1786–1788.

Ziegler T, Hemphill ML, Ziegler ML, Perez-Oronoz G, Klimov AI, Hampson AW, Regnery HL, Cox NJ. 1999. Low incidence of rimantadine resistance in field isolates of influenza A viruses. *J Infect Dis* 180:935–939.

4

Strategies for Controlling Avian Influenza in Birds and Mammals

OVERVIEW

To address the threat that avian influenza (AI) poses to human health, it is necessary to recognize its broader agricultural and economic implications and to integrate this knowledge into disease control strategies. This chapter focuses on the global phenomenon of avian influenza, its impact on the poultry industry, and potential means to control influenza transmission among birds and mammals.

The chapter begins with a review of the activities of the Office International des Épizooties (OIE; also known as the World Organisation for Animal Health), an international and intergovernmental organization at the forefront of animal disease control. The OIE is developing influenza surveillance guidelines that encompass birds, domestic mammals, wildlife, and humans. The OIE recently initiated cooperation between its global network of reference laboratories and that of the World Health Organization (WHO); the partners plan to exchange scientific information on avian influenza, share viral isolates, and may eventually manufacture human vaccines against avian viral strains.

While avian influenza is an uncommon disease of poultry in the United States, the U.S. Department of Agriculture (USDA) recognizes the international importance of the disease and has developed considerable animal health policies to detect, prevent, and control avian influenza. These strategies are presented, along with background information on the biology, ecology, and epidemiology of avian influenza, by David Swayne and David Suarez of the USDA. They review evidence that supports intervention and surveillance focused on the subset of avian influenza viruses that pose significant risk of infecting humans, including certain viruses of low pathogenicity in poultry. The chapter concludes with an example of a low-pathogen avian influenza outbreak in a group of commercial poultry farms and the steps the industry took to contain further spread of the virus, minimize the risk of exposure, and monitor and prevent further infections.

STANDARDS AND ACTIVITIES OF THE OIE RELATED TO AVIAN INFLUENZA

Dewan Sibartie

Scientific and Technical Department
World Organisation for Animal Health (OIE)

Introduction

Preventing the spread of animal diseases and zoonoses through international trade is one of the primary objectives of the World Organisation for Animal Health (OIE). This is accomplished by establishing international standards that facilitate trade while minimizing the risk of introducing infectious animal diseases and zoonoses. The OIE was founded in 1924, as a result of an outbreak of rinderpest in Belgium. Initially 28 countries united with a mandate to share information on animal disease outbreaks to allow the Member Countries to take the appropriate control measures to protect themselves and to prevent further spread of the disease. A total of 167 countries now form part of the OIE, and providing a mechanism for prompt reporting of disease outbreaks and occurrences is still one of the OIE's primary roles.

Over the years, the OIE has been strongly committed to convincing national policy makers and international donors that the cost of strengthening veterinary services to provide better surveillance, early warning systems, and management of epizootics, including zoonoses, is negligible compared to the economic losses resulting from introduction of infectious animal diseases and zoonoses.

The OIE objectives and activities for the prevention and control of infectious animal diseases and zoonoses are focused on the following areas:

- **Transparency in animal disease status worldwide**
  Each Member Country is committed to reporting to the OIE on its health status regarding significant animal diseases and diseases transmissible to humans. The OIE then disseminates the informa-

tion to all Member Countries to enable them to take appropriate actions to protect themselves.

- **Collection, analysis, and dissemination of veterinary information**
  Using its network of internationally recognized scientists, the OIE collects, analyzes, and publishes the latest scientific information on important animal diseases, including those transmissible to humans, especially regarding their prevention and control.
- **Strengthening of international coordination and cooperation in the control of animal diseases**
  The OIE provides technical expertise to Member Countries requesting assistance with animal disease control and eradication programs, particularly in developing countries. These activities are performed in coordination with other international organizations responsible for supporting and funding the eradication of infectious animal diseases and zoonoses.
- **Promotion of the safety of world trade in animals and animal products**
  The OIE develops standards for application by Member Countries to protect themselves against disease incursions as a result of trade in animals and animal products, while avoiding unjustified sanitary barriers. These standards are developed by experts from Member Countries and from the OIE's network of more than 160 Collaborating Centers and Reference Laboratories.

In 1995 the standards developed by the OIE were formalized as international standards by the Agreement on the Application of Sanitary and Phytosanitary Measures (SPS Agreement) of the World Trade Organization (World Trade Organization, 1995). In order to harmonize SPS measures and remove unjustifiable sanitary or health restrictions on international trade, the Agreement states that governments should follow these international standards, guidelines, and recommendations. The goal of the Agreement is to minimize the risk of disease transmission and remove unjustifiable sanitary or health restrictions on international trade. The Agreement states that it is the sovereign right of a country to provide an appropriate level of animal and public health protection at its borders. However, this sovereign right is not to be misused for protectionist purposes: An importing country can only apply sanitary measures to imports if a similar level of protection is applied to all imports and internally by the importing country. Member Countries can introduce standards providing a higher level of protection than that provided by the OIE standards if there is a scientific justification, but these standards must be based on a science-based risk analysis.

The OIE recognizes highly pathogenic avian influenza (HPAI) as an

OIE list A[1] disease having the potential for very serious and rapid spread, irrespective of national borders, which can be of serious socioeconomic and public health consequences and which is of major importance to the international trade of poultry and poultry products. Since 1996 it has become clear that avian influenza viruses may be important pathogens capable of infecting humans directly without reassortment. This has been observed during the recent outbreaks of AI in southeast Asia. However, like other organizations also concerned with human health, the OIE is highly concerned about the possibility that the virus can undergo genetic reassortment and become transmissible within humans, resulting in a pandemic capable of claiming millions of lives, as was the case during the so-called Spanish flu of 1918. Firmly convinced that the best way to reduce human exposure to the virus is to eliminate the virus at source—that is, from animals, including wild birds—the OIE strives to assist Member Countries in providing expertise particularly in the following areas: disease surveillance, early detection, early warning and notification, quality and evaluation of veterinary services, diagnosis, surveillance, control strategies, and international trade in poultry and poultry products.

OIE Reference Laboratories and Experts

The OIE is coordinating a worldwide network of some 150 Reference Laboratories and 13 Collaborating Centers and more than 300 experts in various animal diseases. For avian influenza, there are currently six Reference Laboratories and eight experts, but the OIE also benefits from the expertise of other internationally renowned scientists in the field of AI who are called on to assist OIE ad hoc groups or to carry out technical missions on behalf of the OIE in countries affected by the disease. The OIE Reference Laboratories played a particularly significant role during the avian influenza outbreaks in southeast Asia caused by H5NI strain of the AI virus. Not only have the experts of those laboratories provided technical advice, but they have, for example, also provided useful diagnostic material such as H5 antigens to laboratories in affected countries to assist them in their diagnosis. The application of the Differentiating Infected from Vaccinated Animals (DIVA) tests developed by the OIE Reference Laboratory in Italy will be particularly useful for countries that will embark on the use of marker vaccines for the control of AI. The OIE Reference Laboratories also conduct training courses for technical staff in the diagnosis of the disease and characterization of the virus. In addition, the OIE Reference Laborato-

---

[1]Diseases to be urgently notified by Member Countries.

ries are arranging cooperation with the network of the WHO Influenza Reference Laboratories for the exchange of scientific information, sharing of viruses for strain characterizations, and if necessary, the manufacture of human vaccines from poultry strains of the virus.

OIE Standards

One of the major activities of the OIE is to develop standards, guidelines, and recommendations for the diagnosis and control of important animal diseases, including zoonoses. OIE standards are science-based and are developed by experts and approved by the OIE International Committee, which has representatives from the 167 Member Countries. The World Trade Organization Agreement on Sanitary and Phyto-Sanitary (WTO-SPS) measures recognizes the OIE as the only international organization for setting standards on animal diseases and zoonoses. Standards concerning terrestrial (nonaquatic) animals are contained in the Terrestrial Animal Health Code (the *Terrestrial Code*) (World Organisation for Animal Health, 2003) and the OIE *Manual of Diagnostic Tests and Vaccines*, or Terrestrial Manual (World Organisation for Animal Health, 2004a). The Terrestrial Code provides the governments and the Chief Veterinary Officers of OIE Member Countries with recommendations for establishing national health measures or rules applicable to the importation of animals and animal products with respect to OIE listed animal diseases in order to avoid importation of pathogens while avoiding unjustified sanitary barriers. The Terrestrial Manual describes the diagnostic methods that are to be used and the methods for the production and control of biological products, including vaccines.

The Terrestrial Code

Definition of avian influenza infection. Chapter 2.1.14 of the Terrestrial Code provides standards for highly pathogenic avian influenza (HPAI). However, in view of the latest scientific advances, especially regarding the potential risks posed by low-pathogenic strains and the ability of the virus to infect humans, a new Chapter (World Organisation for Animal Health, 2004b) has been proposed by an OIE ad hoc group of experts and is being studied by OIE Member Countries. A new definition of notifiable avian influenza has been proposed as follows:

> For the purposes of this Terrestrial Code, notifiable avian influenza (NAI) is defined as an infection of poultry caused by any influenza A virus of the H5 or H7 subtypes or by any AI virus with an intravenous pathogenicity index (IVPI) greater than 1.2 (or as an alternative at least 75 percent mortality) as described below. NAI viruses can be divided into highly

pathogenic notifiable avian influenza (HPNAI) and low-pathogenicity notifiable avian influenza (LPNAI):

1.   HPNAI viruses have an IVPI in 6-week-old chickens greater than 1.2 or, as an alternative, cause at least 75 percent mortality in 4- to 8-week-old chickens infected intravenously. H5 and H7 viruses, which do not have an IVPI of greater than 1.2 or cause less than 75 percent mortality in an intravenous lethality test, should be sequenced to determine whether multiple basic amino acids are present at the cleavage site of the hemagglutinin molecule (HA); if the amino acid motif is similar to that observed for other HPNAI isolates, the isolate being tested should be considered as HPNAI.

2.   LPNAI are all influenza A viruses of H5 and H7 subtypes that are not HPNAI viruses.

Disease notification.   The current Terrestrial Code provides for countries to report HPAI within 24 hours. If the proposed Chapter is approved, countries would start notifying all NAI as defined above. Countries also need to report a provisional diagnosis of HPAI if this represents important new information of epidemiological significance to other countries. The OIE in turn forwards this information to other countries in order for countries at risk to take appropriate precautions. Following outbreaks of AI in southeast Asia, the OIE collaborated with other international organizations to provide expertise to countries in the region to improve their disease reporting systems. Thanks to the "rumours tracking system," the OIE has been able to query some countries about rumours of the possible occurrence of AI in those countries. This system proved effective in that at least two countries that had not reported the disease to the OIE then confirmed the presence of the disease. In view of the zoonotic importance of the disease, the OIE is working in close collaboration with WHO on the notification of all important zoonoses. As a result there is constant and instant sharing of information between the two organizations about the occurrence of AI in animals and humans.

Evaluation of veterinary services.   The Terrestrial Code provides guidelines for the quality and the evaluation of veterinary services (which include public and private components) in Member Countries. This is important to assert the credibility of the services because it enhances the international acceptance of the certification of exports and facilitates the risk analysis process of an importing country. The results of this evaluation can help provide the importing country the assurance that information on sanitary/zoosanitary situations provided by the veterinary services of an exporting country is objective, meaningful, and correct. Evaluation of veterinary services has gained further importance since the ban on imports of poultry and poultry products from several southeast Asian countries following the avian influenza crisis. For countries to resume their trade, especially with Europe, the veterinary services must demonstrate efficiency in terms of diagnosis, surveillance, and certification for exports. The Terrestrial Code spells out the procedures for an independent and reliable certification free from political or other commercial considerations.

International trade of poultry and poultry products. As mentioned earlier, the OIE provides standards, guidelines and recommendations to assure the sanitary safety of international trade in animals and animal products to avoid the transfer of agents pathogenic for animals or humans while avoiding unjustified sanitary barriers. In this context, the OIE is fully aware of the constraints faced by countries wishing, for example, to export fresh poultry meat. These constraints relate mainly to vaccination, surveillance, and zoning/compartmentalization. The new proposed Chapter attempts to solve some of these constraints, especially in the light of the outbreaks in southeast Asia, Europe, and North America. During a meeting of AI experts jointly organized by the Food and Agriculture Organization of the United Nations (FAO), the OIE, and WHO, held in February 2004 in Bangkok, Thailand, the three organizations agreed that due to ethical, social, economic, and environmental reasons, the stamping-out policy may not be appropriate for some countries in the region. Thus they recommended that vaccination, which has proved to reduce morbidity, mortality, and virus shedding, can provide an additional useful tool in those countries provided that the vaccines used comply with the standards of the OIE Terrestrial Manual and that vaccines are administered under the supervision of the official veterinary services. The veterinary services should have the necessary expertise and resources to ensure that appropiate and adequate surveillance is carried out to avoid possible problems caused by vaccination, the main one being the difficulty in differentiating infected from vaccinated animals by serology.

The proposed Code Chapter allows the export of live birds from countries, zones, or compartments that have been vaccinated provided details of the vaccines and the vaccination programs are stated. In order to assist well-managed enterprises with a high level of biosecurity to export, the Chapter proposes that the concept of compartmentalization be adopted. The Code defines "compartmentalization" as "one or more establishments under a common biosecurity management system containing an animal subpopulation with a distinct health status with respect to a specific disease for which required surveillance, control, and biosecurity measures have been applied for the purpose of international trade." This concept will enable countries having integrated and well-managed poultry enterprises to export under certain conditions even if the rest of the country is infected.

The new Chapter also proposes that a country or zone/compartment may be considered free from NAI when it has been shown that NAI infection has not been present for the past 12 months. If infected poultry are slaughtered, this period shall be 3 months (instead of 6) after the slaughter of the last infected poultry and disinfection of all affected premises. This would encourage countries wishing to resume exports to carry out stamping-out whenever feasible and apply strict biosecurity measures.

The OIE has already put at the disposal of Member Countries relevant expertise to help them improve the production and quality control of vaccines. Such help is also available for the establishment of OIE Reference Laboratories on AI.

Surveillance and monitoring of animal health. The Terrestrial Code has a generic chapter outlining the general requirements for a country to carry out surveillance and monitoring of animal health. The fundamental principles described in that Chapter also apply to avian influenza. However, an OIE ad hoc group of experts will soon be working on a specific Chapter on surveillance guidelines for avian influenza, taking on board the latest scientific knowledge on AI. In the meantime the new proposed Chapter on AI spells out certain general ideas on serological surveillance in flocks, especially in the presence of vaccination. The DIVA tests developed by an OIE Reference Laboratory will prove helpful to countries using marker vaccines. The principle of this test is accepted by the OIE, and further work on its applicability to other animal diseases is in progress in some OIE Reference Laboratories.

Information provided by the exporting country's surveillance and monitoring program is considered to be a key component of the risk analysis conducted by an importing country. OIE has provided and will continue to provide expert assistance to southeast Asian countries to improve surveillance and monitoring systems to control the disease. The OIE advises that countries establish programs to monitor high-risk avian populations, such as live bird markets, fighting cocks, and other markets selling wild birds. This should decrease the risk of AI transmission through trade.

The Terrestrial Code also provides detailed procedures for conducting a risk analysis that also applies to AI. Member Countries are allowed under the WTO-SPS Agreement to apply a higher level of SPS measures provided there is a scientific justification and it is supported by a risk analysis.

The Terrestrial Manual

The Terrestrial Manual is a companion volume to the Terrestrial Code and provides a uniform approach to the diagnosis of HPAI. Its purpose is also to facilitate international trade in animals and animal products by describing internationally agreed-on laboratory methods for avian influenza diagnosis and requirements for the production and quality control of AI vaccines. The methods described also form the basis for effective avian influenza surveillance and monitoring. The serological techniques described include the hemagglutination-inhibition and agar gel immunodiffusion tests. The immunodiffusion test is a group-specific test that can detect all strains of avian influenza virus and is appropriate for a monitoring program. The Chapter also mentions the use of commercial Enzyme Linked Immunosorbent Assay (ELISA) kits that detect antibody against the nucleocapsid protein. Such tests have usually been evaluated and validated by the manufacturer, and it is essential that the manufacturer's instructions be followed. Although not specifically mentioned in the Chapter on HPAI, the importance of marker vaccines and the DIVA test are well recognized by the OIE. Virus isolation techniques and virus characterization techniques for the confirmation of HPAI are also described in detail.

Stamping-Out and Carcass Disposal

The OIE continues to rely on the principle that stamping-out remains the method of choice for the rapid elimination of the virus and thus its spread to humans, but is fully aware that this method is not applicable to certain countries for reasons stated earlier. For this reason, the OIE has an ad hoc group that has formulated recommendations for the mass slaughter of animals during an emergency and the safe disposal of carcasses. These methods vary depending on the available resources, equipment, and infrastructure. Work is progressing by an OIE ad hoc group on carcass disposal, and the OIE will finalize details of the methods applicable in different situations.

Food Safety

In pursuance with one of its missions to ensure safety of food of animal origin, OIE experts have conducted research on the possible contamination of humans through the consumption of poultry meat or products. This has been particularly important during the recent influenza outbreaks in southeast Asia, when consumption of these commodities fell drastically, threatening millions of farmers who depend almost entirely on subsistence animal farming for their livelihoods. Therefore it was important to restore consumer confidence in poultry products. OIE experts have concluded that humans can only be infected while in contact with infected birds and that the main mode of transmission in humans in the context of this Asian epizootic is by the respiratory route. In addition, they have demonstrated that when poultry products are cooked to an internal temperature of at least 70°C, the virus is destroyed.

The Role of Wildlife

The role of wildlife in the transmission and spread of AI has been widely discussed by the international scientific community. In a February 2004 meeting, the OIE experts in the Working Group on Wildlife Diseases reviewed the available literature and other relevant documentation and made the following salient observations:

- Virtually all H and N combinations have been isolated from birds.
- Wild birds, particularly those associated with aquatic environments, are the reservoirs of viruses of low virulence for poultry.
- Viruses may become virulent following transmission and cycling in commercial poultry.
- There is current concern about the lack of knowledge on the prevalence of viruses of H5 and H7 subtypes in bird populations.
- Outbreaks of disease in commercial poultry have been linked to a close association between commercial poultry and waterfowl on many occasions.
- Isolation of virus from other wild birds is completely overshadowed by the number, variety, and distribution of influenza viruses isolated from waterfowl. The highest rate of detection of influenza virus is from ducks.
- The concentration of ducks, their potential to excrete high levels of virus and its ability to remain viable in an aquatic environment means that "large" areas of the environment will be contaminated.
- Different virus subtypes can be identified simultaneously within a single bird.
- The predominant subtype isolated from domestic ducks varies from year to year.
- Natural protection of ducks does not provide cross-protection between influenza A subtypes.
- Influenza viruses can sweep through bird populations without having any signs of disease present.
- Studies indicate that the viruses identified in Eurasia and Australia are genetically distinct from those in North America. This most likely reflects the distinct flyways of each hemisphere.
- There is an "avian influenza season" (at least in temperate countries) in the fall/winter.
- Surveillance programs of wild birds when outbreaks of poultry influenza have occurred often find little or no signs of infection.

Therefore, they recommend that as far as practically possible, wild birds should be separated from commercial poultry. Surveillance programs should also be conducted in wild birds, placing more emphasis on ducks and using sentinel birds to detect presence of the disease; in temperate zones, surveying should be concentrated in young birds in the fall/winter. They also emphasized that surveillance is of global interest because this type of information in one country is important for other countries to know.

However, the Working Group is of the unanimous opinion that the role of wild birds in occurrences of virulent influenza A in poultry and in humans is widely misunderstood. Virulent strains of these viruses seldom have been found in wild birds, even in association with outbreaks in poultry. The Working Group does not contest the possibility that the co-cycling of more than one influenza strain within a so-called "mixing vessel" host such as the pig may result in genetic exchanges and genetic shift. Such events could result in the evolution of highly pathogenic viral strains with rapid passaging and spread, especially within and between intensively farmed poultry houses, and with high risk of "cross-over" infection to humans. Control programs for virulent strains of avian influenza viruses therefore should be focused on biosecurity of poultry populations and protection of humans exposed to poultry.

Continual OIE Involvement

The OIE continues to monitor the worldwide AI situation closely, paying particular attention to southeast Asia, where the disease has far more economic and possibly more public health impact. Relevant information is posted continuously on the OIE website (http://www.oie.int) to update Member Countries on the prevailing situation. On March 19, 2004, the OIE again alerted countries on the unjustified optimism being displayed by certain countries on the perception that the epidemic is over. The OIE has appealed to Member Countries to maintain vigilance because the virus is still circulating and eradication is a long way ahead. This has been proven to be true as outbreaks of highly pathogenic avian influenza have again been recently recorded in some countries of southeast Asia that thought they had successfully overcome the outbreaks.

Since January 27, 2004, the OIE has been alerting international donors about the pressing need to provide assistance to countries in southeast Asia affected by the disease. Assistance also should be provided to strengthen veterinary services and to improve surveillance and early response to diseases. There cannot be any delay in this assistance not only because of economic reasons, but because no opportunity should be given to that virus to undergo genetic reassortment in human beings and thus create a new human influenza pandemic.

U.S. STRATEGIES FOR CONTROLLING AVIAN INFLUENZA IN AGRICULTURAL SYSTEMS

David E. Swayne and David L. Suarez

U.S. Department of Agriculture, Agriculture Research Service, Southeast Poultry Research Laboratory, Athens, Georgia

Abstract

Strategies to control avian influenza virus are developed to prevent, manage, or eradicate the virus from a country, region, state, county, or farm. These strategies are developed using various aspects of five components: (1) biosecurity, (2) diagnostics and surveillance, (3) eliminating poultry infected with AI virus, (4) decreasing host susceptibility to the virus, and (5) education. Avian influenza in U.S. commercial poultry is uncommon. Prevention of AI is the preferred strategy and is practiced primarily by reducing the risk of introduction or exposure. The primary risks for introduction into commercial poultry include: (1) direct access to wild birds infected with AI viruses, (2) the drinking water source being untreated surface water contaminated with AI viruses, (3) location in the same geographic region as pigs infected with endemic swine influenza virus (turkey breeder hens only), and (4) epidemiologic links to a live poultry marketing system. Vaccines are uncommon and used only in areas of high risk. The USDA licenses all AI vaccines. However, both the USDA and state veterinarian determine when licensed vaccines can be used in the field.

Background on Avian Influenza

Avian influenza is a disease of birds caused by type A orthomyxovirus (Swayne and Halvorson, 2003). Avian influenza viruses are pleomorphic and have eight segments of single-stranded, negative-sense RNA that code for 10 proteins. These proteins include two surface glycoproteins, the hemagglutinin (HA) and neuraminidase (NA), and internal proteins such as the matrix (M) and nucleoproteins (NP). Serologic reaction in the agar gel immunodiffusion (AGID) test to the M and NP is the basis for speciation or classification of all AI viruses as type A influenza viruses (influenza A viruses). Furthermore, serologic reaction to the HA and NA are the basis for subtyping into 15 HA (H1-15) and 9 NA (N1-9) subtypes, respectively.

Avian influenza viruses are grouped into two broad pathotypes based on virulence in chickens: (1) viruses of low virulence, that is, low-pathogenicity AI (LPAI); and (2) viruses of high virulence, that is, high-pathogenicity AI (HPAI) (Swayne and Halvorson, 2003; Swayne and Suarez, 2000). The

LPAI viruses can be any of the hemagglutinin (H1-15) and neuraminidase (N1-9) subtypes. The LPAI viruses cause various clinical problems ranging from clinically in apparent infections to drops in egg production and mild respiratory disease with low mortality rates. However, more severe respiratory disease and higher mortality rates may be seen when such infections are accompanied by secondary viral or bacterial pathogens. By contrast, HPAI viruses have all been of the H5 or H7 hemagglutinin subtypes and produces severe, often fatal, systemic disease affecting multiple internal organ systems. In birds raised on the ground, the infection spreads rapidly, but in poultry houses where birds are caged, the infection may spread more slowly. Infections with HPAI may present with depression, decreased feed consumption, and possibly neurological signs. Lesions seen may include edema-to-necrosis of comb and wattles, edema of the head and legs, subcutaneous hemorrhages of feet, petechial hemorrhages on surface of viscera, and pulmonary edema, congestion, and hemorrhage. For regulatory purposes, AI viruses are classified as high pathogenicity (HP) when they cause 75 percent or greater mortality in intravenously inoculated chickens (all HA subtypes) or have a deduced amino acid sequence at the hemagglutinin proteolytic cleavage site compatible with HPAI virus (H5 or H7 only).

Type A influenza viruses are continually changing either through random mutation in the genome (drift) or through rearrangement of gene segments between two different influenza viruses (shift). The latter results in hybrid or reassortant viruses.

Several detailed reviews have been published in the general area of AI (Swayne and Halvorson, 2003) and HPAI (Swayne and Suarez, 2000), ecology and epidemiology of AI (Swayne, 2000; Webster et al., 1992), AI vaccines (Swayne, 2003), AI control in the United States (Swayne and Akey, 2004), and immunology of avian influenza (Suarez and Schultz, 2000).

Ecology and Epidemiology

Avian influenza viruses exist in five discrete ecosystems (Swayne, 2000). The reservoir for genes of all type A influenza viruses circulate in wild bird populations, principally waterfowl (Order: Anseriformes) and shorebirds (Order: Charadriiformes), but to a lesser frequency in other wild birds, especially in aquatic habitats (Kawaoka et al., 1988; Slemons et al., 1974). The virus appears to be well adapted to these species, causing only an asymptomatic enteric infection with large amounts of virus being shed into the environment. For ducks, such as mallard or pintail ducks, the highest incidence of infection is usually in the fall, when large numbers of young naïve ducks congregate before flying south for the winter. The incidence of infection typically drops to low levels in the winter months, but virus can often be isolated all year long. The wild bird population therefore remains a reservoir source of virus that cannot be practically controlled (Stallknecht and Shane, 1988). Most AI viruses isolated from wild birds are low pathogenicity (LP), but a few have been HP, especially when isolated from wild birds trapped on poultry farms affected with HPAI.

Common poultry species, including chickens and turkeys, are not natural hosts for avian influenza viruses (Hopkins et al., 1990; Suarez, 2000). If chickens are experimentally infected with wild duck isolates, typically the viruses will replicate at low levels, not be transmitted efficiently from bird to bird, and cause little to no disease (Lee et al., 2004). In this situation, the virus will typically fail to maintain itself in the poultry population with or without human intervention. However, through captivation and domestication, humans have altered the natural ecosystems and created four new and different ecosystems where AI viruses may exist and cause avian infections: (1) backyard (village) and recreational poultry (fighting cocks), (2) live poultry market system, (3) outdoor-reared semi-commercial to industrial poultry (ducks and geese, meat turkeys, and "organic" chickens), and (4) indoor-reared industrial poultry (broilers [meat chickens], meat turkeys, egg-laying chickens, breeders, and ducks). However, the risk for AI virus introduction and maintenance varies with each ecosystem. The ecosystems with the highest risk for AI virus infections are 1, 2, and 3 because they may have direct or indirect exposure to wild birds that carry AI viruses. Mixing of poultry species on a farm increases the opportunity for crossing species and adaptation.

Species Adaptation and Transmission

Influenza viruses adapt and have optimal replication in a single animal species with common and easy intraspecies transmission. However, interspecies transmission within the same class is occasionally reported, such as pig to human or wild mallard to domestic turkey. Most rarely, transmission has occurred interspecies and interclass, such as bird to human and bird to pig. Such interspecies transmission is usually inefficient and produces self-limiting infections. However, the influenza A viruses can adapt to the new host species through circulation as low-level infections within a population and, through random mutations in the viral genome, gradually adapt to the new species with increased efficiency of replication and transmission. Alternatively, an existing influenza A virus can reassort with another influenza A virus, producing a hybrid influenza A virus with the resulting eight gene segments being a combination of those from the two viruses. This type of change produced the human pandemic viruses of 1957 and 1968, and the H3N2 swine influenza viruses reported recently in the past 20 years around the world.

Risk Factors for Introduction of Influenza Virus A into Poultry

There are several recognized risk factors for the introduction of influenza A viruses into domestic poultry. The first is direct access of poultry to wild birds infected with AI viruses, especially wild ducks. A good example of this is turkeys in Minnesota that were raised outdoors ("on range") in the 1980s and early 1990s (Halvorson et al., 1985). Outbreaks of multiple subtypes of avian influenza occurred routinely in the fall, when infected ducks had the opportunity to commingle with turkeys. Once the virus was introduced onto a turkey farm, the virus could become adapted to turkeys and spread to other turkey farms by the movement of infected birds and contaminated materials. In the late 1990s, the practice of range-rearing turkeys was greatly diminished in favor of confinement rearing. This management change reduced the exposure of turkeys to wild ducks, and the incidence of avian influenza outbreaks was greatly reduced.

A second risk factor has been infection through AI virus-contaminated drinking water. For some poultry operations, the birds' drinking water comes from surface sources, such as a lake, where wild birds often have free access. If the drinking water is not properly purified, avian influenza virus could be introduced by this source. The use of raw drinking water was suggested to be the source of AI outbreaks in the United States, Australia, and Chile (Sivanandan et al., 1991; Suarez et al., 2004).

A third risk factor has been exposure of turkeys to pigs infected with the swine influenza virus. Turkeys are susceptible to swine influenza viruses, and having a turkey farm and swine farm in close proximity is a risk factor for the introduction of swine influenza to turkeys. Infections with both classical H1N1 swine influenza and the more recent reassortant H1N2 and H3N2 swine influenza viruses have been reported (Suarez et al., 2002; Wright et al., 1992).

A fourth risk factor for the introduction of AI viruses into commercial poultry is the live bird marketing system, which is found in many countries around the world, including the United States. Live bird markets offer a variety of birds that can be slaughtered and used for human food consumption. Historically, this system was used as a way to maintain the freshness of the product before refrigeration was available. However, in the United States today, the live poultry markets cater to consumers who enjoy the variety of birds, including several types of chickens, quail, pheasant, ducks, geese, and other birds, and the freshness offered by the markets. These markets are extremely popular with certain ethnic populations, and the consumer pays a premium price for the live bird compared to purchase of a chilled or frozen bird from a supermarket. However, this system provides an ideal environment to introduce and maintain avian influenza viruses into the U.S. poultry population. Domestic waterfowl, primarily ducks, are often raised on ponds where exposure to wild birds, including ducks, is common. This provides a high risk for domestic ducks to be infected with avian influenza. These infected ducks are often sold in the live bird marketing system, where there is close contact with chickens, quail, and other gallinaceous birds. These birds can become infected and will typically stay in the markets for a few days before being slaughtered and sold, providing an opportunity for the virus to infect the naïve birds that are being introduced into the market periodically. Many live bird markets are never free of birds, and a continuous cycle of infection can be maintained, with the virus continuing to become better adapted to chickens. The virus in the live bird market system, although generally believed to be separate from our commercial poultry system, has been a nidus of infection for spread to our commercial poultry sector. One example is the H7N2 AI virus that has been circulating in the northeast United States since 1994 and has been associated with at least five different outbreaks in industrialized poultry in seven states (Spackman et al., 2003). Another example is the H5N1 HPAI in Hong Kong, where the associated risk of domestic waterfowl introducing avian influenza to chickens and other gallinaceous birds has prompted the Hong Kong government to segregate gallinaceous birds, and ducks and geese from being sold together. Additionally, the Hong Kong government instituted periodic market closures to try to break the cycle of infection within the market. These changes have appeared effective in reducing the incidence of infected birds in the markets.

Basic Strategies for Avian Influenza Control

AI control strategies are designed to achieve one of three goals or outcomes (Swayne and Akey, 2004): (1) prevention—preventing introduction of AI, (2) management—reducing losses by minimizing negative economic impact through management practices, or (3) eradication—total elimination of AI. These goals are achieved through specific control strategies developed through incorporation and use of five universal components: (1) biosecurity (exclusion and inclusion), including quarantine, (2) diagnostics and surveillance, (3) elimination of AI virus-infected poultry, (4) decreasing host susceptibility to the virus (vaccines and host genetics), and (5) education of all personnel on infectious diseases and their control. Various combinations of these five components will determine whether the outcome of a control program will be prevention, management or eradication.

With HPAI, the U.S. Department of Agriculture has legal jurisdiction over the outbreak and can declare an animal health emergency. This sets into motion a cooperative state and federal eradication program as established in the Avian Influenza Emergency Disease Guidelines (U.S. Department of Agriculture, 1994) and supplemental documents. By contrast, LPAI is a less severe disease of poultry and is under the control of the animal health authority in each state, but some H5 and H7 LPAI viruses have exhibited the ability to mutate from LP to HP after circulation in domestic poultry. The USDA is developing a control program that will make all H5 and H7 AI viruses eradicable in the United States. Internationally, the OIE establishes the animal health standards for trade in poultry and poultry products, and HPAI is a legitimate non-tariff trade barrier. However, control of H5 and H7 LPAI has become an international issue and the OIE is developing new AI standards that will include control of H5 and H7 LPAI.

Surveillance for Avian Influenza in Poultry

Surveillance can be active or passive. Active surveillance is based on statistical sampling of a population to determine the presence or absence of AI infection and typically has utilized detection of AI-specific antibody. However, during an AI outbreak within an infected zone, surveillance for the AI virus in poultry is necessary. By contrast, passive surveillance, usually in the form of diagnostic investigations of respiratory, reproductive, or high-mortality diseases, is based on clinical submissions and looks for the etiological cause of the disease either by isolating the agent or by detecting specific nucleic acids or proteins, in this case, for AI virus. Passive surveillance is used to detect the first HPAI cases in an AI-free area and for identifying additional cases within an infected zone. Passive surveillance—that is, lack of clinical cases—cannot be used as the criteria to demonstrate eradication of HPAI or freedom from AI infections. Active and passive surveillance for antibodies or AI virus is conducted in individual state veterinary diagnostic laboratories and the National Veterinary Services Laboratories (Ames, Iowa). A national active surveillance program for H5 and H7 AI is under development for meat chickens and turkeys with sampling at all slaughter plants and for all egg-laying chickens on the farm. Poultry products from this new program will be certified H5 and H7 AI free.

In the United States, AI is an uncommon disease of commercial poultry and AI virus infections are equally uncommon. In a nationwide survey of commercial poultry through the National Poultry Improvement Plan in 1997 (Personal communication, Andy Rorer, National Poultry Improvement Plan, U.S. Department of Agriculture, April 28, 2001), no AI virus infections were identified in meat chicken (broilers) or meat turkey flocks (Table 4-1). Antibodies to AI virus were detected in turkey breeders of North Carolina, but these antibodies were the result of vaccination with H1N1 vaccine and not from AI virus infections (Table 4-1). Infections to AI viruses were detected in chickens on ten and two egg-type chicken farms in Pennsylvania and Virginia, respectively. The 10 affected farms represented 3 percent of the total egg-layer farms in Pennsylvania and the virus was an

TABLE 4-1 Results of the 1997 U.S. National Survey for Avian Influenza Virus (AIV) Infections by Antibody Detection

Poultry Group	Total Production		Negative Tests	Positive Flocks
	Birds	Flocks		
Broiler breeders (U.S.)	54,668,743	3,972	265,960	0
Broilers (U.S.)	7,608,400,000	47,553	201,321	0
Turkey breeders (U.S.)	5,876,522	765	60,197	31
North Carolina	1,524,698	203	12,555	31[a]
Meat turkeys (U.S.)	300,495,000	8,265	96,613	0
Commercial layers (U.S.)	258,166,000	3,969	61,662	12
Pennsylvania	22,605,000	348	53,644	10[b]
Virginia	3,463,000	53	248	2[c]

[a]Antibodies to AIV resulted from vaccination with inactivated H1N1 vaccine.
[b]H7N2 AIV was linked epidemiologically and genetically to live poultry markets.
[c]Antibodies to AIV resulted from H1N1 AIV infection.
SOURCE: Andy Rorer, National Poultry Improvement Plan, U.S. Department of Agriculture, 4/28/2001.

H7N2 LPAI virus that spread from the live poultry market system. The two affected farms represented 4 percent of the total egg-layer farms in Virginia and the virus was an H1N1 LP swine influenza virus.

By contrast, the live poultry market system has had LPAI viruses isolated from birds beginning in 1986, with the current H7N2 LPAI virus appearing in 1994 (Mullaney, 2003). The infection rate of the 123 retail markets in the northeast United States has been as high as 60 percent, but control programs have reduced the rate to between 0 and 5 percent. The live poultry market system continues to be a major source of AI viruses and risk for introduction to the commercial poultry operations.

Avian Influenza Vaccines

The AI vaccines provide protection from clinical signs and death, but protection is hemagglutinin subtype specific such that H5 AI vaccines only protect against the H5 subtype, and so on. In addition, AI vaccines can be helpful in decreasing the number of AI virus-infected birds, reducing environmental contamination with the AI virus, preventing spread of AI viruses between farms, and minimizing economic losses. With HPAI, vaccination may help bring an uncontrolled outbreak into a manageable situation, but eradication can only be accomplished if vaccination is accompanied by enhanced biosecurity, active and passive surveillance, education, and elimination of infected poultry as additional components within the control strategy.

In U.S. commercial poultry production, AI is not an endemic disease and vaccination is uncommon. The principal preventive strategy is avoidance of infection by minimizing the risk for AI virus exposure. However, in some areas of the country with high risk of LPAI exposure, limited amounts of vaccine have been used. In 2001, 2,797,000 doses of H1N1 or H1N2 inactivated AI vaccine was used in turkey breeders to prevent infection by swine influenza viruses (Table 4-2) (Swayne, 2001). In layers, 677,000 doses of inactivated H6N2 AI vaccine were used on one egg-laying chicken farm in California (Table 4-2). Vaccine was only used when necessary to prevent an economic animal health issue and was funded by the farmer or production company. Inactivated AI vaccine averages 5 to 7 cents per dose plus 5 to 7 cents to administer each dose.

In the United States, AI vaccines must be licensed by the USDA's Center for Veterinary Biologics, under one of three authorities, before they can be used. Three types of licenses are issued: autogenous, conditional, and full licensure. Full license has been granted for recombinant fowlpox with H5 AI gene insert (1998) and inactivated H5 (1999) vaccine, but they have not been used in United States. Conditional or autogenous licenses have been granted for various hemagglutinin subtypes, including H6 and H7. Vaccines for H5 and H7 require approval from the USDA and the state veterinarian before use, while all other subtypes only require approval by the state veterinarian for use. Worldwide, Mexico, Guatemala, and El Salvador have used more than 1.3 billion doses of inactivated H5N2 AI vaccine since 1995 and 850 million doses of recombinant fowlpox since 1997. In addition, Pakistan has used inactivated H7N3 AI virus vaccine since 1995. Throughout the Middle East, H9N2 LPAI is endemic, and vaccination with inactivated H9N2 vaccine is commonly practiced.

TABLE 4-2 Avian Influenza Vaccine Usage in United States from July 1, 2000, to June 30, 2001

State	Doses	Subtype	Bird Type
California	677,000	H6N4	Single layer farm
Illinois	79,000	H1N1	Turkey breeders
Michigan	118,000	H1N1	Turkey breeders
Minnesota	51,000	H1N1	Turkey breeders
Missouri	100,000	H1N2	Turkey breeders
North Carolina	1,949,000	H1N1	Turkey breeders
Ohio	500,000	H1N1	Turkey breeders
Total	3,474,000		

Public Health Risk for Avian Influenza

AI viruses have rarely produced infections in humans, and these infections rarely result in human-to-human transmission. In addition, not all AI viruses have the same ability to cross the species barrier and infect humans, and AI viruses that are HP for chickens does not predict their ability to infect humans and cause severe disease. In a previous mouse model study using seven H5 HPAI viruses, only the H5N1 HPAI viruses from Hong Kong during 1997 caused high mortality and significant weight loss in BALB/c mice (Table 4-3) (Dybing et al., 2000). One other H5 HPAI virus caused weight loss, but not high mortality (Table 4-3). By comparison, examination of two H7N2 LPAI viruses from the United States in the BALB/c mouse model (Mx-1 influenza-susceptible mice) showed no lethality and more limited infection of the respiratory infection as compared to the highly lethal Hong Kong H5N1 HPAI virus (Table 4-4) (Henzler et al., 2003). Furthermore, in the CAST/Ei mice (Mx+1 influenza-resistant mice), infection with H7N2 LPAI virus was not detected, but H5N1 was still highly lethal for the mice. These studies suggest that some, but not all, AI viruses have the ability to infect mammalian model systems, and intervention strategies should be focused on reducing the risk for those AI viruses with significant risk of infecting humans.

Finally, the H5N1 HPAI viruses of Asia have been the primary focus as the next potential pandemic influenza viruses. However, we must remember that the previous three pandemics (1918, 1957, and 1968) resulted from reassortment of LPAI with human influenza A viruses and not from HPAI viruses. From that viewpoint, the next pandemic virus could be an H9N2, H6N2, H2N2, or any of a number of hemagglutinin and neuraminidase subtypes. Active surveillance in poultry is a critical issue, and signifi-

TABLE 4-3 Differences in Virulence of Seven HPAI Viruses for a BALB/c Mouse Used to Predict Human Infection and Disease (Dybing et al., 2000)

Virus	Mortality	% Change in Body Weight
A/chicken/Italy/97 (H5N2)	0/8	−3
A/chicken/Scotland/59 (H5N9)	0/8	5
A/turkey/England/91 (H5N1)	1/8	−18
A/chicken/Queretaro/20/95 (H5N2)	0/8	−2
A/human/Hong Kong/156/97 (H5N1)	8/8	−26
A/chicken/Hong Kong/220/97 (H5N1)	8/8	−25
A/human/Hong Kong/728/97 (H5N1)	6/8	−10
Sham	0/8	7

TABLE 4-4 Data on Virus Replication and Mortality in BALB/c and CAST/Ei Mice Following Intranasal Inoculation with Two Low- and One High-Pathogenicity AI Viruses

	Mouse Strain							
	BALB/c			CAST/Ei				
	Mortality[a]	Virus Isolation[b]		Mortality[a]	Virus Isolation[b]			
Groups		Trachea	Lung		Trachea	Lung		
Control	0/2	0/2	0/2	0/2	0/2	0/2		
PA/1767/97 (H7N2)	0/5	$1/2(10^{2.5})$	0/2	0/5	0/2	0/2		
PA/19241/97 (H7N2)	0/5	$2/2(10^{6.2})$	$2/2(10^{5.2})$	0/5	0/2	0/2		
HK/156/97 (H5N1)	5/5	$2/2(10^{6.0})$	$2/2(10^{7.8})$	5/5	$2/2(10^{4.0})$	$2/2(10^{7.2})$		

[a]Number of deaths/total mice observed for 10-day period.
[b]Number of positive mice/number of mice with virus isolation attempts (titer of AI virus isolated in EID_{50}/ml), samples were taken on day 4 postinoculation.
SOURCE: Henzler et al. (2003).

cant veterinary diagnostic and regulatory infrastructure improvements are needed in the developing world to accomplish this goal. These aspects in a global control strategy are lacking in most developing countries, especially Asia. This inability to detect and eliminate AI infections prior to human infections and reassortment are the real threats that may lead to the next world pandemic.

LOW-PATHOGENICITY AVIAN INFLUENZA OUTBREAKS IN COMMERCIAL POULTRY IN CALIFORNIA

Carol Cardona, DVM, PhD, dipl. ACPV

University of California, Davis

Outbreak of H6N2 Avian Influenza in California

California has experienced a number of outbreaks of avian influenza in commercial poultry over the years. Most of these outbreaks have been in turkeys and have previously been reported (Ghazikhanian et al., 1981; McCapes et al., 1986). Beginning in 2000, an outbreak of H6N2 avian influenza began in commercial egg-laying chickens in southern California (Webby et al., 2003; Woolcock et al., 2003). Initially, the infecting virus caused no disease or clinical signs; however, by 2001, the virus seemed to be more adapted to growth in chickens in that it seemed to spread more easily, and was associated with decreased egg production and decreased egg quality in infected flocks (Kinde et al., 2003). The outbreak expanded to new areas of the state and to new types of poultry over a period of 2 years. Because the strain of this virus was not H5 and not H7, there were no regulations or plans in place to control this virus. Eventually, the poultry industry of California was able to control this outbreak with a voluntary plan they developed, but it was not before a great deal of damage had been done.

The H6N2 low-pathogenicity strain of avian influenza virus, which infected commercial poultry in California, is not a strain regulated by either the California Department of Food and Agriculture (CDFA) or the USDA. Most American trading partners and, therefore, regulatory agencies, focus on H5 and H7 viruses. This is completely understandable because these are the viruses that may mutate to become highly pathogenic strains (Easterday et al., 1997). After our experience in California, we believe that low-pathogenicity strains of all types can cause significant losses for commercial poultry producers. And the same connections between farms that would spread an H5 or an H7 strain would also result in the spread of a virus of any H or N type. Although state and federal regulatory agencies have focused on specific viruses for a very good reason, this is a rather arbitrary decision and one that has limited the study of the AI viruses that are the most prevalent among avian species.

The Spread of AIV Among Commercial Poultry Farms

Commercial poultry companies are first and foremost businesses. They are streamlined to reduce production and processing costs, while maximizing profit margins. Many of the practices involved in the modern production of poultry also support the spread and amplification of disease agents such as AI virus.

In California's experience with avian influenza, one such practice was the movement of eggs from the farm to the processing plant. Eggs are collected from the flocks that produced them, then brought to processing plants, where they are cleaned and packed for stores. This proved to be an important way in which avian influenza was transmitted from farm to farm. Eggs are packed on reusable flats in the chicken house. Those flats are then placed onto pallets or racks, which go to the processing plant. Most eggs that are packed are clean, but some may be contaminated by fecal material. That fecal material is often transferred to the reusable plastic flats, where it becomes mixed with other organic material such as broken eggs. The reusable flats are emptied at the plant, washed (less than perfectly), returned to pallets or racks, and then returned either to the farm they came from or to another unrelated farm. When flats and racks are sent to different farms, they carry infectious material from their farm of origin, resulting in the spread of disease. We suspect that AI virus spread among many egg-laying farms by this means. Other practices that probably played a part in the spread of AI virus in California include moving live birds to slaughter; moving manure off infected farms; rendering pickups of dead birds; sharing equipment; and using common transporters and service crews. These practices alone are not unsafe and would not be suspect if farms were distant from each other, but they were not.

Poultry farms, like many other types of animal agriculture, are frequently located near each other to take advantage of shared resources. These resources include feed mills, rendering plants, slaughter facilities, and markets. The result has been that in parts of California, Georgia, Arkansas, Iowa, North Carolina, and other states with large poultry industries, there are local regions with dense populations of poultry. These dense populations, if infected with AI virus, can serve to exponentially expand the virus in a relatively small region, resulting in the infection of both commercial and noncommercial poultry.

Concentrations of commercial poultry support the growth of population sectors, which in turn support animal agriculture. The large numbers of low-paying, low-skill positions in animal agriculture often attract new immigrants as workers. These new immigrants are frequently also engaged in activities that involve live birds, such as cockfighting and the purchase of birds for food at live bird markets. The former has been implicated in the spread of the exotic Newcastle disease virus in California and the latter has been implicated in the spread and maintenance of H7N2 avian influenza virus in the northeastern United States (Bulaga et al., 2003). Both of these populations, the game fowl and the birds produced for live bird markets, have the potential to become reservoirs of virus for commercial poultry populations. Unfortunately, in California and in other parts of the country, neither of these populations is surveyed regularly for disease, and few markets utilize veterinary services.

The Control of Low-Pathogenicity Avian Influenza in California

Once the commercial companies involved in the California outbreak realized they could not economically live with this virus, they developed a voluntary control plan that required surveillance and biosecurity, and placed limits on the movements of infected flocks. The first part of the plan required participants to **minimize the risk of exposure** with the following biosecurity practices:

Transportation of birds

1. Minimize the movement of birds
   a. Use on-site composting or cremation if possible to dispose of carcasses after euthanasia
2. Move birds safely, if they must be moved
   a. Avoid driving near other poultry facilities
   b. Test flocks 2 weeks prior to movement
   c. Birds with clinical disease should never be moved
   d. Clean, disinfected trucks should be used
   e. Principles of biosecurity should be closely followed
3. Move infected birds only to slaughter
   a. Actively shedding birds should not be moved to another facility
   b. Previously infected birds are strongly discouraged from movement except to slaughter

Movement of manure

1. Manure trucks must be tarped before they leave any facility
   a. They must follow routes that avoid contact with other poultry traffic

2. Multiple pickups from different farms on the same day are not allowed
3. Manure should be pushed to the edge of the property for pickup
    a. Traffic patterns should be established that avoid interaction between manure trucks and other farm traffic
    b. Scheduling should be done to avoid clean traffic
4. Manure should not be spread or stored close to any other poultry

Marketing of eggs

1. Dedicated racks and flats will be used for each ranch
2. Racks and flats from different ranches will not be commingled
3. Flats will be washed and disinfected at the processing plant
4. Rack washing at the processing plant is strongly encouraged

Feed mills and feed delivery

1. Feed trucks should be cleaned and disinfected at the feed mill
    a. They should be kept away from "clean" areas of the production facility
    b. They should be cleaned and disinfected again when they enter a facility
2. Drivers should be either kept away from "clean" areas or provided with protective clothing
3. All trucks and equipment leaving a facility should be cleaned and disinfected before exiting the facility if suspect or positive flocks are present

Movement of crews

1. A representative of the poultry company will monitor all work performed by crews to ensure that the following rules are observed:
    a. Protective clothing and footwear provided by the ranch must be worn
    b. Hand washing is required before handling birds
    c. Crew vehicles should be cleaned and disinfected before they enter a facility or, preferably, they should be left off site

Mortality disposal

1. Onsite cremation or composting are the preferred methods of mortality disposal
2. Use renderers safely, if they must be used
    a. Tarp trucks
    b. Put mortality pickup at the edge of the property
    c. Coordinate the routing of the truck to avoid "clean" farm traffic

Shared employees

1.   Employees should not be shared by poultry companies
2.   Employees are required to wear clean clothes to work
3.   Employees are required to disinfect their footwear before entering production facilities
4.   Clean rooms for changing and clean clothes should be provided for employees
5.   Shower facilities are optimal, but are not required

Shared equipment

1.   Equipment should not be shared between poultry facilities
2.   If it is shared, it should be cleaned and disinfected at both ends

Physical proximity

1.   Communicate with neighbors to avoid behaviors that endanger each other's flocks
2.   Control vectors (rodents and insects) as much as possible
3.   Communication of disease status between neighbors is required

Common vendors (propane, utility, supplies, etc.)

1.   Keep unnecessary visitors off the farm
2.   Visitors should wear protective clothing to enter the facility
3.   A consistent visitor policy should be established for all premises
4.   Keep a logbook of visitors

The producer participants in the plan were also required to **Monitor for new infections** with the following surveillance of their flocks:

1.   When there is little risk of infection, flocks will be tested at slaughter
2.   During times when there is a risk of infection:
     a.   20 birds will be tested for AI by AGID monthly
     b.   Flocks must be checked daily for:
          1.   Decreases in egg production
          2.   Increased mortality
          3.   Clinical signs of disease

The next critical step is to determine what should happen with a positive flock. Because there was no money for the indemnification of their losses, depopulation of the flocks was not considered an option. However, the producers selected another strategy, controlled marketing, which has been highly successful in controlling AI in turkeys in Minnesota (Halvorson et al., 1986). The California plan required the following to *Control the virus—making a responsible response to AI virus infection:*

1.   Negative flocks (never infected with avian influenza virus) have no restrictions on movement
2.   Virus-negative flocks (previously positive but no longer shedding virus):
     a.   Move to slaughter
     b.   Pullets (young hens) may be moved to a positive lay ranch
3.   Suspect flocks
     a.   Get a diagnosis as soon as possible
          1.   Contact your veterinarian, and/or
          2.   Submit birds to the diagnostic laboratory
     b.   Notify your neighbors
     c.   Self-quarantine
4.   Positive flocks (currently infected and shedding avian influenza virus)
     a.   Notify neighboring poultry farms
     b.   Self-quarantine
          1.   Do not move birds until the flock is no longer shedding virus
          2.   Coordinate movement of the flock to minimize risk
               a.   Document route and time of travel and let other producers know

or

          3.   Euthanize and dispose of the flock on site (composting or cremation)
               a.   Limit exposure of carcasses to predators and other mechanical vectors

The final step in the California control plan is how to **Prevent infection in future flocks.** In this step, the California producers relied heavily on the use of a killed autogenous vaccine. The use of vaccine allowed them to stop the cycle of infection in multi-age farms, which have a continuous flow of new birds entering the infected farm. Vaccination was highly successful for most farms, but only when implemented in conjunction with biosecurity practices.

1.   Clean and disinfect the farm
     a.   Leave sufficient downtime before repopulation (at least 2 weeks)

2. Use of vaccine in flocks at risk of infection
    a. Fulfill all CDFA/USDA requirements for biosecurity and flock plans

Using this voluntary plan, California controlled and eradicated H6N2 AI virus from commercial poultry flocks. The producers in the state soon learned that not telling each other about AI virus infections resulted in the spread of the outbreak. The outbreak was stopped when more communication began among all types of producers. This seems like a simple lesson to have learned, but the poultry producers and processors in California are no different from other small business owners in that they do not usually share confidential information with their competitors. To achieve the level of communication that resulted in the eradication of AI virus in California, all participants had to agree not to use infection status to gain a competitive advantage.

Exposure of Humans to Poultry in the United States

The U.S. commercial poultry industry protects public health by focusing its efforts on preventing poultry infections with AI viruses. This goal of prevention is both economically rewarding for the poultry business and a sound public health practice. However, because natural AI virus reservoirs are widely dispersed, this strategy does not always work, as was the case in California. When AI virus infections occur, it is important to understand where and how the general public interacts with poultry in order to assess and minimize risk of spread.

Many people envision poultry production as it was 100 years ago, as a dozen chickens on the family farm. However, today, poultry production occurs on large farms that house dense populations of chickens or turkeys. The industrialization of food production has meant that the general public is not exposed to the processes by which they are fed. The work force that produces all the food we need to survive is small and in the case of poultry, includes workers in poultry facilities and slaughterhouses, bird haulers, vaccination crews, manure haulers, renderers, and veterinarians. These workers are the most likely to be exposed to poultry pathogens infecting commercial poultry flocks.

In many parts of the world, poultry for consumption are purchased live, allowing the consumer to assess the bird's health and fitness. Live bird markets also exist in the United States, on the east coast, in the midwest, and in the major immigrant centers on the west coast (Los Angeles and San Francisco). Live bird markets all over the world are an important part of daily commerce and represent both a mixing pot of avian and mammalian disease agents and a steady stream of human traffic. The transmission of avian influenza to humans in Hong Kong in 1997 (Mounts et al., 1999; Shortridge et al., 2000; Subbarao et al., 1998) and in other parts of Asia (Webster, 2004) has raised the profile of live bird markets. Although surveillance has been increased, disease control measures have been established in only a few locations (Mullaney, 2003), primarily because they have been difficult to conceive and implement. Today, in the United States and all over the world, these markets remain a key location where the public is in direct contact with poultry that are sometimes actively shedding AI virus.

Perhaps the most intensive contact between poultry and people in the United States occurs among those individuals who own poultry for hobby purposes or keep them as a continuing source of eggs or fresh meat. These individuals come from a wide variety of cultural backgrounds and socioeconomic strata. However, these individuals—including cockfighters, 4H participants, poultry fanciers, and backyard flock owners—have one thing in common: few of them take their birds to veterinarians. This is partially due to a lack of interest in poultry on the part of most practicing veterinarians and partly because these owners do not want to spend money for veterinary care. Because they rarely see veterinarians, AI virus infections in these types of flocks usually go undetected and unreported. This lack of care combined with the level of contact between flock owners and hobby or backyard chickens make these human and poultry interactions some of the most important to public health.

So, while the general public is largely limited in its exposure to poultry by intensive farming and biosecurity practices, there are a number of exceptions through which humans may be intensively exposed to poultry. These scenarios are where disease prevention in poultry flocks is limited by a lack of contact with veterinarians and a lack of poultry husbandry knowledge that public health may be critically at risk. Unfortunately, many of the people most intensively exposed to these small populations of poultry are also underserved by human health professionals.

In California, the outbreak of H6N2 avian influenza in densely populated poultry regions resulted in the exposure of many small flocks to AI virus. How many were infected or their types are not known. However, we suspect that some of these noncommercial flocks are now persistently infected manmade reservoirs for the virus. These types of reservoirs have been implicated in the spread of disease to commercial flocks, but their roles in public health have been largely invisible.

Conclusions

The fact that California's low-pathogenicity strain of avian influenza virus was of the H6N2 type did not prevent it from spreading to many commercial poultry flocks or from causing disease and production losses in infected chickens and turkeys. In addition, the fact that this virus was not of the H5 or H7 types does not limit its potential to donate genetic material to potential pandemic strains. The interaction of animal agriculture and the public is complex and dynamic, and we do not fully understand the risks associated with the various types of contacts between humans and birds. We do not know where or how the next pandemic influenza virus will arise, but that lack of knowledge should not limit the surveillance we conduct in birds or in the public.

Low-pathogenicity strains of AI virus are the most prevalent strains among all species of birds, including commercial poultry. Non-H5 and -H7 low-pathogenicity AI viruses have contributed genetic material to the highly pathogenic viruses currently circulating in Asia (Chin et al., 2002), and one has infected humans (Lin et al., 2000). Our knowledge of where the next pandemic virus will arise is too premature to eliminate as irrelevant the non-H5 or -H7 avian influenza strains.

REFERENCES

Bulaga LL, Garber L, Senne D, Myers TJ, Good R, Wainwright S, Trock S, Suarez DL. 2003. Epidemiologic and surveillance studies on avian influenza in live-bird markets in New York and New Jersey, 2001. *Avian Diseases* 47(Suppl):996–1001.

Chin PS, Hoffmann E, Webby R, Webster RG, Guan Y, Peiris M, Shortridge KF. 2002. Molecular evolution of H6 influenza viruses from poultry in Southeastern China: Prevalence of H6N1 influenza viruses possessing seven A/Hong Kong/156/97 (H5N1)-like genes in poultry. *J Virol* 76:507–516.

Dybing JK, Schultz Cherry S, Swayne DE, Suarez DL, Perdue ML. 2000. Distinct pathogenesis of Hong Kong-origin H5N1 viruses in mice as compared to other highly pathogenic H5 avian influenza viruses. *J Virol* 74:1443–1450.

Easterday BC, Hinshaw VS, Halvorson DA. 1997. Influenza. In: Calnek BW, Barnes HJ, Beard CW, McDougald LR, Saif YM, eds. *Diseases of Poultry*. 10th ed. Ames, IA: Iowa State University Press. Pp. 583–605.

Ghazikhanian GY, Kelly BJ, Dungan WM, Bankowski RA, Reynolds B, Wichman RW. 1981 (April 22–24). *Avian Influenza Outbreaks in Turkey Breeder Flocks from 1979 to 1981*. Presented at the First International Symposium on Avian Influenza, Beltsville, MD.

Halvorson DA, Kelleher CJ, Senne DA. 1985. Epizootiology of avian influenza: Effect of season on incidence in sentinel ducks and domestic turkeys in Minnesota. *Applied Environ Microbiol* 49:914–919.

Halvorson DA, Karunakaran D, Abraham AS, Newman JA, Sivanandan V. 1986. Efficacy of vaccine in the control of avian influenza. In: *Proceedings of the Second International Symposium on Avian Influenza*. Athens, GA: United States Animal Health Association. Pp. 264–270.

Henzler DJ, Kradel DC, Davison S, Ziegler AF, Singletary D, DeBok P, Castro AE, Lu H, Eckroade R, Swayne D, Lagoda W, Schmucker B, Nesselrodt A. 2003. Epidemiology, production losses, and control measures associated with an outbreak of avian influenza subtype H7N2 in Pennsylvania (1996–98). *Avian Diseases* 47:1022–1036.

Hopkins BA, Skeeles JK, Houghten GE, Slagle D, Gardner K. 1990. A survey of infectious diseases in wild turkeys (*Meleagridis gallopavo silvestris*) from Arkansas. *J Wildl Dis* 26:468–472.

Kawaoka Y, Chambers TM, Sladen WL, Webster RG. 1988. Is the gene pool of influenza viruses in shorebirds and gulls different from that in wild ducks? *Virology* 163:247–250.

Kinde H, Read DH, Daft BM, Hammarlund M, Moore J, Uzal F, Mukai J, Woolcock P. 2003. The occurrence of avian influenza A subtype H6N2 in commercial layer flocks in Southern California (2000–02): Clinicopathologic findings. *Avian Diseases* 47:1214–1218.

Lee CW, Senne DA, Linares JA, Woolcock PR, Stallknecht DE, Spackman E, Swayne DE, Suarez DL. 2004. Characterization of recent H5 subtype avian influenza viruses from U.S. poultry. *Avian Pathol* 33:288–297.

Lin YP, Shaw M, Gregory V, Cameron K, Lim W, Klimov A, Subbarao K, Guan Y, Krauss S, Shortridge K, Webster R, Cox N, Hay A. 2000. Avian-to-human transmission of H9N2 subtype influenza A viruses: Relationship between H9N2 and H5N1 human isolates. *Proc Natl Acad Sci U S A* 97:9654–9658.

McCapes RH, Bankowski RA, West GBE. 1986 (September 3–5). *Avian Influenza in California. The Nature of Clinical Disease 1964–1985.* Presented at the Second International Symposium on Avian Influenza, University of Georgia, Athens, GA.

Mounts AW, Kwong H, Izurieta HS, Ho Y, Au T, Lee M, Buxton Bridges C, Williams SW, Mak KH, Katz JM, Thompson WW, Cox NJ, Fukuda K. 1999. Case-control study of risk factors for avian influenza A (H5N1) disease, Hong Kong, 1997. *J Infect Dis* 180:505–508.

Mullaney R. 2003. Live-bird market closure activities in the northeastern United States. *Avian Diseases* 47:1096–1098.

Shortridge KF, Gao P, Guan Y, Ito T, Kawaoka Y, Markwell D, Takada A, Webster RG. 2000. Interspecies transmission of influenza viruses: H5N1 virus and a Hong Kong SAR perspective. *Vet Microbiol* 74:141–147.

Sivanandan V, Halvorson DA, Laudert E, Senne DA, Kumar MC. 1991. Isolation of H13N2 influenza A virus from turkeys and surface water. *Avian Diseases* 35:974–977.

Slemons RD, Johnson DC, Osborn JS, Hayes F. 1974. Type-A influenza viruses isolated from wild free-flying ducks in California. *Avian Diseases* 18:119–124.

Spackman E, Senne DA, Davison S, Suarez DL. 2003. Sequence analysis of recent H7 avian influenza viruses associated with three different outbreaks in commercial poultry in the United States. *J Virol* 77:13399–13402.

Stallknecht DE, Shane SM. 1988. Host range of avian influenza virus in free-living birds. *Vet Res Commun* 12:125–141.

Suarez DL. 2000. Evolution of avian influenza viruses. *Vet Microbiol* 74:15–27.

Suarez DL, Schultz CS. 2000. Immunology of avian influenza virus: A review. *Dev Comp Immunol* 24:269–283.

Suarez DL, Woolcock PR, Bermudez AJ, Senne DA. 2002. Isolation from turkey breeder hens of a reassortant H1N2 influenza virus with swine, human, and avian lineage genes. *Avian Diseases* 46:111–121.

Suarez DL, Senne DA, Banks J, Brown IH, Essen SC, Lee CS, Manvell RJ, Mathieu-Benson C, Moreno V, Pedersen JC, Panigrahy B, Rojas H, Spackman E, Alexander DJ. 2004. Recombination resulting in virulence shift in avian influenza outbreak, Chile. *EID* 10:693–699.

Subbarao K, Klimov A, Katz J, Regnery H, Lim W, Hall H, Perdue M, Swayne D, Bender C, Huang J, Hemphill M, Rowe T, Shaw M, Xu X, Fukuda K, Cox N. 1998. Characterization of an avian influenza A (H5N1) virus isolated from a child with a fatal respiratory illness. *Science* 279:393–396.

Swayne DE. 2000. Understanding the ecology and epidemiology of avian influenza viruses: Implications for zoonotic potential. In: Brown CC, Bolin CA, eds. *Emerging Diseases of Animals.* Washington, DC: ASM Press. Pp. 101–130.

Swayne DE. 2001. Avian influenza vaccine use during 2001. In: *Proceedings of the 104th Annual Meeting of the U.S. Animal Health Association, Hershey, Pennsylvania, October 9-14, 2001.* Richmond, VA: U.S. Animal Health Association. Pp. 469–471.

Swayne DE. 2003. Vaccines for list A poultry diseases: Emphasis on avian influenza. *Developments in Biologics (Basel)* 114:201–212.

Swayne DE, Akey B. 2004. Avian influenza control strategies in the United States of America. In: Koch G, ed. *Proceedings of the Wageningen Frontis International Workshop on Avian Influenza Prevention and Control.* Wageningen, The Netherlands: Kluwer Academic Publishers. Pp. 129–146.

Swayne DE, Halvorson DA. 2003. Influenza. In: Saif YM, Barnes HJ, Fadly AM, Glisson JR, McDougald LR, Swayne DE, eds. *Diseases of Poultry.* 11th ed. Ames, IA: Iowa State University Press. Pp. 135–160.

Swayne DE, Suarez DL. 2000. Highly pathogenic avian influenza. *Rev Sci Tech Off Int Epiz* 19:463–482.

U.S. Department of Agriculture. 1994. *Avian Influenza Emergency Disease Guidelines.* Hyattsville, MD: Animal Plant Health Inspection Service, U.S. Department of Agriculture.

Webby RJ, Woolcock PR, Krauss SL, Walker DB, Chin PS, Shortridge KF, Webster RG. 2003. Multiple genotypes of nonpathogenic H6N2 influenza viruses isolated from chickens in California. *Avian Diseases* 47:905–910.

Webster RG. 2004. Wet markets—a continuing source of Severe Acute Respiratory Syndrome and influenza? *Lancet* 363:234–236.

Webster RG, Bean WJ, Gorman OT, Chambers TM, Kawaoka Y. 1992. Evolution and ecology of influenza A viruses. *Microbiol Rev* 56:152–179.

Woolcock PR, Suarez DL, Kuney D. 2003. Low-pathogenicity avian influenza virus (H6N2) in chickens in California, 2000–02. *Avian Diseases* 47:872–881.

World Organisation for Animal Health (OIE). 2003. *Terrestrial Animal Health Code.* 12th ed. Paris, France: OIE.

World Organisation for Animal Health (OIE). 2004a. *Manual of Diagnostic Tests and Vaccines for Terrestrial Animals.* 5th ed. Paris, France: OIE.

World Organisation for Animal Health (OIE). 2004b. Highly Pathogenic Avian influenza. In: *Terrestrial Animal Health Code.* 12th ed. Paris, France: OIE.

World Trade Organization. 1995. *Agreement on the Application of Sanitary and Phytosanitary Measures.* [Online]. Available: http://www.wto.org/english/tratop_e/sps_e/spsagr_e.htm [accessed December 8, 2004].

Wright SM, Kawaoka Y, Sharp GB, Senne DA, Webster RG. 1992. Interspecies transmission and reassortment of influenza A viruses in pigs and turkeys in the United States. *Am J Epidemiol* 136:488–497.

5

Emerging Technical Tools

OVERVIEW

A trend that has long been recognized is that people who have had influenza may have less severe symptoms when subsequently infected with immunologically distinct viruses. Immunization with the virus of one influenza A subtype has been shown to reduce morbidity and mortality in animals infected with virus of a different subtype, a phenomenon known as heterosubtypic immunity. In the first contribution to this chapter, Suzanne Epstein describes animal studies on the various means of inducing heterosubtypic immunity and explores the possibility of taking advantage of conserved features among influenza viruses to reduce mortality in a pandemic until a matched vaccine became widely available. Routine immunization could potentially be used to induce heterosubtypic immunity in advance of a pandemic, and the vaccine could also be offered early in a pandemic to those who had not received it.

An even more ambitious strategy is presented in the next contribution, which describes the engineering of influenza A-resistant chickens that combines (1) RNA interference, (2) genes that block the expression of incoming viral genomes, and (3) RNA decoys, short sequences that mimic the binding sites of RNA proteins and thereby act as competitive inhibitors for transcription. Although researchers pursing this strategy recognize the many logistical and scientific roadblocks in their path, they nonetheless envision the elimination of a major pandemic threat through global repopulation with influenza-resistant transgenic chickens.

Rapid detection techniques are critically needed for a quick diagnosis of the pathogen. The faster the pathogen is detected, the faster the outbreak can be controlled. The chapter continues with a description of several novel approaches for rapid early detection, including the most promising assay, real-time fluorescent polymerase chain reaction, as well as some other techniques: antigen capture/enzyme-linked immunosorbent assay, mass spectrometry, and restriction fragment length polymorphisms. The development of these techniques for detection will enable a quick diagnosis of the agent and faster development of vaccines.

The chapter concludes with mathematical modeling of pandemic preparedness plans, showing the consequences on health economic outcomes of possible intervention strategies. This modeling helps to determine the costs and benefits of different strategies and gauges the public health benefits of optimized preparedness.

CONTROL OF INFLUENZA VIRUS INFECTION BY IMMUNITY TO CONSERVED VIRAL FEATURES

Suzanne L. Epstein[1,2]

Office of Cellular, Tissue and Gene Therapies, Center for Biologics Evaluation and Research, Food and Drug Administration

Influenza has circulated among humans for centuries and kills more people than many newly emerging diseases. The present methods for control of influenza are not adequate, especially for dealing with a pandemic. In the face of a rapidly spreading outbreak, a race to isolate the virus and prepare a vaccine would probably not succeed in time to avoid great losses. Thus, additional anti-infection strategies are needed. Broad cross-protection against widely divergent influenza A subtypes is readily achieved in animals by several means of immunization. How does cross-protection work in animals, and can we apply what we have learned about it to induce broad cross-protection in humans?

[1]Suzanne L. Epstein, PhD, Chief, Laboratory of Immunology and Developmental Biology, Division of Cellular and Gene Therapies, HFM-730, Office of Cellular, Tissue and Gene Therapies, Center for Biologics Evaluation and Research, Food and Drug Administration, 301-827-0450, fax: 301-827-0449, e-mail: epsteins@cber.fda.gov.
[2]SLE acknowledges grant support from the National Vaccine Program. I thank Steven Bauer, Ira Berkower, Mark Tompkins, Zi-Shan Zhao and Chia-Yun Lo for critical review of various versions of the manuscript.

Background: Influenza Virus, Immunity, and Vaccination

If an influenza pandemic began, emergency efforts to isolate the pandemic virus strain and prepare a vaccine from it would begin, while the pandemic spread. Should we pin our hopes on that race? On antiviral drugs? Or are there vaccines that could be made in advance and offer some degree of protection? Current vaccines focus on variable, strain-specific epitopes of circulating influenza virus strains and new viral strains require new vaccines. Here, a different approach will be considered, vaccination based on shared epitopes as an anti-infective measure that could provide broad protection against even new pandemic strains.

This review will draw together relevant observations from animal studies and from human epidemiology. In the venerable influenza field, some of the older literature is highly relevant to current questions in ways that were not considered at the time, so it must be revisited. After providing background on influenza infection and immunity, the review will focus on broad cross-protection against influenza A subtypes. It will explore the mechanisms of cross-protection in animals, the induction of cross-protection by vaccines of different types and their ability to protect against challenge with potential pandemic subtypes, such as H5N1. Finally, it will consider the possibility of broad immune cross-protection in humans and the public health implications for control of epidemics and pandemics.

Influenza remains a major public health problem. The World Health Organization (WHO) estimates that in a typical year, 10 to 20 percent of the world's population is infected with influenza, resulting in 3,000,000 to 5,000,000 severe illnesses and 250,000 to 500,000 deaths (World Health Organization, 1999). In the United States, there are tens of thousands of deaths each year and the problem will increase due to the aging of the population and the susceptibility of the elderly.

During pandemics, the losses are even greater. The 1918 influenza pandemic was the most extreme, causing two billion cases, 20 to 40 million deaths worldwide and 500,000 in the United States, and killing with great speed. Young, healthy adults were not spared and approximately 80 percent of the U.S. Army's World War I deaths were due to influenza (Wright and Webster, 2001). Pandemics in 1957 and 1968 also caused widespread disease and excess deaths. For further historical information, see Kilbourne (1975).

Vaccination is a highly successful strategy for controlling infectious diseases. It is cost-effective and population-wide campaigns are feasible. However, the pathogens against which vaccination has been most successful (e.g., smallpox and polio) have viral types that are few in number and genetically stable. With influenza virus, extensive genetic variation leads to the problem that different dominant viral strains circulate in the human population each year (Figure 5-1). The current vaccine system involves

257

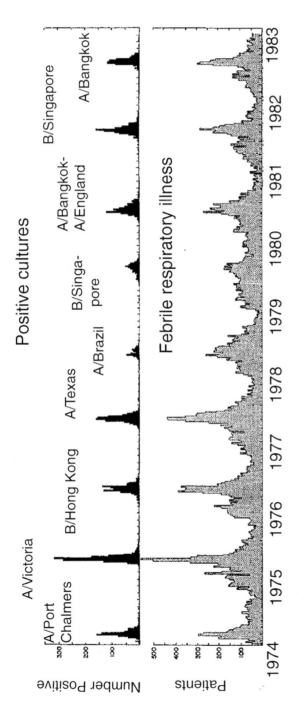

FIGURE 5-1 Periodic outbreaks of influenza in a surveillance study in Texas. Lower panel shows number of persons with acute febrile respiratory illness, upper panel shows number of persons with positive cultures for influenza virus. Strain names are of predominant viruses only. Note that different viral strains dominate in different years. Adapted from Figure 1 in Glezen et al. (1984). Reprinted with permission from Elsevier, Oxford, UK.

worldwide surveillance, predictions of strains likely to circulate during the next season and manufacture of new vaccines. This system is cumbersome, imperfect in effectiveness due to the guesswork involved and rushed in timing. Delays in vaccine derivation and manufacture can lead to shortages, as occurred in 2000 (CDC, 2000). A vaccination strategy that included broad cross-protection in addition to strain-specific protection could have a major public health impact; therefore, the potential of such an approach needs to be thoroughly explored.

There are three major influenza virus types, A, B and C. Infection with influenza C virus is relatively mild clinically (Murphy and Webster, 1990) and will not be discussed here. Influenza A and B viruses are distantly related but not cross-reactive or -protective against each other in animals (de St. Groth and Donnelley, 1950), even during mixed simultaneous infection (Liang et al., 1994). The influenza virus A and B genomes each consist of eight separate RNA segments. Point mutations lead to "antigenic drift" (small, incremental changes). Reassortment of entire segments of the genome is an additional source of antigenic variation and, in the case of influenza A, can lead to "antigenic shift" (sudden, large change) corresponding to a change in subtype.

Influenza virus and its components are shown diagrammatically in Figure 5-2. Hemagglutinin (HA) and neuraminidase (NA) are the components that vary the most. Subtypes of influenza A virus are defined serologically by their HA and NA antigens. The nomenclature for influenza A reflects this, for example, H3N2 refers to HA of subtype 3 and NA of subtype 2. There are 15 HA subtypes and nine NA subtypes (Wright and Webster, 2001). All these subtypes infect aquatic birds, and human pandemic viruses have arisen from avian viruses by reassortment (Webster, 2002). Emergence in humans of subtypes they have not previously encountered can lead to pandemics, for example, the emergence of H1N1 in 1918, H2N2 in 1957 and H3N2 in 1968 (Kilbourne, 1975). Small outbreaks of novel subtypes in humans occur more often than pandemics, for example, H5N1 in Hong Kong in 1997 (Claas et al., 1998), H9N2 in Hong Kong in 1999 (Saito et al., 2001), or an isolated case of H7N7 in The Netherlands in 2003 (van Kolfschooten, 2003).

Immunization with the virus of one influenza A subtype can protect animals against challenge with virus of a different subtype. This cross-protection has long been studied in animal models (Schulman and Kilbourne, 1965). In this review, it will be called heterosubtypic immunity or Het-I, to use the abbreviation of Gerhard (Liang et al., 1994) (it has also been called heterotypic immunity by some authors). This form of immunity does not generally prevent all infection by the heterosubtypic virus but it leads to more rapid viral clearance and to reduction in morbidity and mortality. In this review, the terms 'protection' and 'protective immunity'

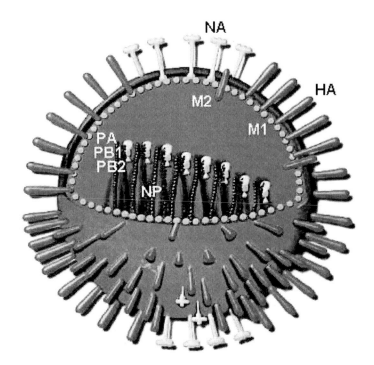

Variable surface glycoproteins (important antibody targets):

HA: Hemagglutinin
NA: Neuraminidase

Conserved proteins (important T cell targets):

M: Matrix encodes M1, M2
NP: Nucleoprotein
PB1: Basic polymerase
PB2: Basic polymerase
PA: Acidic polymerase
NS: "Nonstructural" encodes NS1, NS2

FIGURE 5-2 Diagram of influenza virus and its components. The core containing the RNA genome and replication machinery is surrounded by a matrix and then an envelope. HA, NA and M2 extend through the envelope to the outside. Diagram adapted from (www.snm.ch/public/sante/prevention/prevention-sommarie.htm). Reproduced with permission from Dr. Herve Zender, La Societe Neuchateloise de Medecine (SNM).

will not imply complete prevention of viral infection, but instead, a reduction in viral titers and protection of the life and health of the host.

Figure 5-3 shows diagrammatically the categories of influenza viruses, their relatedness, the terms for describing immunity to various challenges and the resulting protection. Relatedness of viral core and envelope proteins is shown by similarity of color. The corresponding relationships in protein sequence are shown in Table 5-1 for the HA and NA proteins, as well as for nucleoprotein (NP) as an important conserved protein.

A variety of birds and mammals can be infected with influenza A and B viruses, naturally or in the laboratory (Kilbourne, 1987). Serological reagents are often produced in ferrets. Influenza viruses can be adapted to

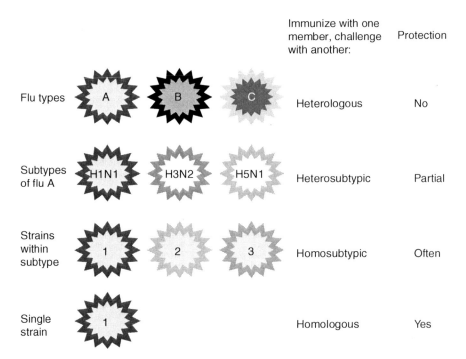

FIGURE 5-3 Categories of influenza viruses and immunity they induce. Colors indicate similarity. For example, influenza virus types A, B and C differ for both internal proteins and the HA and NA external glycoproteins. Within the influenza A type, subtypes have major differences in HA and NA but only subtle differences in internal proteins. Within an influenza A subtype, for example, H1N1, the HA and NA differ in more subtle ways shown by the more similar colors. Note that the term 'heterologous' immunity is also used to refer to immunity induced by one virus and reactive with an unrelated virus (Selin et al., 1994) but the term will not be used that way in this review.

TABLE 5-1 Influenza Viruses: Nomenclature and Relatedness

Influenza Viruses	Percent Amino Acid Homology in Hemagglutinin (HA)	Percent Amino Acid Homology in Neuraminidase (NA)	Percent Amino Acid Homology in Nucleoprotein (NP)
Types Influenza A, B, C	24-40% A vs. B, C unrelated[a]	26-29% A vs. B[a]	A vs B, 38% A vs. C, 22%[a]
Subtypes H1-H15, N1-N9 Example: H1N1	25-80%[a,b] Examples: H1 vs. H3, 25-40% H2vs. H5, 80%	42-57%[a]	Example: H1N1 vs H3N2, 92-97%[c]
Strains within a subtype	>90%[a]	>90%[d] (N2's)	Close to 100%

NOTES: [a]Murphy and Webster, 1990; [b]Scholtissek, 1983; [c]Altmuller et al., 1989; [d]Xu et al., 1996.

mice and in them cause disease with many of the characteristics of human influenza: upper respiratory infection, tracheobronchitis and pneumonia (Yetter et al., 1980; Renegar, 1992). They provide an affordable animal model with a short generation time and many reagents defining surface markers on important cellular populations. In addition, there are numerous recombinant and congenic strains, and more recently transgenic and knock-out strains of immunological significance. Thus, much work on immunity to influenza virus infection has been performed in mice. Results in an animal model do not predict in every particular what will happen in humans, but they provide a valuable information base that can help design future studies in humans and novel approaches to vaccine development.

Immunity to Influenza Virus Infection

How to Analyze Mechanisms of Immunity in Animal Models

The complexity and redundancy of the immune system is good for defense against pathogens but hard on those trying to interpret experiments. Any response that is measured was likely accompanied by other concurrent responses that were not. Thus, correlation of a response with protection does not prove that it mediates the protection. Passive transfer of antibody or T-cells helps by showing that an effector is capable of mediating an outcome, but does not mean that it always does. The adoptive transfer may use unnatural doses and the transferred components may not localize normally.

Mice with a targeted gene disruption ('knockout') can be used to test whether the corresponding component is required for a certain outcome. Keep in mind however, that a component not required under one set of conditions may still play a role and it may be required under other circumstances. Note also that a knockout animal lacks the component from birth and may compensate for its absence by other biological changes.

Another approach to analysis is depletion of certain immune cells *in vivo* (often CD4+ or CD8+ T-cells). If animals were intact when primed and are depleted only during the period of viral challenge infection, then depletion is informative about effector functions. It is imperfect in that residual cells could lurk at tissue sites not tested or at levels not detectable. However, depletion has the advantage that it can be performed acutely, not leaving much time for compensation by other changes in the animal.

Multiple approaches are necessary if we are to accumulate a realistic view of immune responses and their potential under various circumstances. No one approach can describe the multifaceted immune response and all its shifting balances.

Immunity to Influenza Virus: B- and T-cell Responses

The immune system clears infection the first time a virus is encountered. It also preserves specific memory of viral antigens, so that it can prevent or at least limit reinfection if the same virus is encountered again. Fundamentals of immune responses (B- and T-cell responses, antigen processing, presentation by major histocompatability complex [MHC] class I and II and epitope dominance) are reviewed elsewhere and will not be covered here.

Antibodies to influenza virus can protect against reinfection and passively transferred antibody can protect naive animals. However, this form of protection is often subtype-specific or even narrowly specific to certain viral strains (Ada and Jones, 1986), failing to protect against mismatched strains (De Jong et al., 2000). Additional immunity is provided by effector T-cells. They play important roles in clearing influenza virus and protecting against challenge, although they can also cause immunopathology (Wells et al., 1981). Doherty's and other groups have provided much evidence for a beneficial role of class I MHC-restricted CD8+ cytotoxic T-lymphocytes (CTLs) in clearing primary influenza virus infection (Doherty et al., 1997) and also in protection against challenge with homologous virus (Lu and Askonas, 1980). The conserved NP viral protein is a major target antigen for CTLs in mice (Yewdell et al., 1985). In some studies of immunizations with NP, immune responses were observed but little or no protection

(Webster et al., 1991; Lawson et al., 1994), while in other cases NP regimens were protective against challenge (Ulmer et al., 1993; Fu et al., 1999). MHC class II-restricted CTL activity specific for influenza virus antigens has also been reported (Taylor and Bender, 1995).

The role of CD8+ CTLs in protective immunity is virus-specific: CTLs only control the virus they recognize. Bystander viruses coinfecting the same lungs are not controlled (Lukacher et al., 1984), ruling out nonantigen-specific mechanisms based on natural killer (NK) cells or soluble mediators such as interferon (IFN), cytokines, or chemokines released when T-cells recognize virus. Topham and colleagues demonstrated that *in vivo* protection by CD8+ cells requires lysis mediated by either perforin or Fas (Topham et al., 1997). Tumor necrosis factor (TNF)-α-mediated killing has also been reported *in vitro* (Liu et al., 1999; Zhao et al., 2001).

Mechanisms of Heterosubtypic Immunity Induced by Infection with Live Virus

Focus will now be placed on Het-I, that is, cross-protection by prior exposure to one influenza A subtype against challenge with a divergent subtype. Respiratory infection with live wild type virus efficiently induces Het-I and will be discussed initially.

Roles of T-cells

T-cells are candidates for contributors to Het-I because they participate in clearing virus from infected tissues and many of them cross-react with all influenza A subtypes. In one study of Het-I, *in vivo* depletion showed that CD4+ and CD8+ T-cells both contributed to control of challenge virus in the nose (Liang et al., 1994). In the lungs, CD4+ cells did not appear to contribute but CD8+ cells did, plus some other mechanism that remained after depletion of both. This study also showed that Het-I against influenza A was immunologically specific in its effector phase; coinfecting influenza B virus replicated unchecked in the same lung tissue (Liang et al., 1994). Thus, like homologous protection by CTLs discussed earlier, Het-I induced by live virus requires specific effector functions of antibodies or T-cells that recognize the virus.

Mice with a targeted disruption of the β2-microglobulin (β2m) gene have been studied as a model lacking class I MHC restricted CD8+ T-cells. They can survive primary influenza virus infection and can mount protective immune responses to homologous and heterosubtypic challenge (Bender et al., 1994; Epstein et al., 1997). β2m$^{-/-}$ mice have multiple immune deficiencies besides a lack of CTLs, but one can at least say from these results that CD8+ CTLs are not required for Het-I (Raulet, 1994; Epstein et al.,

2000). Confirmatory evidence comes from CD8 knockout mice, which also have deficient class I-restricted CTL and retain Het-I (Nguyen et al., 2001).

Can T-cell responses alone protect against influenza? Immunoglobulin (Ig)$^{-/-}$ knockout mice lacking antibodies and mature B-cells have been used to study this question, including μMT mice (targeted disruption of the membrane exon of μ heavy chain), JHD mice (disruption of the heavy chain joining segments, thus no Ig gene rearrangement) and DI mice (disruption of JHD segments and also κ light chain constant regions). Several studies have shown that such mice could clear primary influenza virus infection but less effectively than normal mice and immunization protected them at least to some extent against homologous challenge (Bot et al., 1996; Topham and Doherty, 1998; Epstein et al., 1998; Graham and Braciale, 1997). What about Het-I? In one study, no Het-I could be demonstrated in μMT mice but under conditions that showed no protection against homologous challenge, either (Nguyen et al., 2001). Indeed, protective immunity is weaker than normal in these mice. Our group has identified conditions under which Het-I could be demonstrated in mice without antibodies. Immunization with H2N2 or H3N2 viruses partially controlled replication of H1N1 challenge virus. This immunity was dependent upon both CD4+ and CD8+ T-cells (Benton et al., 2001).

There is a caveat to interpretation of these results: Ig$^{-/-}$ mice have an immune defect besides absence of antibodies. In a variety of pathogen systems, naive B-cells can restore their ability to clear an infection but not via antibody production (Elkins et al., 1999; Mozdzanowska et al., 2000). These findings suggest a role for B-cells as antigen-presenting cells (APCs).

Role of Antibodies

Antibodies had been suggested as a mediator of Het-I because foster nursing on immune mothers transferred protection to the pups (Mbawuike et al., 1990) and absence of CD8+ CTLs did not abrogate Het-I. What type of antibodies could be involved? IgG dominates in immune serum and reaches mucosal sites, including the lungs by transudation. IgA is found in the lungs along with IgG, and IgA dominates in the nose where it is thought to be especially important. Since mucosal immunization is highly effective, secretory antibodies have been a focus of study and polymeric IgA has been shown to mediate protection against influenza virus (Renegar and Small, 1991). Polymeric IgA can cross the epithelium of the lung and other organs by transcyrosis dependent upon the poly-Ig receptor and can interfere with viral infection as it crosses the infected cells (Mazanec et al., 1992; Mazanec et al., 1995). Certain IgA monoclonal antibodies (mAbs) to core proteins protect against rotavirus infection, although they do not neutralize virus (Burns et al., 1996; Schwartz-Cornil et al., 2002); these results suggested that during transcytosis antibody interferes with intracellular virus assembly. Antibody to conserved antigens, as required for Het-I, could mediate such a mechanism.

To resolve questions about IgA's role in control of infections, Harriman and colleagues derived an IgA knockout mouse (Harriman et al., 1999). These mice could clear a primary influenza virus infection and a subunit vaccine protected them against lethal challenge (Mbawuike et al., 1999). We later showed that IgA$^{-/-}$ mice were capable of Het-I under two sets of conditions, lethal challenge infection of the total respiratory tract (TRT) and nonlethal challenge restricted to the upper respiratory tract (URT) (Benton et al., 2001). Thus, Het-I can be effective in the absence of IgA. There may, however, be quantitative defects in control of virus by IgA$^{-/-}$ mice.

Anatomic Compartments and Heterosubtypic Immunity

The influence of routes of immunization on the resulting antiviral responses was demonstrated in 1950 by de St. Groth (de St. Groth and Donnelley, 1950). Immunization of mice with live virus via respiratory tract infection was far more effective than intraperitoneal or subcutaneous immunization in protecting against challenge with homologous virus. In one case, the difference in effectiveness was on the order of a hundred million-fold! The superiority of immunization via mucosal sites presumably reflects viral replication in the respiratory tract and induction of local as well as systemic immunity.

The importance of the anatomic sites in which priming takes place was also highlighted in a study by Nguyen and colleagues. Live virus was given by intraperitoneal or intravenous routes, or by TRT or URT infection (Nguyen et al., 1999). TRT immunization generated better CTL responses than the other routes. It also generated heterosubtypic protection, while the other routes did not. Any of the routes generated cross-reactive CTLs in the spleen and some in the cervical lymph nodes. However, only the TRT route induced CTLs in the mediastinal lymph nodes which drain the lungs and from which CTLs are recruited to the lungs during infection. Depletion of CTLs was not performed to prove they mediated the observed protection, so roles of other local immune responses in Het-I were not ruled out.

Heterosubtypic Immunity Induced by Vaccines Against Influenza A Subtypes Common or Novel in Humans

The previous section explored Het-I induced by wild type virus infection. How can we induce it more safely? This section will explore the ability of various vaccines to induce Het-I. Challenge viruses will include subtypes

in human circulation currently, as well as potential future pandemic subtypes. The studies use different vaccine formulations, virus strains, doses,
routes of administration and measures of protection. Since the vaccine
candidates have not been compared side by side, general conclusions and
comparisons are not yet possible. The details are crucial. This or that
preparation may induce cross-protection but how efficiently, at what dose,
by what route of administration and against what challenge?

The 1997 outbreak of H5Nl in humans in Hong Kong raised fears that
this subtype could spread and perhaps cause a pandemic. Preparation of
reassortant vaccine strains was difficult and took over a year (WHO, 2003),
while recombinant H5 protein proved not very immunogenic (Nicholson et
al., 2001; Treanor et al., 2001). Fortunately, there was no human-to-human
transmission and the outbreak subsided. Vaccine candidates face new problems in that pathogenesis of H5N1 infection is different from that of H1N1
and H3N2. H5N1 viruses are extremely virulent in chickens, causing systemic spread, replication in various organs and rapid death (Suarez et al.,
1998; Subbarao et al., 1998). Some H5N1 strains spread to nonrespiratory
organs in mice and cause symptoms within 24 h and deaths earlier than
H1N1 and H3N2 viruses (Gao et al., 1999; Lu et al., 1999). Thus, it was
not clear whether immunizations inducing heterosubtypic immunity effective against H1N1 and H3N2 viruses would work against H5N1 infection.
Several types of heterosubtypic immunizations have given encouraging
results with H5N1 challenge and a few with H9N2 challenge, as will be
described in the following sections. These approaches could provide a first-
line of defense against a pandemic virus, until antigenically-matched HA-
based vaccines could be prepared.

Protein and Peptide Vaccines

A variety of peptide and protein vaccines based on conserved sites
confer heterosubtypic protection in animal models, mediated by antibody
and/or T-cells. Only a few examples can be mentioned. Despite the generally inefficient entry of exogenous proteins into the class I MHC antigen-
presentation pathway, peptides and proteins are able to induce CTL responses to some extent. For example, a fusion protein consisting of part of
NS1 fused to the C-terminal part of the HA2 domain of subtype H1 was
shown to induce antibody and CTL to influenza virus. It protected mice
against challenge with either H1N1 or H2N2 but not H3N2. Depletion of
either CD4+ or CD8+ cells partially abrogated this protection (Mbawuike
et al., 1994).

Another protein vaccine is based on matrix (M)2. M2 is a conserved
protein that spans the virion membrane with a portion exposed on the
outside and is a target of protective antibodies. Recombinant M2 protein

has been shown to induce protective immunity against lethal challenge (Slepushkin et al., 1995). Recently Neirynck and colleagues showed that a highly conserved N-terminal peptide of M2 fused to a carrier protein protected mice against homologous and heterosubtypic challenge. This protection was passively transferred by serum antibodies (Neirynck et al., 1999).

Note that vaccines based on peptides or minigenes chosen as dominant T-cell epitopes are unlikely to be effective in responders of all MHC types. Whole genes or proteins providing multiple potential epitopes seem more promising than individual peptides for inducing T-cell immunity in the outbred human population.

DNA Vaccines

Like viral infection, DNA immunization results in endogenous expression of antigens. Thus, in addition to generating antibody responses, it efficiently delivers viral proteins to the antigen-presentation pathways favorable for inducing CTL responses. Extensive studies of DNA vaccination against influenza have used various antigens and routes of administration. Most relevant to Het-I is DNA vaccination with conserved components, such as NP and M. NP DNA induces antibody and T-cell responses and protects against heterosubtypic challenge (Ulmer et al., 1993; Rhodes et al., 1993). Using NP or both NP and M DNA, protection against heterosubtypic challenge was shown to be mediated by both CD4+ and CD8+ cells (Epstein et al., 2000; Ulmer et al., 1998).

In addressing control of infection with H5 viruses, NP DNA gave only modest protection in chickens that was viewed as inadequate (Kodihalli et al., 2000). Nonetheless, we tested the potential of DNA vaccination in mice, using NP and M genes from an H1N1 virus (Epstein et al., 2002). NP + M DNA vaccination protected against lethal challenge with the H5N1 strain HK/156 and reduced lung virus titers approximately 500-fold. NP + M DNA vaccination protected partially against a modest dose of the virulent strain A/HK/483, while DNA vaccination plus viral boosting protected effectively against a higher dose. These results encourage further exploration of DNA vaccination to induce broad cross-protection, with or without viral boosting.

Efforts are being made to improve the potency of DNA vaccination by use of re-engineered plasmids (codon modification to increase expression, optimization of immunostimulatory signals), additional viral antigens, DNA prime-recombinant viral boost strategies, adjuvants and targeting of antigens to favorable antigen presentation pathways. Similar to some other vaccines, DNA vaccines could be prepared in advance and used off the shelf. DNA vaccines have the additional advantage over viruses that they do not require a cold chain. They are currently expensive but if mass produced, would come down in cost and might become practical for use in parts of the world where the need for refrigeration limits use. Even if DNA vaccination does not turn out to be a method of choice, it provides an analytical technique to test antigenic components separately and optimize the contribution of each to the response.

Inactivated Virus and Subunit Vaccines

Inactivated virus had long been thought relatively ineffective at inducing Het-I, based on studies giving it by systemic routes, such as intramuscularly (Webster and Askonas, 1980). Several recent reports, however, challenge this view and suggest new uses of inactivated vaccines.

In one study (Takada et al., 1999), Takada and colleagues tested as vaccines several inactivated H5 viruses given intranasally. Unexpectedly, a mismatched control virus (inactivated H3N1) given intranasally also protected against lethal H5N1 challenge, suggesting that the new route of administration allowed inactivated vaccine to induce broad protection across a subtype difference.

Tumpey and coworkers studied protection against H5N1 by formalin-inactivated H3N2 virus and analyzed its immune mechanisms (Tumpey et al., 2001). Inactivated virus plus adjuvant given intranasally but not subcutaneously protected mice against lethal H5N1 challenge. The protection was not abrogated by depletion of both CD4+ and CD8+ cells. In addition, the protection was seen in $\beta2\mu^{-/-}$ but not Ig$^{-/-}$ mice. The caveat discussed above, that they have an APC defect, limits the interpretation of the results in the Ig$^{-/-}$ mice. However, in addition, IgG and IgA antibodies reactive with both H3 and H5 HA were detected in the serum and lungs of normal mice immunized intranasally but not subcutaneously. The antibodies neutralized H3N2 but not H5N1 virus. All together, the results suggested a non-neutralizing antibody mechanism of Het-I that is inducible by mucosal but not systemic vaccination with inactivated virus.

These findings were recently extended by Takada and colleagues using inactivated vaccines of HA subtypes H1, H2, H3, H5, and H9 (Takada et al., 2003). When given intranasally, all of these protected mice against challenge with the virulent H5N1 virus, HK/483. IgG antibodies crossreactive with HK/483 viral antigens were detected in the serum and lung wash samples, while IgA was preferentially detected in nasal washes. As in the Tumpey study, antibodies neutralized homologous virus but not H5N1 virus.

Inactivated virus incorporated into ISCOMS (immunostimulating complex [adjuvanted particles]) (Morein et al., 1984) has also been shown to induce Het-I in mice. H1N1 influenza ISCOMS protected mice against lethal challenge with H1N1, H2N2 and H3N2 and reduced lung titers of

H5N1 and H9N2 (Sambhara et al., 2001). In monkeys, flu-ISCOMS failed to protect across the smaller divergence of a drift variant (Rimmelzwaan et al., 2001).

The Takada and Tumpey studies delivered the vaccines under general anesthesia, which would not be a practical method of human vaccination. However, getting antigen to the lungs might be achieved by other means, such as a small particle aerosol. These findings give hope for induction of Het-I with existing vaccines.

Live Attenuated Virus

Use of live attenuated viruses (H5 and H9, for example) as vaccines of potential pandemic subtypes has been proposed by some investigators (Chen et al., 2003; Subbarao et al., 2003; WHO, 2003) but entails some risk. The HA gene of the new subtype could reassort with a nonattenuated virus in the community, leading to release of an infectious, nonattenuated virus of the new subtype. Such an approach would be too risky unless a pandemic were already spreading rapidly in the area and had a high death rate. Since cleavability of HA is related to virulence (Hatta et al., 2001), removing this site by genetic engineering would help by reducing potential pathogenicity.

Live attenuated influenza vaccines of circulating strains (A/H1N1, A/H3N2 and B) have long been used in Russia, were recently approved for marketing in the USA and have a good safety record. Can live attenuated, cold-adapted vaccines given mucosally induce Het-I and thus protect against potential pandemic subtypes? Recall that wild type virus infection given by TRT exposure in mice induces Het-I but virus infection confined to the URT does not (Nguyen et al., 1999). Cold-adapted vaccine strains infect the URT but replicate poorly in the warmer environment of the lungs of humans or mice. Whether the lower respiratory tract infection they produce is adequate to induce Het-I efficiently is unknown. If they induce Het-I well, these vaccines will not only have a role in controlling annual influenza epidemics but may also have a role in pandemic prevention.

The Possibility of Het-I in Humans

Human immunity to influenza has often been said to be subtype-specific and any heterosubtypic immunity dismissed as ineffective (Murphy and Coelingh, 2002). However, some cross-protection in humans has been reported during consecutive or overlapping epidemics, with reduction both in susceptibility to a second virus and intensity of symptoms (Sonoguchi et al., 1985). During a pandemic, human populations are exposed to an influenza subtype to which they have no prior exposure. If humans have Het-I of even partial effectiveness and short duration, it could make a major public health contribution.

As discussed above, CTLs are one important mechanism of defense against influenza revealed in the animal studies. Humans have cross-reactive CTLs, too. In human volunteers challenged with H1N1, a cross-reactive memory CTL response correlated with control of infection, even in those individuals with no anti-H1N1 antibody (McMichael et al., 1983a). CTL immunity to influenza in humans has been reported to wane over a period of about 3 to 5 years (McMichael et al., 1983b) but that does not mean we should dismiss its significance.

At the time of the pandemics of 1957 and 1968, enough was known about influenza virus for recorded observations to include virological testing and analysis. The pandemic of 1968 involved a switch only in the HA, so antibodies to NA could have helped control infection. In 1957, however, both the HA and the NA were changed with the switch from H1N1 to H2N2, so this pandemic provides a situation with special potential for analyzing Het-I. In one study of the 1957 pandemic (Slepushkin, 1959), approximately 15,000 workers in a Russian factory were monitored by self-reporting. Influenza-like illness in the spring before emergence of H2N2 gave a 2.2-fold reduction in attacks during the summer when H2N2 began circulating and a 1.6-fold reduction in attacks during the fall. This suggests an impact of prior immunity on susceptibility to the new virus subtype. However, influenza infections were not confirmed by laboratory tests in this study.

Many studies of the 1957 pandemic noted that the incidence of influenza was much higher in children than in adults and declined progressively with age among adults. One active surveillance study, the Cleveland family study, was carried out from 1947 to 1957 and was especially informative for several reasons. The population consisted only of families with young children and thus all the adults were exposed to children as vectors. Furthermore, influenza virus infections were confirmed by culturing of swabs, not just based on symptoms. In this population, the incidence of culture-confirmed influenza was much higher in children than in adults (Jordan et al., 1958). The difference between adults and children was much less pronounced in 1950, 1951 and 1953, during the H1N1 era. This argues against the idea that children are inherently different in some other way, such as behavior or physiology. Thus, the data suggest an effect of prior immunity accumulated over time and exposures. At the time Jordan and colleagues pointed out that serum antibody was not the explanation because sera of their study participants did not inhibit the 1957 virus in HA1 tests (Jordan et al., 1958). They suggested 'unknown factors'. What has been learned about immunity since then from studies of animal models suggests that cross-reactive mucosal immunity to viral epitopes conserved between subtypes could be the unknown factor.

If humans have Het-I, we need ways to induce it with safe vaccines. CTL and secretory antibodies are candidates for mediating cross-protection, as in animals. Human CTL recognize a wide variety of influenza antigens, with some epitopes subtype-specific and some cross-reactive (Jameson et al., 1998). Which vaccines induce CTL? Clinical trials of inactivated and live attenuated vaccines, plus the combination of both, are reviewed extensively elsewhere (Couch et al., 1997; Murphy and Coelingh, 2002). Trials are often monitored serologically but the vaccinations that best induce serum antibodies are not always the ones best at inducing CTL or mucosal IgA. Some trials have measured T-cell memory, for example, a trial of inactivated vaccine with and without ISCOMS (Ennis et al., 1999) but clearly some key questions remain to be asked.

Efficacy trials in humans have not been informative about Het-I; they are monitored for prevention of infection with the same subtype(s) as the vaccine, either strain-matched or in some years drift variants. One clinical study raised the question of Het-I in order to see whether it would interfere with subsequent vaccination with a live attenuated virus of a different subtype (Steinhoff et al., 1993). Results showed that prior exposure to wild type virus or cold-adapted vaccine of one influenza A subtype did not interfere with subsequent vaccination with a different cold-adapted vaccine subtype. However, that study was done in young children (6–36 months old). The hints in the historical evidence leave room for the possibility that adults have accumulated a type of immunity that is weaker or more transient in children and thus that Het-I might have potential for public health impact.

The Future: Vaccines and Pandemic Planning

Given the extensive evidence in animals and the hints in humans, the potential of Het-I to reduce morbidity and mortality from a new pandemic strain should be explored. Strainmatched vaccines would probably not be available in time in the case of a rapidly spreading pandemic, even with new technologies for vaccine production. Thus, other anti-infective measures for pandemic intervention are needed, both antiviral drugs and, if continued investigation justifies it, vaccines inducing Het-I. Vaccination strategies using conserved components and experimentally determined to be efficient at inducing Het-I could be used routinely and vaccine could also be offered early in a pandemic to those who had not received it before. It would be intended to offer partial protection as a first line of defense, to be followed by strain-matched vaccines when available. This approach might also be useful to address concern about use of influenza virus as a bioterrorism threat, because this type of protection does not require prediction of what virus is coming.

An active clinical surveillance study could provide evidence for or against the idea that human Het-I is of a useful magnitude. The study population would be monitored for respiratory illnesses and suspected influenza would be confirmed by viral culture. The vaccination history of participants would also be recorded. Over a period of years, as new viral strains would enter the community, susceptibility could be examined in relation to prior history of influenza virus infections and vaccinations. If a pandemic should occur, the records would be available and the machinery in place to assess the impact of prior infections and vaccinations of different types on susceptibility to the new virus. More likely than a pandemic would be localized outbreaks of novel subtypes (for example, avian viruses transmitted to humans). If such an outbreak occurred in the study population, it might provide an opportunity to evaluate the effects of cross-protection.

Pandemic planning to date has relied mainly on proposals for emergency strain identification, preparation of new vaccines from the pandemic virus and use of antiviral drugs. Additional strategies are required. If heterosubtypic immunity could even partially control infection and thus reduce the morbidity and mortality due to a spreading pandemic, we need to study how best to induce and make use of this type of immunity.

Five-Year View

Many vaccine candidates will be compared in animal models for their ability to protect against potential pandemic subtypes of influenza. Meanwhile, the use of live attenuated vaccines will increase and surveillance of its effectiveness will continue. Besides protecting individuals, this will also increase herd immunity and thus contribute to protection of those who are not vaccinated or who do not respond optimally, such as the elderly. Clinical trials of additional vaccine candidates will assess their potential and, in some cases, the role of immunity to conserved components in protection.

Expert Opinion

Current influenza vaccination practices need improvement, given the high toll of disease. Besides studies of vaccines, clinical surveillance studies are needed to determine the consequences of prior infections and vaccinations in humans as new strains emerge. The potential of heterosubtypic immunity (broad cross-protection) to help control a pandemic has been largely ignored until recently but should be investigated systematically. A large number of vaccine candidates with different advantages and disadvantages are under study. Their ability to induce broad cross-protection should be one of the elements assessed as they move through clinical trials and into use.

Key Issues

•   Cross-protection against multiple influenza A subtypes can be induced in animals by prior infection or vaccination. Multiple viral antigens and multiple immune effector mechanisms can participate.
•   Mucosal vaccination induces different immune responses than systemic vaccination and is more effective at inducing broad cross-protection to multiple influenza A subtypes in animals.
•   Broad cross-protection in humans is of unclear potency and duration, but epidemiological data suggest that it may have an impact.
•   A variety of vaccines may induce broad cross-protection if administered appropriately.
•   Imperfect vaccine protection is worth having, especially for a virus causing an acute (not latent) infection. It could provide a first line of pandemic defense, to be augmented by subtype- or strain-specific vaccines when available.

Information Resources

•   www.flu.lanl.gov/review/epitopes.html
"*Known Influenza Virus Antigenic Peptides Listed by Restricting Major Histocompatibility Complex Molecules,*" Suzanne L Epstein, Jonathan W Yewdell, Jack R Bennink.
•   www.cdc.gov/ncidod/diseaseslflu/fluvirus.htm
Centers for Disease Control and Prevention influenza website
•   www.who.int/health-topics/influenza.htm
World Health Organization fact sheet on influenza

GENERATION OF TRANSGENIC CHICKENS RESISTANT TO AVIAN INFLUENZA VIRUS

Laurence Tiley

Department of Veterinary Medicine,
University of Cambridge, United Kingdom

and
Helen Sang

Roslin Institute, Midlothian, United Kingdom

Summary

Recent developments in transgenic technologies and inhibitory strategies offer a real opportunity for generating disease-resistant livestock. The domesticated chicken provides an ideal test-bed for investigating the feasibility of achieving this goal in a relevant species. Avian influenza virus presents an attractive target. This disease poses an extremely serious public health threat and is a major economic burden on the poultry industry. Research is underway to determine the most effective transgenic approaches to suppressing influenza virus replication in chickens and to perhaps one day eradicate the disease in this species.

Introduction

Influenza virus is an accomplished species jumper. The natural reservoirs for the virus are aquatic birds such as ducks, geese, and shore birds (Hinshaw et al., 1981; Kawaoka et al., 1988), which contain all of the known subtypes of influenza A. Within these hosts it is usually a relatively benign and genetically stable agent (Webster et al., 1995). Other species are inevitably exposed to these viruses, but usually this does not result in a successful propagative infection. The virus needs to adapt to succeed in the altered environment of a new host. Influenza virus replication readily generates the genetic diversity required for rapid evolution in response to such diversifying selective pressure. Periodically (as in the case of H5N1 in Hong Kong 1997 and subsequent events [Sims et al., 2003]), the virus manages to successfully infect a new host, in this case humans. In common with many emerging viruses, this can result in high case fatality rates among those infected individuals. The crucial adaptation that is needed for full emergence as a new pandemic virus is the ability to transmit efficiently from one individual to another. Fortunately this happened to only a very limited extent with H5N1 in 1997 (Buxton Bridges et al., 2000). However, the three pandemics of human influenza in the 20th century are clear evidence that the virus has succeeded in doing so in the past.

Although in principle it is possible that a new strain of influenza could emerge as a consequence of direct transmission from a wild bird to a human, the evidence suggests that this is extremely unlikely. It is much more likely that an intermediate or bridging host will be involved. Intensively reared domestic livestock such as pigs and poultry are the prime candidates as they are permissive for avian influenza viruses, and can act as amplifier hosts. This results in the massive and prolonged exposure of humans to novel and evolving strains of virus, thus increasing the probability of successful transmission to humans. Reassortment between human and avian strains of virus, either in pigs (which are susceptible to both

[Scholtissek et al., 1985]) or in humans (Claas and Osterhaus, 1998), provides a further means for rapid adaptation to the human host. The level and extent of exposure from infected chickens should not be underestimated. The 2004 epidemic of H5N1 was the largest outbreak of highly pathogenic avian influenza (HPAI) on record and this resulted in at least 34 human cases, 23 of which were fatal. However, there is no reason to expect that the next pandemic strain must be derived from an HPAI. The human pandemic strains H1N1, H2N2, and H3N2 all resemble low-pathogenicity avian influenza (LPAI) viruses. LPAI is prevalent in chickens throughout the world (Alexander, 2003; Senne, 2003).

Nothing can be done to eliminate the small threat of direct transmission from wild birds to humans. However, the major threat posed by the intermediate host species can be tackled in a number of ways, including improved farming/trading practices, vaccination, and biosecurity. A more radical approach, which has now become technically feasible, is to replace these animals with transgenic animals that are resistant to influenza virus. Eliminating avian influenza in chickens internationally would be beneficial on three fronts: It would reduce the risk of cross-species transmission to humans; it would eliminate the economic impact of controlling the disease in poultry; and it would improve the welfare of the animals by reducing the morbidity associated with the disease.

The Time Is Ripe

Basic scientific research into the molecular biology of influenza virus has uncovered several strategies that show great promise for inhibiting influenza replication. Some of these have been known about for many years, but lacked a suitable approach to deliver them.

Mx

The Mx genes were first discovered through their ability to confer a potent antiviral state in mice carrying functional alleles in response to Type I interferons (Haller et al., 1979; Staeheli et al., 1984). In the case of the mouse Mx1 gene, this response is restricted to orthomyxoviruses. Interferon-induced antiviral responses to other viruses (such as Vesicular Stomatitis Virus (VSV) and encephalomyocarditis virus (EMCV)) in mice are independent of Mx1 (Haller et al., 1981). Mx1 alone is both necessary and sufficient to confer this protection, that is, no other IFN-responsive genes are required (Staehli et al., 1986). By contrast, the Mx2 gene of mice is active against VSV and hantaviruses, but inactive against influenza virus (Zurcher et al., 1992). Mx gene homologues have been identified in many other vertebrate species, including humans (Aebi et al., 1989) and avians

(Bernasconi et al., 1995). Human Mx (MxA) has a broad antiviral specificity and is active against influenza virus, measles virus (Schnorr et al., 1993), Semliki Forest virus (Landis et al., 1998), and VSV, among others. The mechanism of action of MxA may be different from that of Mx1, as they have distinct subcellular localizations and antiviral specificities (Dreiding et al., 1985; Pavlovic et al., 1992). For reasons that are not readily apparent, many extensively in-bred lines lack functional Mx genes. This is true for the chicken Mx gene, which has recently been identified (Ko et al., 2002). Mx from most breeds of commercial chickens have a serine amino acid at position 631 and lack antiviral properties whereas functional chicken Mx proteins have asparagine at this position (Ko et al., 2004). The full properties of the chicken Mx gene product have yet to be published, but it appears to follow the MxA pattern of broad efficacy against influenza virus and VSV.

Despite many years of study, the mechanism of action of Mx proteins is still poorly understood. The proteins are all closely related, and all have high levels of homology to dynamin (Obar et al., 1990) and possess consensus GTP-binding domains (Aebi et al., 1989) and a C-terminal leucine zipper (Melen et al., 1992). The broad activity of some Mx proteins suggests an intracellular target intersecting a range of viral pathways. With regard to influenza virus, Mx1 apparently blocks primary transcription of incoming viral genomes (Krug et al., 1985) whereas MxA blocks viral protein synthesis and genome replication, but does not affect primary transcription (Pavlovic et al., 1992). It has been proposed that Mx specifically interacts with the viral polymerase, and evidence exists suggesting this may involve the PB2 (Huang et al., 1992) and/or NP proteins (Turan et al., 2004).

Prospects for Using Mx Genes in Birds

Mouse Mx1 has potent antiviral properties even when transferred into non-murine cell lines lacking endogenous Mx activity (Garber et al., 1991). Chick embryo fibroblast cell lines expressing Mx1 were refractory to influenza virus replication, showing reduced plaquing efficiency, multicycle yield, and viral gene expression. The avian Mx gene inhibits influenza virus and VSV replication when transfected into Mx-negative mouse cell lines (Ko et al., 2004). Either murine or avian Mx genes appear to be promising candidates for introduction into chickens. Restoring Mx function to chickens is likely to be beneficial in controlling influenza, but is unlikely to be sufficient on its own—after all, humans have functional MxA genes, but we still suffer from the flu. This may reflect the fact that Mx is induced by interferon and influenza virus can disrupt interferon responses (one function of the viral NS1 protein [Talon et al., 2000]). Placing the Mx gene under the control of a constitutive promoter would get around this problem, but may in turn affect the viability of the chicken. Constitutive expression of MxA has been found to promote cell death in response to apoptotic stimuli (Mibayashi et al., 2002). The optimal strategy for expression of Mx needs further investigation.

Decoys (DIs)

RNA decoys are short RNA molecules expressed at high levels that mimic the binding sites for specific RNA-binding proteins. By sequestering these proteins, they act as competitive inhibitors and prevent the normal function of the proteins concerned. Natural decoys exist and are responsible for the formation of defective interfering particles common to certain RNA viruses such as influenza and vesicular stomatitis virus. DI particles are virus particles that contain viral genomes with substantial deletions. By replicating more efficiently than the wild-type virus, they out-compete for host and viral intracellular resources and thus lower the resultant yield of wild-type virus. Natural DIs need to be packaged into virions if they are to persist in cell culture. Therefore, they must contain the signals required for replication and packaging. Synthetic decoys need only to mimic the binding site of the protein. The influenza virus RNA polymerase is a sequence-specific RNA-binding protein complex composed of three viral proteins, PB1, PB2, and PA (Tiley et al., 1994). The complex binds with high affinity to the first 11 bases at the 5′ end of the viral genome (vRNA) (Figure 5-4, boxed sequence). These sequences are absolutely conserved in all segments of all subtypes of influenza A virus (Robertson, 1979) and play several key roles in the control of replication, transcription, and packaging (Li and Palese, 1992; Parvin et al., 1989; Seong and Brownlee, 1992; Hagen et al., 1994; Cianci et al., 1995; Neumann and Hobom, 1995; Lee et al., 2003; Fodor et al., 1994, 1995; Luytjes et al., 1989; Odagiri and Tashiro, 1997). The polymerase also binds to the terminal 10-11 bases at the 5' end of the complementary replication intermediate (cRNA). These too are extremely well conserved across subtypes.

Experiments *in vitro* have demonstrated that the interaction of the polymerase with these terminal RNAs is very stable, and decoys based on these sequences have been shown to be potent competitive inhibitors of the polymerase (Luo et al., 1997). Decoy concentration will be a critical factor in the effectiveness of this strategy *in vivo*. In practice it has been found that the most effective decoys are composed of both the 5' and 3' end sequences expressed as a single RNA molecule (so-called panhandle decoys) (Figure 5-4). This may reflect the concentration of decoy achievable in the cell. Panhandle decoys being partially double stranded may be more resistant to intracellular RNAses and thus able to accumulate to higher levels. Alterna-

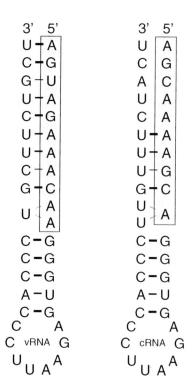

FIGURE 5-4 Typical decoy RNA sequences based upon conserved 5′ and 3′ terminal sequences of influenza virus vRNA and cRNA. Shaded boxes indicate the high affinity polymerase binding site located at the 5′ end of the viral RNAs.

tively, the level of expression provided by the delivery vector alone may be insufficient to achieve significant inhibition. Panhandle decoys contain all the sequences necessary and in the appropriate context for them to be replicated by the influenza virus polymerase. This could result in the decoy levels being amplified by the viral polymerase to levels that impact on virus replication. Clearly this question is crucial to the design of the most efficient decoys. Figure 5-5 shows the effectiveness of a flu-specific RNA decoy in comparison to RNAi-mediated (RNA interference or RNAi) inhibition (see below) using a cell culture-based viral transcription/replication assay. Both approaches can produce substantial levels of inhibition.

Decoy RNAs exploit an interaction between two very highly conserved viral components, the viral polymerase and the terminal sequences of the eight viral genome segments. Thus it is very unlikely that the virus will succeed in circumventing the effect of the decoy by mutation. Should the polymerase mutate such that it has an altered binding specificity, it would

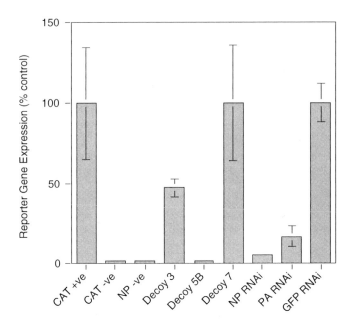

FIGURE 5-5 Inhibition of influenza virus replication by RNA decoys and RNAi. 293T cells were transfected with plasmids expressing influenza virus PB1, PB2, PA, and NP proteins and a plasmid that expresses an RNA corresponding to a negative sense chloramphenicol acetyltransferase (CAT) gene bounded by the 5′ and 3′ termini of vRNA. Transcription of the –ve sense CAT reporter RNA by the influenza virus polymerase leads to the production of CAT protein that can be quantitated by Enzyme Linked Immunosorbent Assay (ELISA). Omission of the CAT reporter (CAT –ve) or polymerase component (NP –ve) ablates CAT gene expression. The effects of various RNA decoy and RNAi expression plasmids are shown. Decoy 3, vRNA sense decoy; Decoy 5B, cRNA sense decoy; Decoy 7, control decoy lacking polymerase binding site; NP and PA RNAi targeting NP and PA mRNA respectively, as reported in Ge et al. (2003); GFP RNAi, irrelevant RNAi targeting the GFP gene.

likely be necessary that each of the termini undergo a compensatory mutation in order to still be recognized. The likelihood of this occurring for all eight segments is very remote.

RNAi

The discovery of the existence of an RNA-mediated gene silencing pathway (RNA interference or RNAi) in a wide range of species, including vertebrates, has already demonstrated enormous potential (for reviews, see

Caplen, 2004; Joost Haasnoot et al., 2003). Short double-stranded RNA molecules 19–21 nucleotides (nt) long, below the threshold for triggering the interferon response, are able to initiate the selective degradation of messenger RNA (mRNA) molecules to which they have the corresponding sequence. Such short interfering RNAs (siRNAs) are unwound and become incorporated into an RNA induced silencing complex (RISC). This complex uses its integral siRNA to recognize and bind to the complementary target mRNA and cleave it in a catalytic reaction using a RISC-associated RNAse. A number of strategies have been developed that allow this system to be exploited using plasmid or viral vector-based approaches. The most versatile so far uses a single strong promoter to drive the expression of a short hairpin RNA (shRNA) that is processed by the cellular protein Dicer into an siRNA suitable for incorporation into the RISC (Paddison et al., 2002). This system mimics the naturally occurring micro RNA (miRNA) system of gene expression control. More sophisticated designs of shRNA modeled closely on the miRNA system are leading to a better understanding of the requirements for effective siRNA molecules (Krol et al., 2004).

RNAi is a catalytic process, and so is less critically dependent on the level of shRNA expression. Design of flu-specific shRNA has concentrated on the highly conserved regions to ensure the RNAis have the broadest range of effectiveness on different subtypes of influenza A virus (Ge et al., 2003). These invariant regions may simply reflect an absence of immune selection, or may be under some other functional constraint of which we are currently unaware. If the former, it is likely that the virus will be able to escape the selective pressure imposed by the RNAi by simply mutating the target site. This has already been demonstrated for RNAi-mediated inhibition of HIV and poliovirus gene expression (Boden et al., 2003; Gitlin et al., 2002). To overcome this it will undoubtedly be necessary to express multiple RNAis against several different targets (akin to combination therapy using antivirals). However, as the number of different siRNAs increases, the efficiency of inhibition by each individual component may decrease as the RISC becomes saturated. This could also have knock-on effects during development. Certain viruses clearly have mechanisms for avoiding RNAi-mediated suppression (Joost Haasnoot et al., 2003). It has been suggested that the influenza virus NS1 protein (an RNA-binding protein itself) is an inhibitor of RNAi (Bucher et al., 2004; Delgadillo et al., 2004; Li et al., 2004). Experimental support for this comes from work on plants and worms, and as yet no evidence for such a function in natural hosts for flu has been reported. RNAi delivered as double-stranded RNA or as shRNA are effective against flu in both cell culture and mice, suggesting that flu is still vulnerable to this approach (Ge et al., 2003; Tompkins et al., 2004).

The Tools Are Now Available

Until very recently, the chief stumbling block to developing influenza-virus resistant chickens was not a lack of ideas, but the lack of a delivery system suitable for engineering the chicken genome. Limited success had been achieved using avian retroviral vectors (Rapp et al., 2003), but the efficiency of transduction was very low, and the levels of transgene expression were poor and not maintained through subsequent generations as a result of transgene silencing. The key breakthrough was the use of lentiviral vectors enveloped in the VSV glycoprotein (G) protein to deliver the transgene package (McGrew et al., 2004). These vectors can be prepared to very high concentrations (10^{10} transduction units per milliliter [ml]), enter virtually any cell type, and successfully infect and integrate into the chromosomes of cells irrespective of whether these cells are undergoing cell division at the time. For reasons that are still not fully understood, most transgenes introduced by lentiviral vectors do not appear to be subject to gene silencing (Kafri et al., 1997; Naldini et al., 1996).

The efficiency with which lentiviral vectors can transduce the chicken germline has been investigated (McGrew et al., 2004). High-titer preparations of vectors derived from equine infectious anemia virus, pseudotyped with VSV-G, were injected into chick embryos in new laid eggs in ovo, then cultured to hatch. The resulting birds were bred to determine the frequency of production of germline transgenic birds: the frequency achieved using high titers of virus vectors approached 100 percent and the transmission rate of the integrated viruses to the next generation was between 4 percent and 45 percent. The integrated viruses were stably transmitted on to the next generation, suggesting that transgenic lines produced using lentiviral vectors will be stable. Analysis of expression of reporter gene constructs carried by the vectors showed a conserved expression profile between individuals that was maintained after transmission through the germline for at least two generations (Figure 5-6). These results suggest that lentiviral vectors may be used to generate transgenic birds at very high frequencies and that the transgenes carried by the vectors will be expressed in a reliable manner when the transgenic birds are bred. These vectors may be easily engineered to carry siRNA, decoy, and Mx expression constructs. Transgenic mice, produced using lentiviral vectors that carry siRNA expression constructs, have been shown to express effective interfering siRNAs (Rubinson et al., 2003).

Future Hurdles

The first attempts to generate influenza-resistant transgenic chickens are currently underway, and more sophisticated vectors carrying all three of the inhibitory components described above are in production. However, there is still a long way to go before this research reaches its final objective. The technical objectives are achievable in the relatively short term (3 to 5 years). More challenging will be the need to demonstrate the long-term efficacy, lack of detrimental effects on the chicken or the environment, and safety for human consumption to the satisfaction of the regulatory bodies and the public at large.

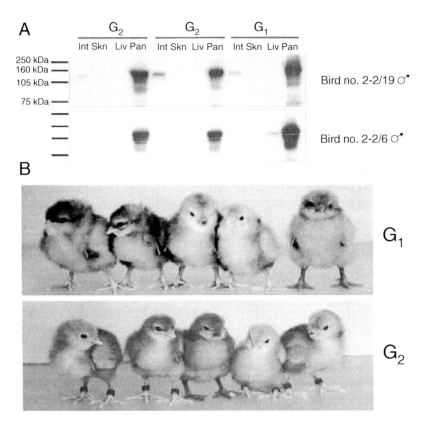

FIGURE 5-6 Reporter gene expression in transgenic birds. A. Western Blot analysis for Lac Z protein extracted from intestine (Int) skin (Skn), liver (Liv), and pancreas (Pan) of G1 cockerels 2-2/19 and 2-2/6 carrying Lac Z expressing lentivector pONY8.0cZ and two G2 offspring from each bird. B. Top panel: five G1 offspring of bird number 4-1. The four birds on the left are transgenic for the green fluorescent protein gene expressed from lentivectors pONY8.0G (all vectors provided by Oxford Biomedica [UK] Ltd). The bird on the right is not transgenic. Lower panel: five G2 offspring from bird number 4-1/66. The bird in the center is nontransgenic.

Is Global Repopulation with Transgenic Chickens Achievable?

Approximately 15 billion chickens are produced each year, so clearly it will take some considerable time, effort, and expense to achieve this goal. For example, approximately sixteen different layer breeds have significant market share worldwide. Each is a three- or four-way cross. Thus, roughly 64 transgenic pure-lines would be required if one wished to reestablish the status quo. Chickens can be bred remarkably quickly. Adult layer stocks produce about 1.8 viable female chicks per week, with an expected viability of more than 90 percent. Replacing the 3 to 4 billion layers would take just 2 to 3 years once the transgenic lines had been made.

Long-Term Efficacy

Transgene expression using lentivectors appears to be very stable, and it is arguable that if transgene expression persists over two generations (as has already been demonstrated in chickens) (McGrew et al., 2004), it is unlikely that it is ever going to suffer from transgene silencing—but time will tell. The selection of resistant mutant viruses is another distinct possibility. By using several independent inhibitory strategies it is hoped that the virus will be unable to overcome the blocks to its replication, thus ensuring the long-term effectiveness of the approach. This is a prerequisite if it is to be worthwhile to move toward the large-scale production of transgenic birds.

Adverse Effects

Because the transgenes are integrated at random in the chicken genome, there is the possibility of deleterious effects in some birds, depending on the location of the integration site. The availability of the chicken genome sequence will make analysis of integration sites quite straightforward, and facilitate the elimination of transgenic birds with the most obviously undesirable gene disruptions. The great advantage of the transgenic approach is that the single desired trait (resistance to influenza virus) can be inserted directly into commercial breeds, obviating the need to introduce the traits by cross-breeding with its associated problems of co-introducing undesirable traits. Once the founder transgenic birds have been fully characterized and shown to be healthy, the birds would be bred normally and subsequent generations would not require repeated genetic modification.

Safety for Humans and the Environment

The strategy used to deliver the transgenes uses a highly efficient and stable delivery vector. The vector has been modified extensively to make it completely devoid of any viral gene products and it is incapable of replication. The transgenes, decoys, and RNAi are under the control of avian promoter sequences and Mx is a naturally occurring avian gene. ShRNA and decoys are short RNA stemloop sequences that are extremely unlikely to pose any risk to anything other than influenza virus itself. It is difficult to conceive of any realistic risk to human health associated with consumption of such transgenic food. Likewise, chickens carrying such transgenes pose no realistic environmental threat.

Public Attitudes

The prevailing sentiment portrayed by the U.K. media regarding genetically modified products is undeniably negative. However, the majority of the U.K. population are not absolutely against genetically modified organisms (GMO) as food. Most hold the correct view that each GMO must be rigorously assessed on a case-by-case basis. The case for developing influenza-resistant chickens is a strong one on economic, public health, and animal welfare grounds. The risks are extremely small and will be thoroughly assessed. Nevertheless, at least for the foreseeable future in the United Kingdom, there would be significant resistance to the introduction of GMO chickens. Other countries are much more pragmatic about GMO food and are likely to welcome such a development more enthusiastically. Eliminating the chicken from the pandemic influenza equation might delay or prevent the next pandemic disaster. Even the most dire GMO scaremongering scenario would seem trivial by comparison to a rerun of the Spanish Lady of 1918.

MOLECULAR DIAGNOSTICS IN AN INSECURE WORLD

Michael L. Perdue[3]

Animal Waste Pathogen Laboratory, Animal and Natural Resources
Institute, U.S. Department of Agriculture,
Agricultural Research Service

---

[3]This proceedings manuscript documents an oral presentation given in the session on Molecular Diagnostics at the Fifth International Symposium on Avian Influenza, April 14–17, 2002, The University of Georgia, Athens, GA.

Summary

As of October 2001, the potential for use of infectious agents, such as anthrax, as weapons has been firmly established. It has been suggested that attacks on a nation's agriculture might be a preferred form of terrorism or economic disruption that would not have the attendant stigma of infecting and causing disease in humans. Highly pathogenic avian influenza virus is on every top ten list available for potential agricultural bioweapon agents, generally following foot and mouth disease virus and Newcastle disease virus at or near the top of the list. Rapid detection techniques for bioweapon agents are a critical need for the first-responder community, on a par with vaccine and antiviral development in preventing spread of disease. There are several current approaches for rapid, early responder detection of biological agents including influenza A viruses. There are also several proposed novel approaches in development. The most promising existing approach is real-time fluorescent PCR analysis in a portable format using exquisitely sensitive and specific primers and probes. The potential for reliable and rapid early-responder detection approaches are described, as well as the most promising platforms for using real-time PCR for avian influenza, as well as other potential bioweapon agents.

Current State of Molecular Diagnostics

Homeland defense has become a new item on everyone's budget request list—including the agricultural world. According to congressional testimonies by D.A. Henderson (2001) and others, rapid detection of introduced biological agents is a critical component in protecting human lives, along with rapid development of vaccines and antimicrobials. While we are all aware that profit margins in poultry production scarcely allow for the kinds of expensive molecular detection equipment that are affordable in the world of human health, the polymerase chain reaction (PCR) as a diagnostic tool has been well established among poultry health professionals for many years (American Association of Avian Pathologists, 1992). Several producers now have their own diagnostic capabilities that include routine PCR analysis for many poultry pathogens. As the market for sophisticated portable detection devices that employ PCR becomes greater, the price of on-site detection for agricultural pathogens will come down. Consequently, it is reasonable to pursue development of detection reagents for high-profile poultry pathogens, particularly the rapidly spreading respiratory pathogens. During an outbreak of a foreign animal disease such as highly pathogenic avian influenza, time is a critical factor in the extent of containment of the disease and the assessment of contamination of surrounding poultry operations and wild bird populations. Fluorescence-based PCR detection can use a single platform for detection of a host of pathogens. Once the fundamental target genes have been identified and sequenced in the laboratory, the designed primers and probes can be transferred directly to the portable machine format. Many commercially available machines can use the same chemistries, and multiple fluorescent wavelengths should eventually allow multiplex analysis for more than one pathogen per reaction. Also, unlike immunologically based detection methods, fluorescent primers and probes can be altered slightly to accommodate known genetic changes, without having to regenerate and revalidate as with serum-based reagents.

Agricultural Biological Threat Agents

Although agriculture does not immediately come to mind when one considers biowarfare or bioterrorism, every nation that has had a biological warfare program has had an anti-animal and an anticrop component (Rodgers et al., 1999; Wilson et al., 2001). Thus a number of potential threats have been identified for both animals and plants. Expert panels have been convened in recent years to determine attributes most likely to contribute to effectiveness of a bioweapon, and oftentimes the agents have then been ranked. Table 5-2 is a working top ten list of animal pathogens that have been used by the Agricultural Research Service in the last 2 years as a guide for developing detection reagents. At least four of these listed organisms (foot-and-mouth disease [FMD] virus, Newcastle disease virus [NDV], hog cholera virus, and Rinderpest) have been weaponized at one time in the past and evaluated under field conditions (Wilson et al., 2000). Since many of the animal commodity groups, including poultry, are clustered in high concentrations in various regions of the country, the possibility of an event of widespread introduction is high. The reasons for potential purposeful introductions are many and varied, and unfortunately it is not difficult to think of scenarios resulting in purposeful introduction of biological agents into the poultry industry. Thus, we must remain vigilant. The regulatory agencies that would respond to introduction of foreign animal diseases are likely capable of handling a single introduction (Ginsburg, 2000), although the recent FMD outbreak in the United Kingdom clearly illustrates the potential devastating effects of just a single entry point of a highly infectious foreign animal disease. A concerted attack on U.S. poultry with multiple introductions would almost certainly paralyze the industry even with the best efforts of the regulatory agencies.

Avian Influenza A Viruses as Potential Bioweapons

Highly pathogenic avian influenza viruses are generally found on all the lists of potential agricultural bioweapons. Like virulent Newcastle disease viruses that have been weaponized in the past, the AI viruses can be highly

TABLE 5-2 Diseases and Animal Pathogens of Concern to the Agricultural Research Service, U.S. Department of Agriculture

Disease	Agent
Foot and mouth disease	Apthovirus
Velogenic viscerotropic Newcastle disease	Paramyxovirus type 1, specific strains
Highly pathogenic avian influenza	Orthomyxovirus, type A, some subtypes H5 and H7
Hog cholera	Pestivirus
Rinderpest	Morbillivirus
Contagious bovine pleuropneumonia	Mycoplasma
Lumpy skin disease	Poxvirus
Blue tongue virus	Orbivirus
African horse sickness	Orbivirus
African swine fever	Asfivirus

and rapidly infectious via respiratory transmission. Unlike Newcastle disease virus, however, they can further be genetically reassorted in the laboratory to combine genes in a grouping that does not exist in nature, either by mating live viruses or rescuing virus from expression plasmids (Fodor et al., 1999; Hoffmann et al., 2000). The latter plasmid-based techniques are amazing technical developments, but they raise the possibility of major genetic manipulation of viruses and introduction of foreign genes into influenza gene backbones. Consequently, zoonotic influenza viruses in general are getting more attention as potential bioweapons (Peters, 2002). Although it seems highly unlikely that anyone would engineer an avian influenza virus for the purpose of attacking the poultry industry, other potential illegal uses that could spread live or engineered viruses exist. For example, anecdotal evidence exists purporting that poultry farmers have used infectious virus collected from an outbreak to infect their own stock, in attempts to vaccinate or in hopes of indemnification as a result of having infected flocks.

Whatever the case, the need for the capability to rapidly and accurately detect avian influenza viruses, as well as other highly infectious poultry pathogens in the environment, is growing, and new research efforts are needed to evaluate the best approaches to put into the hands of early responders to a purposeful introduction. Availability of validated, rapid, and reliable tests that would supplement the use of slower culture-based detection and immunological subtyping of avian influenza strains would be most useful.

Rapid Detection and Diagnosis

In the face of a scenario where multiple purposeful introductions of avian influenza virus into the poultry industry have occurred, rapid and accurate evaluation of environmental contamination becomes critical, especially if a zoonotic virus is encountered. In such a case the following prioritized attributes of a detection assay would be 1) speed and accuracy, 2) simplicity, 3) common platform for both environmental detection and diagnosis of infected animals, and 4) cost. There are nearly as many approaches to rapidly detecting pathogens and diagnosing disease as there are companies and laboratories developing the technologies. The term diagnostics is widely used to refer to both pinpointing a disease based on the presence of the organism in the host and simply detecting the agent where it should not be. In the veterinary world, generally speaking, the early responders will be state or company veterinarians who will see the disease first, then regulatory agencies that will seek to evaluate the extent of presence or spread. In the case of a zoonotic agent, of course, the public health agencies would become involved quickly. In the case of an agricultural pathogen that does not affect human health, contingency plans are in place to control the spread of disease that depend on the nature of the outbreak. Everyone agrees that the faster the pathogen is detected and the extent of contamination of the environment ascertained, the faster the outbreak can be controlled.

The long-sought, magic, 5-min test for detection is most closely approximated by the antigen capture/enzyme-linked immunosorbent assay (ELISA) based approach, where a sample is loaded onto a filter to which specific antibody is bound and a secondary reporter reagent gives colorimetric verification of presence of an antibody-antigen complex. The Directigen® Flu kit (Becton Dickinson, Franklin Lakes, NJ) is currently being used as a screening tool in disease outbreaks for the detection of any influenza A virus. This technology is rapid and has been used for both humans and poultry for years. It is based on detection of the influenza A nucleoprotein and is not suitable for subtyping strains. The sensitivity of such immunologically based tests is generally lower than nucleic acid based tests, and costs are such that individual bird samples must be pooled before screening.

A number of novel rapid detection approaches employ mass spectrometry (MS) to measure ionization and ion capture profiles following treatment of samples (Donlon and Jackman, 1999). The idea is that environmental samples containing pathogens when treated will yield signature patterns that will instantaneously identify the presence of the pathogen. One of these methods, matrix assisted laser desorption ionization time-of-flight (MALDI-TOF) spectroscopy employs a laser to ionize the sample and then a measuring chamber to measure the characteristics of the ions as they speed through the chamber. These instruments are continuously being made smaller and smaller, and suitcase size versions are currently being evaluated. Speed of detection is the advantage here if the problems associated with dirty environmental samples can be overcome by preselecting the pathogen out of its native matrix. The procedure will also lend itself to chip-based microarray technology since the laser could move over the array and the time of flight measurements made virtually instantaneously. The future success of such a device in the hands of the early responder will depend on working out the problems associated with preparing the environmental sample for clean measurements by the mass spectrometer. Further, while it is likely that an influenza A virus would provide a characteristic or signature MS profile, the possibilities for obtaining strain-specific characteristics are unknown but would seem very unlikely.

Nucleic-acid based detection and diagnostics will ultimately provide the most information to early responders, scientists, and the regulatory agencies. Just as in DNA forensic analysis in humans, characteristic genetic profiles or gene sequences of microbes can be obtained for each individual species and any strain of that species. Rapid detection of pathogens using PCR amplification of specific genes has been employed for many years, but it requires preparation of an electrophoretic gel run with molecular weight standards to identify and quantify the production of the amplicons. For eukaryotes and DNA containing pathogens, restriction fragment length polymorphisms (RFLPs) and many variations on that idea have been used to unequivocally identify organisms. The same approach can be taken with RNA viruses such as influenza viruses (Offringa et al., 2000), and there are commercially available mobile labs that exploit this approach, such as mobile molecular laboratory (model MML-0150, MJ Research, Waltham MA). Ultimately, small scale, suitcase size nucleic acid sequencers will be available, and this will provide the most information of all to identify environmental pathogens. But this technology is not yet available and is certainly not affordable.

There is one nucleic acid based detection approach for which portable platforms are commercially available and which is becoming accepted by early responders (Fatah, 2001) as a way to identify environmental pathogens, fluorescent real-time/PCR analysis (FRT/PCR). The fundamental chemistry and reaction conditions for this approach have actually been around for years (Heid et al., 1996; Livak et al., 1995) and was originally termed Taqman® PCR (Grove, 1999). Many technological variations of the Taqman chemistry have been developed, including Fret probes and molecular beacon probes, but all use fluorescent probes coupled to PCR for the detection of a wide variety of pathogens. The TAQMAN reaction is extremely specific, more so than other PCR, in that it requires correct alignment of three separate stretches of sequences in the target pathogen. Like PCR, two primers are designed based on specific target sequences and these amplify a short region of the genome in the regular hot/cool cycle of the PCR. In addition, a probe is designed to bind specifically to the amplicons, and this probe contains a fluorescent molecule on one end and a quencher molecule on the other end. The native exonuclease activity of the polymerase in the PCR cleaves this fluorescent molecule during the reaction releasing its fluorescence from the quenching molecule. So as more amplicon is produced, more probe is bound and more fluorescence is released in real time.

What has happened in the last couple of years is the emergence of commercially available portable machines that can use this technology for a host of pathogens. In addition, the availability of dried or packaged re-agents for a variety of pathogens will allow early responders to prepare a sample in the field and run FRT/PCR in place. We have prepared a number of primers and probe reagents that are specific for avian influenza viruses, and these are reported and described by Spackman et al. in this publication.

The advantages of this new technology and reagents are multiple. One is that the reaction is dead end; that is, after the amplification and measure-ment, the unopened reaction tube is thrown away, reducing the potential for cross contamination. Second, there are now a variety of fluorescent tags of different wavelengths so that the possibility exists for multiplex analysis within the same reaction tube using different wavelength filters to discern positive reactions. Finally, subject matter experts can analyze the reactions in real time in a format that allows for immediate evaluation over the Internet, since web-enabled software is available for some of the portable systems.

Two commercially available portable systems currently exploit these reactions. They are the Idaho technology ruggedized advanced pathogen identification device (RAPID®) system and the Cepheid Corporation SmartCycler®. Benchtop laboratory versions of each are also available from science supply companies. Each portable machine has desirable fea-tures that make it different from the other, but rather than go through those here, I refer the reader to the websites for each company: www.idahotech.com and www.cepheid.com. One feature of the RAPID system that makes it particularly attractive is its web-enabled software and potential for wireless transmission that allows transmission of data in real time from the field back to a command center. An epidemiologic tracking system developed in concert with the U.S. Air Force, lightweight epidemiology advanced detec-tion and emergency response (LEADER) uses the RAPID system and allows a central command point to be connected to several machines at once deployed at remote sites at considerable distances apart. So, in terms of potential for early responders, these kinds of systems provide a lot of promise. With standardized reagents and extraction protocols and communications with a central command post, evaluation of environmental contamination and infection of animals can be quickly evaluated for the regulatory decision makers.

Figure 5-7 illustrates two handheld instruments that use the real-time rapid PCR format and are still in evaluation stages. Efforts continue to miniaturize the detection process such that the technology can be made available to early responders, who would presumably be screening for a single agent to evaluate contamination and spread on the spot. Whether use of these will become a reality in the near future is anyone's guess. Several hundred of the portable RAPID and SmartCycler machines have been sold to various agencies, such as the National Guard and police departments, but the question is whether dried or prepackaged reagents with long enough shelf lives can be made available. FRT/PCR reagents for other RNA viruses similar to influenza A virus have worked in the prepackaged format, so getting from RNA to real-time analysis is certainly possible. Data presented

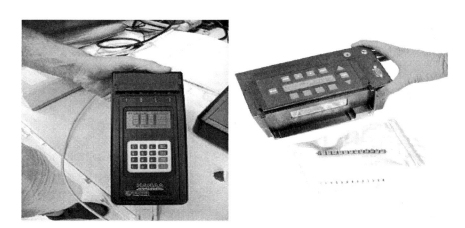

FIGURE 5-7 Handheld PCR devices. Two next generation fluorescent real-time PCR devices. On the left is the handheld advanced nucleic acid analyzer (HANAA), a prototype device developed by Lawrence Livermore Laboratories. The device is battery operable and has four cycling chambers to hold PCR reaction tubes. The unit on the right is Idaho Technology's RAZOR system, which cycles temperatures for the reaction by moving reaction mixtures back and forth in the plastic tubes between fixed temperature chambers and can run 12 reactions simultaneously. In each case, the nucleic acid has to be first extracted from the sample matrix before running the FRT/PCR. With the RAZOR system a set of prepackaged extraction reagents is provided in syringes, and the final sample is injected into the blue plastic receiver tubes. Photos courtesy of Jim Higgins (left) and Idaho Technology (right).

in this symposium have shown that sensitivity of the FRT/PCR approach for avian influenza viruses could be improved, but specificity is very good and costs promise to be cheaper than the immunologically based detection kits. More research is certainly needed to provide prepackaged reagents that could be used by early responders to detect influenza viruses in the environment. However, given the commercial success of this technology, which was used quite extensively during the anthrax attack in the fall of 2001, it is definitely worth pursuing avian influenza specific primer and probe development and validation of assays in real-world settings, such as those described in this symposium.

MODELING PANDEMIC PREPAREDNESS SCENARIOS: HEALTH ECONOMIC IMPLICATIONS OF ENHANCED PANDEMIC VACCINE SUPPLY

Jeroen K. Medema,[4,5] *York F. Zoellnerb,*[6] *James Ryan,*[7] *Abraham M. Palachea*[8]

Abstract

Influenza pandemic planning is a complex, multifactorial process, which involves public health authorities, regulatory authorities, academia and industry. It is further complicated by the unpredictability of the time of emergence and severity of the next pandemic and the effectiveness of influenza epidemic interventions. The complexity and uncertainties surrounding pandemic preparedness have so far kept the various stakeholders from joining forces and tackling the problem from its roots. We developed a mathematical model, which shows the tangible consequences of conceptual

---

[4]Corresponding author: tel: +31-294-477000; fax: +31-294-431164; e-mail: jeroen.medema@solvay.com.

[5]Business Group Influenza, Solvay Pharmaceuticals BV, P.O. Box 900, Weesp 1380 DA, The Netherlands.

[6]Department of Health Economics, Solvay Pharmaceuticals GmbH, P.O. Box 220, Hannover 30002, Germany.

[7]Mapi Values, The Adelphi Mill, Bollington, Macclesfield, Cheshire SK105JB, UK.

[8]The authors like to thank James Piercy of Mapi Values for the health economic support during development of the model and Professor Kristin L. Nichol of the University of Minnesota Medical School for her valuable comments on the manuscript.

plans by linking possible pandemic scenarios to health economic outcomes of possible intervention strategies. This model helps to structure the discussion on pandemic preparedness and facilitates the translation of pandemic planning concepts to concrete plans. The case study for which the model has been used shows the current level of global pandemic preparedness in an assumed pandemic scenario, the health economic implications of enhanced pandemic vaccine supply and the importance of cell culture-based influenza vaccine manufacturing technologies as a tool for pandemic control.

Introduction

Influenza is an acute respiratory disease, which can often lead to serious and life-threatening complications in several populations, like the elderly and chronically ill. It occurs in annual epidemics in regions of temperate climates with illness attack rates of 10–20%, leading to an average of 114,000 hospitalizations and 20,000 excess deaths in the United States alone (Strikas et al., 2002). In addition to these annual epidemics, type A influenza viruses have caused pandemics, i.e., sudden global epidemics in all age groups with higher attack and mortality rates. These pandemics are caused by a newly emerging virus subtype in the human population, resulting from reassortment of gene segments between influenza viruses with different host susceptibility (e.g., human, swine and avian strains) or by direct transmission of non-human virus subtypes to humans.

The last century has seen three influenza pandemics, the "Spanish Flu" in 1918–1919, the "Asian Flu" in 1957 and the "Hong Kong Flu" in 1968. The first, one of the most severe events in human history in terms of cases and deaths, was responsible for an estimated 2 billion cases and 20–50 million deaths worldwide (Potter, 1998; Davies, 2000). The latter two were less severe; the 1957 pandemic led to over 1 million deaths worldwide and 70-80,000 in the United States, whereas the "Hong Kong Flu" was reported as relatively mild with peak mortality rates similar to 1957 (Potter, 1998; Strikas et al., 2002). As the influenza virus was only discovered in 1933, influenza diagnosis was poor before that date; hence the corresponding clinical cases have neither been identified nor documented as such before the twentieth century. Analysis of historical documentation, however, clearly indicates that influenza pandemics have occurred at irregular intervals over many centuries and there are no reasons to doubt they will occur again.

The increased awareness of the societal burden of annual influenza epidemics since the mid-1990s led to an increasing awareness of the pandemic threat we are facing. Furthermore, the emergence of two new influenza viruses—subtype H5N1 in 1997 and subtype H9N2 in 1999—in humans in the Hong Kong area, which seem to be transmitted directly from avian species made this threat real and imminent. The events following 11 September 2001 have further contributed by drawing the general public's attention to the hazard of biological threats.

The increased awareness on influenza pandemics has led to discussions by public health authorities, regulatory authorities, academia, and industry on what our society can and should do to prepare for the next pandemic. This has resulted amongst others in the founding of the Influenza Vaccine Supply (IVS) Taskforce, a new pandemic discussion and collaboration platform in which all major influenza vaccine manufacturers are represented. Increased awareness has also resulted in governmental pandemic preparedness plans on national and regional levels, such as the "Influenza Pandemic Preparedness Action Plan for the United States" and "A pandemic influenza planning guide for state and local officials" by the Centers of Disease Control and Prevention (Strikas et al., 2002; Patriarca et al., 1999) and the "Canadian contingency plan for pandemic influenza" (Health Canada, 2000). Several attempts are undertaken to bring pandemic planning to multinational or even global level, such as the November 2001 conference on "Preparedness planning in the EU: Influenza and other health threats" and the WHO influenza pandemic preparedness plan (World Health Organization, 1999). Although some regions, e.g. the Canadian province of Ontario, are quite well advanced in pandemic planning and implementation, most of both national and international plans are not completed, let alone realized.

Pandemic planning is a multifactorial process with a consequent high complexity. It is further complicated by the unpredictability of the next pandemic; its time of emergence, spread and severity cannot be foreseen and the efficacy of interventions available for annual influenza epidemics cannot be extrapolated per se to a pandemic situation. Both the complexity and the uncertainties surrounding pandemic preparedness have so far kept the various stakeholders from joining forces and tackling the problem from its roots. The complexity of preparedness planning must be simplified by dividing it into several "sub-projects", which should be addressed separately to bring pandemic planning from abstract concepts to the desired concreteness.

We developed a mathematical model which shows the tangible consequences of conceptual plans by linking possible pandemic scenarios to health economic outcomes of possible intervention strategies. This model helps to structure the discussion on pandemic preparedness by calculating costs and benefits, gauges the public health benefits of optimized preparedness, and facilitates the translation of pandemic planning concepts to concrete plans.

Materials and Methods

A computer-based simulation model has been developed by MAPI Values (Macclesfield, United Kingdom) and Solvay Pharmaceuticals (Weesp, The Netherlands, and Hannover, Germany), which allows for epidemiological, cost and efficacy inputs as well as manufacturing constraints. The model combines a vaccine production model with an adapted and revised cost-effectiveness model of influenza intervention strategies, based on that developed by Scuffham and West (2002).

Inputs for Pandemic Scenarios

The model inputs for the pandemic scenarios determine the characteristics of the pandemic to which the several intervention strategies can be directed; these input parameters are the attack and mortality rate of that particular pandemic virus, the time of emergence of the pandemic virus and the time for the pandemic to spread and end.

Inputs for Intervention Scenarios

The model inputs for intervention scenarios determine the availability of possible interventions, e.g., pandemic vaccine and antivirals, such as amantadine or the new neuraminidase inhibitors. These input parameters include specific vaccine production inputs, such as time to produce a suitable pandemic virus seed time to produce a batch of vaccine, availability of eggs for egg-based vaccine production and available vaccine manufacturing capacity. They do not include specific antiviral production inputs, as it is assumed that if antivirals are selected as intervention strategy, they will be stockpiled and readily available. Intervention scenario inputs also include parameters, such as pandemic vaccine potency and dosing regime. It is assumed that all manufactured vaccines are used.

Inputs for Intervention Effectiveness

Inputs for intervention effectiveness include parameters such as reduction of influenza-like illness (ILI) cases, reduction in primary care physician (PCP) visits for ILI symptoms, reduction of hospitalizations due to influenza and pneumonia, other respiratory illnesses and congestive heart failure.

Health Economic Inputs

The model allows direct costs, from the perspective of the health care system, to be put in. Parameters for direct costs include all medical costs of the burden of the pandemic and for the intervention strategy selected. The medical costs for the burden of the pandemic include input parameters like costs of PCP consultations, costs of hospitalization due to influenza and pneumonia, other respiratory illnesses and to congestive heart failure. By combining average costs with resource use (PCP consultations, hospitalizations, etc.), the total medical costs for that particular pandemic can be calculated. The medical costs for the intervention strategy include the vaccine and vaccination cost as well as the costs of antiviral prophylaxis or therapy.

The model allows for a series of secondary input parameters, such as the probability of having an antiviral prescribed during a PCP visit with ILI symptoms, proportion of PCP visits undertaken at home and days off work per case.

Approach

One way of giving structure to conceptual pandemic preparedness plans is to evaluate these plans from a health economic perspective. Therefore the developed model is used to calculate the costs and benefits of certain intervention scenarios for different pandemic scenarios. The strength of the model is its ability to visualize different pandemic scenarios and different preparedness strategies, which is reinforced by assuming the pandemic threat is imminent, rather than taking place at an unknown point in time decades from now. Hence we assumed the next pandemic strain emerges 1 January, 2004, in order to show the current level of pandemic preparedness and how the model can visualize this.

We assumed that the pandemic scenario caused by the "2004 pandemic" virus is based on the 1918–1919 pandemic with influenza attack rates of 20–50% depending on region and a case fatality rate of 1.5% in two pandemic waves (Potter, 1998). For the "2004 pandemic" an average 1918-1919 attack rate of 35% in a single wave with a case fatality rate of 1.87% (Scuffham and West, 2002) are put into the model as pandemic scenario parameters.

Health economic parameters put into the model are based on average data obtained in the elderly in the United Kingdom in recent annual influenza epidemics (Scuffham and West, 2002). For the "2004 pandemic" case study it is assumed that health services utilization during the influenza pandemic are comparable to those during annual epidemics; increased absenteeism of health care workers and societal disruption by the pandemic are not taken into account. It is acknowledged that health care costs and health economical consequences of influenza in the United Kingdom cannot be translated to other countries, especially not to developing countries. Therefore, the latter are left out of this case study and the results that come from this study only visualize the level of preparedness of the developed countries. The total population of the developed countries is estimated at 1 billion. The key input parameters for the model including vaccination efficacy, are listed in Table 5-3.

Results

The outputs of the model that show the burden of the assumed "2004 pandemic" on developed countries are listed in Table 5-4 under the no intervention scenario. These data show that the no intervention scenario leads to 350 million cases and 22.2, 48.2 and 6.55 million influenza-related PCP consultations, hospitalizations and excess deaths, respectively. Total direct medical care costs add up to € 166.6 billion, with hospitalizations costs of € 165.2 billion as the major contributor.

To visualize the current level of pandemic preparedness, the intervention strategies that can he launched to decrease the burden of the "2004 pandemic" are based on existing egg-based influenza vaccine technologies. Currently, the estimated Northern Hemisphere influenza vaccine usage is 230 million trivalent doses, which translates to a global influenza vaccine manufacturing capacity of 22 million monovalent doses (i.e., 15 μg of pandemic strain antigen) per week. Two main starting materials are needed to manufacture the pandemic vaccine with the current technology: a sufficient amount of embryonated hen's eggs bred under controlled conditions and a seed of the virus strain to which the vaccine is directed. Preparation of the latter is performed by WHO collaborating centers and takes 1.5–2.5 months for annual epidemic strains. For the assumed "2004 pandemic" seed preparation time is unknown and unpredictable; we assumed a seed preparation time of 3 months, which means that pandemic vaccine manufacture can start 1 April 2004. This is within the regulated annual influenza vaccine manufacturing season, which means that the eggs are readily available for pandemic vaccine manufacture. We assumed that the applied "2004 pandemic" vaccine will be 7.5 μg monovalent given in two doses and should be administered within 6 months after emergence of the "2004 pandemic" virus.

The results of the assumed intervention strategy on the "2004 pandemic" are listed in Table 5-4 as intervention scenario 1. These data show that the current level of pandemic preparedness in the assumed egg-derived scenario leads to vaccination of 17% of the population, which avoids 29.8 million influenza cases, 1.74 million PCP visits, 267 million hospitalizations and 556,000 deaths compared to a scenario of no vaccination. The intervention strategy costs add up to € 2.2 billion, but as this strategy leads to a reduction of € 9.3 billion medical care costs, the saving on direct costs of the "2004 pandemic" is € 7.1 billion.

TABLE 5-3 Key Input Parameters Used Within the Model

Vaccine production	
Month of pandemic strain	January 2004[a,b]
Month egg seed released by WHO	April 2004[a]
Month last vaccine required in market	July 2004[a,b]
Number of weeks to produce a vaccine	5[a,b]
Weeks cell seed released before egg seed	9[b]
Size of (trivalent) vaccine unit (μg)	45[a,b]
Number of shots required per person	2[a,b]
Dose per shot (μg)	7.5[a,b]
Annual manufacturing capacity	230,000,000[a,b]
Demographics	
Overall population	1,000,000,000[a,b]
Target population	1,000,000,000[a,b]
Influenza attack rate (%)	35[a,b]
Years per life lost	5[c]
Event probabilities	
PCP consultations (for influenza)	6.34[d]
Hospitalization rates due to:	
Influenza + pneumonia	2.52[d]
Other respiratory disease	9.34[d]
Congestive heart failure	1.9[d]
Mortality rate	1.87[d]
Vaccine effectiveness	
Vaccine efficacy (%)	53[e]
Reduction in GP visits (%)	46[f]
Reduction in hospitalizations due to:	
Influenza + pneumonia (%)	39[f]
Other respiratory disease (%)	32[f]
Congestive heart failure (%)	27[f]
Reduction in mortality (%)	50[f]
Unit costs and economic parameters	
PCP consultation (€)	28.6[c]
Influenza vaccine price (€)	10[a,b]
Influenza vaccine service and administration(€)	3.1[c]
Discount rate	5[c]
Hospitalization for:	
Influenza + pneumonia (€)	3,585[c]
Other respiratory disease (€)	3,362[c]
Congestive heart failure (€)	3,556[c]
Average hospital cost per bed per day (€)	261[c]

[a]Authors' assumption for egg-based vaccine intervention strategies.
[b]Authors' assumption for cell culture-based vaccine intervention strategies.
[c]Scuffham and West (2002).
[d]Derived from Scuffham and West (2002).
[e]Govaert et al. (1994).
[f]Nichol et al. (1998).

TABLE 5-4 Burden of Different Intervention Scenarios in the Assumed Pandemic

	No Intervention	Intervention Scenario 1 Egg-Based Vaccine Manufacture	Intervention Scenario 2 Cell Culture-Based Vaccine Manufacture
Vaccination coverage (%)	0	17	37
Number vaccinated	0	170,000,000	370,000,000
Number of cases (influenza)	350,000,000	320,250,000	285,250,000
PCP visits for treatment (influenza)	22,190,000	20,454,742	18,413,262
Hospitalizations	48,160,000	45,491,663	42,352,443
Excess deaths	6,545,000	5,988,675	5,334,175
Discounted years per life lost	25,640,894	23,461,418	20,897,328
PCP visit costs vaccinations (€)	0	2,227,000,000	4,847,000,000
PCP visit costs treatment (€)	1,007,181,910	928,420,285	835,759,549
Hospitalization costs (€)	165,170,880,000	156,010,312,598	145,233,174,478
Strategy costs (€)	0	2,227,000,000	4,847,000,000
Medical care costs (€)	166,647,295,200	157,371,272,130	146,458,303,811
Total direct costs (€)	166,647,295,200	159,598,272,130	151,305,303,811

The question for pandemic planners is if the level of pandemic preparedness can be improved and which intervention strategies should be selected to achieve this. As vaccination is the most cost effective intervention, an improved intervention strategy from a health economic perspective would be to produce more pandemic vaccine in the available time frame. This can be achieved by increasing the time period for vaccine manufacture, by increasing the vaccine manufacturing capacity or preferably by a combination of the two.

An earlier availability of a suitable seed virus would increase the time frame for pandemic vaccine manufacture and hence improve the intervention strategy. The new cell culture-based influenza vaccine manufacturing technology likely facilitates seed preparation, as mammalian cell culture may require less adaptation of viruses and shows containment of more pathogenic pandemic viruses without prior decrease of their virulence (see Section 4[9]). To visualize this we calculated the level of pandemic preparedness with an intervention scenario of cell culture-based vaccine manufacturing, assuming that preparation of a cell culture-based seed virus takes 1 month and assuming that the current global weekly manufacturing capacity of 22 million monovalent doses is cell culture-based instead of egg-based. The results of this assumed intervention strategy on the "2004 pandemic" are listed in Table 5-4 as intervention scenario 2.

These results show that, compared to no intervention scenario, the cell culture-based intervention strategy avoids 75 million influenza cases, 3.78 million PCP consultations for influenza treatment and, respectively, 5.81 million and 1.21 million influenza-related hospitalizations and excess deaths. Compared to the assumed egg-based vaccine intervention with 17% vaccine coverage, the cell culture-based intervention strategy leads to vaccination of 37% of the population, avoiding an additional 35 million influenza cases, 2.04 million PCP consultations for influenza treatment, 3.14 million influenza-related hospitalizations and 654,500 excess deaths. The cell culture-based intervention strategy costs add up to € 4.9 billion, but as this strategy leads to a reduction of € 20.2 billion medical care costs, the saving on direct costs of the "2004 pandemic" is € 15.3 billion, an additional € 8.3 billion compared to the egg-based intervention scenario.

The years per life lost gained are € 2.56 million, whereas the cost per life year gained is € 3198. The cost per case, hospitalization and death averted are, respectively, € 234, € 2612 and € 12,530.

Discussion

The "2004 pandemic" case study is based on numerous assumptions. Each can be challenged and, indeed, such uncertain variables are discussed by pandemic planners to challenge preparedness concepts. However, the assumed parameters are only inputs to the presented model and not part of the model itself. Therefore, questioning these assumptions is not questioning the model itself. The model is only a tool to visualize the consequences and effectiveness of a number of planning concepts, to which it lends struc-

---

[9]Editor's note: Section 4 refers to the Discussion.

ture and logic. Moreover, a sensitivity analysis of the model can be used to set priorities within pandemic planning discussions: the more sensitive the model is to a given assumption, the higher the effect of that particular input on the level of pandemic preparedness.

A sensitivity analysis of the "2004 pandemic" case study shows that the model is most sensitive to the pandemic scenario in terms of attack and mortality rates, as well as to the intervention scenarios in terms of effectiveness and available amounts of pandemic vaccine. It is less sensitive to medical care costs and relatively insensitive to pandemic vaccine price. The total direct medical costs of € 166.6 billion are remarkably close to the € 166.5 billion calculated by the CDC for a pandemic with 35% attack rate (Meltzer et al., 1999). However, these are for the United States alone with 89 million cases, 734,000 hospitalizations and 207,000 excess deaths on a smaller population than in the model presented here. Although the CDC model is similar, the inputs are based on U.S. data, explaining the higher costs.

Pandemic Scenario

The assumptions put into the model to derive the presented "2004 pandemic" scenario have been based on the 1918–1919 pandemic in terms of spread and severity. The first cases were reported in March 1918, leading to a first wave that was not severe. It took about 5–6 months before the pandemic evolved into a second wave with the particular characteristics of high attack and mortality rates, in the age groups at risk for epidemic influenza as well as other age groups, like children and young adults (Potter, 1998). This pandemic shows that everybody can be at risk for pandemic influenza and means that at that time intervention in all age groups at risk should have taken place in these 6 months between emergence and actuality of the pandemic. However, both knowledge and surveillance of circulating influenza viruses have been well established over the last 50 years, enabling an earlier identification of potential pandemic viruses and consequently an earlier onset of intervention programs compared to 1918. Furthermore, improved influenza diagnosis and the availability of intervention enable us to significantly reduce pandemic virus spread. On the other hand, the increased globalization and international travel in current times are likely to speed up spread of pandemic viruses to a large extent. As these phenomena counteract, we assumed for the "2004 pandemic" the same time frame between emergence and spread of the pandemic virus as in 1918.

The severity of a pandemic is reflected in the model by attack rate and event probabilities, such as influenza-related PCP consultations, hospitalizations and case fatality rate. For the "2004 pandemic" we assumed a higher attack rate to reflect a higher severity compared to annual epidemics. All event probabilities for the "2004 pandemic" are based on annual epidemic UK event probabilities for the elderly, which are higher than for other age groups. However, the higher attack rate implies that during the "2004 pandemic" other age groups are affected as well and extrapolation of high event probabilities in the elderly to these age groups also reflects a more severe event.

Egg-Based Vaccine Intervention Scenario

Health economic studies on annual influenza epidemics have shown that influenza vaccination is by far more cost-effective than prescription of antivirals for prophylaxis or therapy (Scuffham and West, 2002). Because the health economic perspective has been used in the model to visualize the current level of pandemic preparedness, vaccination has been selected as the pandemic intervention strategy in the current case study as well. The case study is limited to the developed world, because the health economic inputs are based on data gathered in a developed country, but pandemics are a global event and the burden in developing countries might be even greater because of lower public health. However, as long as global pandemic preparedness plans have not been realized, the world will face a limited availability of interventions. These will be made available to developed countries first at the cost of the developing world.

The intervention scenario input parameters are based on current influenza vaccine manufacturing technologies. We assumed that the applied "2004 pandemic" vaccine will be 7.5 µg monovalent given in two doses, as the human population is immunologically naive to the pandemic strain and will need a booster-dose to elicit a protective immune response. Clinical studies in unprimed individuals indeed indicate that a two dose regime is needed (Nicholson et al., 1979), but that this may be achieved with a lower, possibly adjuvanted dose (Nicholson et al., 2001; Hehme et al., 2002).

The next pandemic is likely to be detected by the WHO global influenza surveillance network and, just as for annual epidemic strains, WHO collaboration centers prepare the pandemic virus seed. Seed preparation time for the next pandemic is unpredictable and cannot be based on experience with epidemic strains: although the H5N1-subtype that emerged in Hong Kong in 1997 appeared only a candidate pandemic virus, a suitable seed is still not available 5 years later. In case of a high pandemic threat the efforts that will be put into seed preparation will be accordingly and preparation times for pandemic seeds suitable for egg-based vaccine manufacture in general is expected to be 2–8 months (internal communication J. Woods of WHO Collaboration Center NIBSC, WHO Experts-IVS Taskforce Meeting, September 26, 2002, Geneva). For the case study we assumed 3 months, leaving 3 months for vaccine manufacture, distribution and vaccination before the "2004 pandemic" would evolve and widely spread.

Field strains circulating in the human population usually do not propagate well on eggs and need to be attenuated for egg-based vaccine manufacture. Therefore, both epidemic and pandemic seed preparation for egg-based technology mainly consists of preparation of so-called high growth reassortants by reassortment of field strains with strains that propagate well on eggs. Additionally, pandemic viruses are more virulent than epidemic strains and need to be attenuated to decrease their virulence to safely propagate such viruses in existing egg-based manufacturing facilities, as these are based on open systems.

On the contrary, cell culture-based vaccine manufacture is performed in closed bioreactor systems, enabling the desired containment to process more virulent pandemic viruses without prior attenuation and hence less laborious seed preparation. Moreover, cell culture-based influenza vaccine manufacturing technologies make use of mammalian cell lines, such as MDCK, which are more closely related to the human host than the avian egg-based technology. MDCK-grown human influenza field isolates indeed are generally more antigenically homogenous and more alike the original field strain than egg-grown isolates (Zambon, 1998), which is probably caused by host cell selection of variants. Mammalian epithelioid cells like MDCK appear to be the most sensitive cell culture system for human influenza viruses to date (Zambon, 1998), whereas some human influenza isolates need to be adapted to growth in the allantoic cavity (Murphy and Webster, 1996). Therefore, cell culture is generally used for primary isolation of human influenza viruses. The probability that human pandemic viruses readily grow in mammalian cells therefore seems higher than in the more distant avian host, thereby making the preparation of high growth reassortants obsolete and decreasing the time for pandemic seed preparation. This favors the preparation of pandemic seeds by propagation of the pandemic strain directly on mammalian cell culture instead of via embryonated eggs. However, for annual epidemic vaccine manufacture the egg-passage is a regulatory obligation; omission of this procedure therefore needs to be cleared by authorities.

As the time period for vaccine manufacture is mainly determined by the time a suitable virus seed is available and the time the pandemic spreads in the population, a potential quicker release of pandemic seed suitable for cell culture enables the production of more vaccines. The more vaccines, the greater the vaccination rate and the greater the opportunity to benefit from both reduced mortality and reduced total costs. This underlines the importance of cell culture-based influenza vaccine manufacturing as tool for increased pandemic preparedness.

By assuming the pandemic virus emerges in January, eggs are readily available for pandemic vaccine manufacture once the seed is available. However, a pandemic virus can emerge all year round, also outside the annual epidemic vaccine manufacturing period. Given that logistics of egg preparation require ordering about 1 year in advance, availability of sufficient eggs outside the planned period certainly can be questioned. Cell culture-based vaccine manufacture however makes long-term advance planning obsolete, as all starting materials are in stock and readily available whenever required. This advantage however is not illustrated in the assumed "2004 pandemic", thereby underestimating the advantageous health economics of cell culture-based over egg-based intervention and thus the importance of cell culture-based vaccine manufacturing as tool for increased pandemic preparedness.

Although the presented model can lend structure and logic to pandemic preparedness discussions, pandemic planning remains a complex process. The efficacy of interventions, such as vaccines and antivirals, during pandemics needs to be studied and proven beforehand as much as possible in order to make such interventions available in time. Regulatory procedures of such interventions need to be harmonized and adapted to the short-time lines available in pandemic situations and logistical systems need to be set up or streamlined to successfully execute the intervention strategy. Pandemic vaccination might be the most cost-effective approach, but will require the availability of a suitable virus seed and adequate manufacturing facilities to process such a seed. In order to manufacture sufficient amounts for an adequate level of pandemic vaccine, manufacturing capacity needs to be increased. As stated by WHO, policy makers need to keep in mind the several years needed to construct new production facilities and significantly increase production capacity (World Health Organization, 2002). This only has an economical incentive if interpandemic vaccine usage is increased, which—just as pandemic preparedness—is a joint responsibility of the public and private sector.

REFERENCES

Ada GL, Jones PD. 1986. The immune response to influenza infection. *Curr Top Microbiol Immunol* 128:1–54.

Aebi M, Fah J, Hurt N, Samuel CE, Thomis D, Bazzigher L, Pavlovic J, Haller O, Staeheli P. 1989. cDNA structures and regulation of two interferon-induced human Mx proteins. *Mol Cell Biol* 9:5062–5072.

Alexander DJ. 2003. Report on avian influenza in the Eastern Hemisphere during 1997–2002. *Avian Diseases* 47:792–797.

Altmuller A, Fitch WM, Scholtissek C. 1989. Biological and genetic evolution of the nucleoprotein gene of human influenza A viruses. *J Gen Virol* 70:2111–2119.

American Association of Avian Pathologists. 1992 (August). *Proceedings of the Symposium on Biotechnology Applications in Avian Medicine*. American Veterinary Medical Association Meeting, Boston, MA.

Bender BS, Bell WE, Taylor S, Small PA Jr. 1994. Class I major histocompatibility complex-restricted cytotoxic T lymphocytes are not necessary for heterotypic immunity to influenza. *J Infect Dis* 170(5):1195-1200.

Benton KA, Misplon JA, La C-Y, Bruckiewicz RR, Prasad SA, Epstein SL. 2001. Heterosubtypic immunity to influenza A virus in mice lacking either IgA, all Ig, NKT cells, or gd T-cells. *J Immunol* 166:7437–7445.

Bernasconi D, Schultz U, Staeheli P. 1995. The interferon-induced Mx protein of chickens lacks antiviral activity. *J Interferon Cytokine Res* 15:47–53.

Boden D, Pusch O, Lee F, Tucker L, Ramratnam B. 2003. Human immunodeficiency virus type 1 escape from RNA interference. *J Virol* 77:11531–11535.

Bot A, Reichlin A, Isobe H, Bot S, Schulman J, Yokoyama WM, Bona CA. 1996. Cellular mechanisms involved in protection and recovery from influenza virus infection in immunodeficient mice. *J Virol* 70:5668–5672.

Bucher E, Hemmes H, de Haan P, Goldbach R, Prins M. 2004. The influenza A virus NS1 protein binds small interfering RNAs and suppresses RNA silencing in plants. *J Gen Virol* 85:983–991.

Burns JW, Siadat-Pajouh M, Krishnaney AA, Greenberg HB. 1996. Protective effect of rotavirus VP6-specific 19A monoclonal antibodies that lack neutralizing activity. *Science* 272:104–107.

Buxton Bridges C, Katz JM, Seto WH, Chan PK, Tsang D, Ho W, Mak KH, Lim W, Tam JS, Clarke M, Williams SG, Mounts AW, Bresee JS, Conn LA, Rowe T, Hu-Primmer J, Abernathy RA, Lu X, Cox NJ, Fukuda K. 2000. Risk of influenza A (H5N1) infection among health care workers exposed to patients with influenza A (H5N1), Hong Kong. *J Infect Dis* 181:344–348.

Caplen NJ. 2004. Gene therapy progress and prospects. Downregulating gene expression: The impact of RNA interference. *Gene Ther* 11:1241–1248.

CDC (Centers for Disease Control and Prevention). 2000. Updated recommendations from the Advisory Committee on Immunization Practices in response to delays in supply of influenza vaccine for the 2000–01 season. *MMWR* 49:888–892.

Chen HL, Subbarao K, Swayne D, Chen Q, Lu X, Katz J, Cox N, Matsuoka Y. 2003. Generation and evaluation of a high-growth reassortant H9N2 influenza A virus as a pandemic vaccine candidate. *Vaccine* 21:1974–1979.

Cianci C, Tiley L, Krystal M. 1995. Differential activation of the influenza virus polymerase via template RNA binding. *J Virol* 69:3995–3999.

Claas EC, Osterhaus AD. 1998. New clues to the emergence of flu pandemics. *Nat Med* 4:1122–1123.

Claas EC, Osterhaus AD, van Beek R, De Jong JC, Rimmelzwaan GF, Senne DA, Krauss S, Shortridge KF, Webster RG. 1998. Human influenza A H5N1 virus related to a highly pathogenic avian influenza virus. *Lancet* 351:472–477.

Couch RB, Keitel WA, Cate TR. 1997. Improvement of inactivated influenza virus vaccines. *J Infect Dis* 176(Suppl 1):S38–S44.

Davies P. 2000. *Catching Cold: 1918s Forgotten Tragedy and the Scientific Hunt for the Virus That Caused It*. Harmondsworth, UK: Penguin Books.

de Jong JC, Beyer WE, Palache AM, Rimmelzwaan GF, Osterhaus AD. 2000. Mismatch between the 1997/1998 influenza vaccine and the major epidemic A(H3N2) virus strain as the cause of an inadequate vaccine-induced antibody response to this strain in the elderly. *Med Viral* 61:94–99.

de St. Groth SF, Donnelley M. 1950. Studies in experimental immunology of influenza. IV. The protective value of active immunization. *Aust J Exp Biol Med Sci* 28:61–75.

Delgadillo MO, Saenz P, Salvador B, Garcia JA, Simon-Mateo C. 2004. Human influenza virus NS1 protein enhances viral pathogenicity and acts as an RNA silencing suppressor in plants. *J Gen Virol* 85:993–999.

Doherty PC, Topham DJ, Tripp RA, Cardin RD, Brooks JW, Stevenson PG. 1997. Effector CD4(+) and CD8(+) T-cell mechanisms in the control of respiratory virus infections. *Immunol Rev* 159:105–117.

Donlon M, Jackman J. 1999. DARPA integrated chemical and biological detection system. *Johns Hopkins APL Technical Digest* 20:320–325.

Dreiding P, Staeheli P, Haller O. 1985. Interferon-induced protein Mx accumulates in nuclei of mouse cells expressing resistance to influenza viruses. *Virology* 140:192–196.

Elkins KL, Bosio CM, Rhinehart-Jones TR. 1999. Importance of B-cells but not specific antibodies, in primary and secondary protective immunity to the intracellular bacterium Franciella tularensis live vaccine strain. *Infect Immun* 67:6002–6007.

Ennis FA, Cruz J, Jameson J, Klein M, Burt D, Thipphawong J. 1999. Augmentation of human influenza A virus-specific cytotoxic T-lymphocyte memory by influenza vaccine and adjuvanted carriers (ISCOMS). *Virology* 259:256–261.

Epstein SL. 2003. Control of influenza virus infection by immunity to conserved viral features. *Expert Rev Anti Infect Ther* 1(4):627–638.

Epstein SL, La CY, Misplon JA, Lawson CM, Hendrickson BA, Max EE, Subbarao K. 1997. Mechanisms of heterosubtypic immunity to lethal influenza A virus infection in fully immunocompetent, T cell-depleted, beta2-microglobulin-deficient, and J chain-deficient mice. *J Immunol* 158:1222–1230.

Epstein SL, La CY, Misplon JA, Bennink JR. 1998. Mechanism of protective immunity against influenza virus infection in mice without antibodies. *J Immunol* 160:322–327.

Epstein SL, Stack A, Misplon JA, Lo CY, Mostowski H, Bennink J, Subbarao K. 2000. Vaccination with DNA encoding internal proteins of influenza virus does not require CD8(+) cytotoxic T lymphocytes: Either CD4(+) or CD8(+) T cells can promote survival and recovery after challenge. *Intl Immunol* 12:91–101.

Epstein SL, Tumpey TM, Misplon JA, Lo CY, Cooper LA, Subbarao K, Renshaw M, Sambhara S, Katz JM. 2002. DNA vaccine expressing conserved influenza virus proteins protective against H5N1 challenge infection in mice. *Emerg Infect Dis* 8:796–801.

Fatah AA. 2001. An introduction to biological agent detection equipment for emergency first responders. U.S. Department of Justice, National Institute of Justice Publication NIJ Guide.

Fodor E, Pritlove DC, Brownlee GG. 1994. The influenza virus panhandle is involved in the initiation of transcription. *J Virol* 68:4092–4096.

Fodor E, Pritlove DC, Brownlee GG. 1995. Characterization of the RNA-fork model of virion RNA in the initiation of transcription in influenza A virus. *J Virol* 69:4012–4019.

Fodor E, Devenish L, Engelhardt OG, Palese P, Brownlee GG, Garcia-Sastre A. 1999. Rescue of influenza A virus from recombinant DNA. *J Virol* 73:9679–9682.

Fu TM, Guan LM, Friedman A, Schofield TL, Ulmer JB, Liu MA, Donnelly JJ. 1999. Dose dependence of CTL precursor frequency induced by a DNA vaccine and correlation with protective immunity against influenza virus challenge. *J Immunol* 162:4163–4170.

Gao P, Watanabe S, Ito T, Goto H, Wells K, McGregor M, Cooley AJ, Kawaoka Y. 1999. Biological heterogeneity, including systemic replication in mice, of H5N1 influenza A virus isolates from humans in Hong Kong. *J Virol* 73:3184–3189.

Garber EA, Chute HT, Condra JH, Gotlib L, Colonno RJ, Smith RG. 1991. Avian cells expressing the murine Mx1 protein are resistant to influenza virus infection. *Virology* 180:754–762.

Ge Q, McManus MT, Nguyen T, Shen CH, Sharp PA, Eisen HN, Chen J. 2003. RNA interference of influenza virus production by directly targeting mRNA for degradation and indirectly inhibiting all viral RNA transcription. *Proc Natl Acad Sci USA* 100:2718–2723.

Ginsburg J. 2000, September 11. Bioinvasion. *Business Week*. Pp. 70–78.

Gitlin L, Karelsky S, Andino R. 2002. Short interfering RNA confers intracellular antiviral immunity in human cells. *Nature* 418:430–434.

Glezen WP, Six HR, Perrotta DM, Decker M, Joseph S. 1984. Epidemics and their causative viruses—Community Experience. In: Stuart Harris CH, Potter CW, eds. *The Molecular Virology and Epidemiology of Influenza.* London, England: Academic Press. Pp. 17–32.

Govaert TM, Sprenger MJ, Dinang GJ, Aretz K, Masurel N, Knotternus JA. 1994. Immune response to influenza vaccination of elderly people. A randomized double-blind placebo-controlled trial. *Vaccine* 12:1185–1189.

Graham MB, Braciale TJ. 1997. Resistance to and recovery from lethal influenza virus infection in B-lymphocyte-deficient mice. *Exp Med* 186:2063–2068.

Grove DS. 1999. Quantitative real-time polymerase chain reaction for the core facility using TaqMan and the Perkin-Elmer/Applied Biosystems Division 7700 Sequence detector. *J Biomol Tech* 10:11–16.

Hagen M, Chung TD, Butcher JA, Krystal M. 1994. Recombinant influenza virus polymerase: Requirement of both 5' and 3' viral ends for endonuclease activity. *J Virol* 68:1509–1515.

Haller O, Arnheiter H, Gresser I, Lindenmann J. 1979. Genetically determined, interferon-dependent resistance to influenza virus in mice. *J Exp Med* 149:601–612.

Haller O, Arnheiter H, Gresser I, Lindenmann J. 1981. Virus-specific interferon action. Protection of newborn Mx carriers against lethal infection with influenza virus. *J Exp Med* 154:199–203.

Harriman GR, Bogue M, Rogers P, Finegold M, Pacheco S, Bradley A, Zhang Y, Mbawuike IN. 1999. Targeted deletion of the IgA constant region in mice leads to IgA deficiency with alterations in expression of other Ig isotypes. *J Immunol* 162:2521–2529.

Hatta M, Gao P, Halfmann P, Kawaoka Y. 2001. Molecular basis for high virulence of Hong Kong H5N1 influenza A viruses. *Science* 293:1840–1842.

Health Canada. 2000 (January 5). *Canadian Contingency Plan for Pandemic Influenza*— Draft. The Laboratory Center for Disease Control, Health Canada, Ottowa.

Hehme N, Engelmann H, Kunzel W, Neumeier E, Sanger R. 2002. Pandemic preparedness lessons learnt from H2N2 and H9N2 candidate vaccines. *Med Microbio Immunol* 191:203–208.

Heid CA, Stevens J, Livak KJ, Williams PM. 1996. Real time quantitative PCR. *Genome Res* 6:986–994.

Henderson DA. 2001. *Hearing on the Threat of Bioterrorism and the Spread of Infectious Diseases.* Statement at the September 5, 2001, hearing of the Committee on Foreign Relations, U.S. Senate. [Online]. Available: http://www.hopkins-biodefense.org/pages/library/spread.html.

Hinshaw VS, Webster RG, Rodriguez RJ. 1981. Influenza A viruses: Combinations of hemagglutinin and neuraminidase subtypes isolated from animals and other sources. *Arch Virol* 67:191–201.

Hoffmann E, Neumann G, Kawaoka Y, Hobom G, Webster RG. 2000. A DNA transfection system for generation of influenza A virus from eight plasmids. *Proc Natl Acad Sci USA* 97:6108–6113.

Huang T, Pavlovic J, Staeheli P, Krystal M. 1992. Overexpression of the influenza virus polymerase can titrate out inhibition by the murine Mx1 protein. *J Virol* 66:4154–4160.

Jameson J, Cruz J, Ennis FA. 1998. Human cytotoxic T-lymphocyte repertoire to influenza A viruses. *Virology* 72:8682–8689.

Joost Haasnoot PC, Cupac D, Berkhout B. 2003. Inhibition of virus replication by RNA interference. *J Biomed Sci* 10:607–616.

Jordan WS Jr, Denny FW Jr, Badger GF, Curtiss C, Dingle JH, Oseasohn R, Stevens DA. 1958. A study of illness in a group of Cleveland families. XVII. The occurrence of Asian influenza. *Am J Hyg* 68:190–212.

Kafri T, Blomer U, Peterson DA, Gage FH, Verma IM. 1997. Sustained expression of genes delivered directly into liver and muscle by lentiviral vectors. *Nat Genet* 17:314–317.

Kawaoka Y, Chambers TM, Sladen WL, Webster RG. 1988. Is the gene pool of influenza viruses in shorebirds and gulls different from that in wild ducks? *J Virol* 163:247–250.

Kilbourne ED. 1975. Epidemiology of influenza. In: Kilbourne ED, ed. *The Influenza Viruses and Influenza.* New York: Academic Press. Pp. 483–538.

Kilbourne ED. 1987. *Influenza.* New York, NY: Plenum Medical Book Co. Pp. 229–232.

Ko JH, Jin HK, Asano A, Takada A, Ninomiya A, Kida H, Hokiyama H, Ohara M, Tsuzuki M, Nishibori M, Mizutani M, Watanabe T. 2002. Polymorphisms and the differential antiviral activity of the chicken Mx gene. *Genome Res* 12:595–601.

Ko JH, Takada A, Mitsuhashi T, Agui T, Watanabe T. 2004. Native antiviral specificity of chicken Mx protein depends on amino acid variation at position 631. *Anim Genet* 35:119–122.

Kodihalli S, Kobasa DL, Webster RG. 2000. Strategies for inducing protection against avian influenza A virus subtypes with DNA vaccines. *Vaccine* 18:2592–2599.

Krol J, Sobczak K, Wilczynska U, Drath M, Jasinska A, Kaczynska D, Krzyzosiak WJ. 2004. Structural features of microRNA (miRNA) precursors and their relevance to miRNA biogenesis and small interfering RNA/short hairpin RNA design. *J Biol Chem* 279(40):42230-42239.

Krug RM, Shaw M, Broni B, Shapiro G, Haller O. 1985. Inhibition of influenza viral mRNA synthesis in cells expressing the interferon-induced Mx gene product. *J Virol* 56:201–206.

Landis H, Simon-Jodicke A, Kloti A, Di Paolo C, Schnorr JJ, Schneider-Schaulies S, Hefti HP, Pavlovic J. 1998. Human MxA protein confers resistance to Semliki Forest virus and inhibits the amplification of a Semliki Forest virus-based replicon in the absence of viral structural proteins. *J Virol* 72:1516–1522.

Lawson CM, Bennink JR, Restifo NP, Yewdell JW, Murphy BR. 1994. Primary pulmonary cytotoxic T-lymphocytes induced by immunization with a vaccinia virus recombinant expressing influenza A virus nucleoprotein peptide do not protect mice against challenge. *J Virol* 68:3505–3511.

Lee MT, Klumpp K, Digard P, Tiley L. 2003. Activation of influenza virus RNA polymerase by the 5' and 3' terminal duplex of genomic RNA. *Nucleic Acids Res* 31(6):1624–1632.

Li WX, Li H, Lu R, Li F, Dus M, Atkinson P, Brydon EW, Johnson KL, Garcia-Sastre A, Ball LA, Palese P, Ding SW. 2004. Interferon antagonist proteins of influenza and vaccinia viruses are suppressors of RNA silencing. *Proc Natl Acad Sci USA* 101:1350–1355.

Li X, Palese P. 1992. Mutational analysis of the promoter required for influenza virus virion RNA synthesis. *J Virol* 66:4331–4338.

Liang S, Mozdzanowska K, Palladino G, Gerhard W. 1994. Heterosubtypic immunity to influenza type A virus in mice: Effector mechanisms and their longevity. *J Immunol* 152:1653–1661.

Liu AN, Mohammed AZ, Rice WR, Fiedeldey DT, Liebermann JS, Whitsett JA, Braciale TJ, Enelow RI. 1999. Perforin-independent CD8+ T-cell mediated cytotoxicity of alveolar epithelial cells is preferentially mediated by tumor necrosis factor-alpha. Relative insensitivity to Fas ligand. *Am Respiratory Cell Mol Biol* 20:849–858.

Livak KJ, Flood SJ, Marmaro J, Giusti W, Deetz K. 1995. Oligonucleotides with fluorescent dyes at opposite ends provide a quenched probe system useful for detecting PCR product and nucleic acid hybridization. *PCR Methods Appl* 4:357–362.

Lu LV, Askonas BA. 1980. Cross-reactivity for different type A influenza viruses of a cloned T-killer cell line. *Nature* 288:164–165.

Lu X, Tumpey TM, Morken T, Zaki SR, Cox NJ, Katz JM. 1999. A mouse model for the evaluation of pathogenesis and immunity to influenza A (H5N1) viruses isolated from humans. *J Virol* 73:5903–5911.

Lukacher AE, Braciale VL, Braciale TJ. 1984. *In vivo* effector function of influenza virus specific cytotoxic T-lymphocyte clones is highly specific. *Exp Med* 160:814–826.

Luo G, Danetz S, Krystal M. 1997. Inhibition of influenza viral polymerases by minimal viral RNA decoys. *J Gen Virol* 78:2329–2333.

Luytjes W, Krystal M, Enami M, Parvin JD, Palese P. 1989. Amplification, expression, and packaging of a foreign gene by influenza virus. *Cell* 59:1107–1113.

Mazanec MB, Kaeczel CS, Lamm ME, Fletcher D, Nedrud JG. 1992. Intracellular neutralization of virus by immunoglobulin A antibodies. *Proc Natl Acad Sci USA* 89:6901–6905.

Mazanec MB, Coudret CL, Fletcher DR. 1995. Intracellular neutralization of influenza virus by immunoglobulin A antihemagglutinin monoclonal antibodies. *J Virol* 69:1339–1343.

Mbawuike IN, Six HR, Cate TR, Couch RB. 1990. Vaccination with inactivated influenza A virus during pregnancy protects neonatal mice against lethal challenge by influenza A viruses representing three subtypes. *Virology* 64:1370–1374.

Mbawuike IN, Dillon SB, Demuth SG, Jones CS, Cate TR, Couch RB. 1994. Influenza A subtype cross-protection after immunization of outbred mice with a purified chimeric NS1/HA2 influenza virus protein. *Vaccine* 12:1340–1349.

Mbawuike IN, Pacheco S, Acuna CL, Switzer KC, Zhang Y, Harriman GR. 1999. Mucosal immunity to influenza without IgA: An IgA knockout mouse model. *J Immunol* 162:2530–2537.

McGrew MJ, Sherman A, Ellard FM, Lillico SG, Gilhooley HJ, Kingsman AJ, Mitrophanous KA, Sang H. 2004. Efficient production of germline transgenic chickens using lentiviral vectors. *EMBO Rep* 5:728–733.

McMichael AJ, Gotch FM, Noble GR, Beare PAS. 1983a. Cytotoxic T-cell immunity to influenza. *N Engl J Med* 309:13–17.

McMichael AJ, Gotch FM, Dongworth DW, Clark A, Potter CW. 1983b. Declining T-cell immunity to influenza, 1977–1982. *Lancet* 2:762–764.

Medema JK, Zoellner YF, Ryan J, and Palache AM. 2004. Modeling pandemic preparedness scenarios: Health economic implications of enhanced pandemic vaccine supply. *Virus Res* 103:9–15.

Melen K, Ronni T, Broni B, Krug RM, von Bonsdorff CH, Julkunen I. 1992. Interferon-induced Mx proteins form oligomers and contain a putative leucine zipper. *J Biol Chem* 267:25898–25907.

Meltzer MI, Cox NJ, Fukuda K. 1999. The economic impact of pandemic influenza in the United States: Priorities for intervention. *Emerg Infect Dis* 5:659–671.

Mibayashi M, Nakad K, Nagata K. 2002. Promoted cell death of cells expressing human MxA by influenza virus infection. *Microbiol Immunol* 46:29–36.

Morein B, Sundquist B, Hoglund S, Dalsgaard K, Osterhaus A. 1984. Iscom, a novel structure for antigenic presentation of membrane proteins from enveloped viruses. *Nature* 308:457–460.

Mozdzanowska K, Maiese K, Gerhard W. 2000. Th cell-deficient mice control influenza virus infection more effectively than Th- and B-cell-deficient mice. Evidence for a Th-independent contribution by B-cells to virus clearance. *J Immunol* 164:2635–2643.

Murphy BR, Coelingh K. 2002. Principles underlying the development and use of live attenuated cold-adapted influenza A and B virus vaccines. *Viral Immunology* 15:295–323.

Murphy BR, Webster RG. 1990. Orthomyxoviruses. In: Fields BN, Knipe DM et al., eds. *Virology*. 2nd ed. New York, NY: Raven Press. Pp. 1091–1152.

Murphy BR, Webster RG. 1996. Orthomyxoviruses. In: Fields BN, Knipe DM, Howley PM, eds. *Fields Virology*. 3rd ed. Philadelphia, PA: Lippincott-Raven. Pp. 1397-1445.

Naldini L, Blomer U, Gage FH, Trono D, Verma IM. 1996. Efficient transfer, integration, and sustained long-term expression of the transgene in adult rat brains injected with a lentiviral vector. *Proc Natl Acad Sci USA* 93:11382–11388.

Neirynck S, Deroo T, Saelens X, Vanlandschoot P, Jou WM, Fiers W. 1999. A universal influenza A vaccine based on the extracellular domain of the M2 protein. *Nature Med* 5:1157–1163.

Neumann G, Hobom G. 1995. Mutational analysis of influenza virus promoter elements *in vivo. J Gen Virol* 76:1709–1717.

Nguyen HH, Moldoveanu Z, Novak MJ, van Ginkel FW, Ban E, Kiyono H, McGhee JR, Mestecky J. 1999. Heterosubtypic immunity to lethal influenza A virus infection is associated with virus-specific CD8+ cytotoxic T-lymphocyte responses induced in mucosa-associated tissues. *Virology* 254:50–60.

Nguyen HH, van Ginkel FW, Vu HL, McGhee JR, Mestecky J. 2001. Heterosubtypic immunity to influenza A virus infection requires B-cells but not CD8+ cytotoxic T-lymphocytes. *Infect Dis* 183:368–376.

Nichol KL, Wuorenma J, von Sternberg T. 1998. Benefits of influenza vaccination for low-, intermediate-, and high-risk senior citizens. *Arch Intern Med* 80:1769–1776.

Nicholson KG, Tyrrell DA, Harrison P, Potter CW, Jennings R, Clark A, Schild GC, Wood JM, Yetts R, Seagroatt V, Huggins A, Anderson SG. 1979. Clinical studies of monovalent inactivated whole virus and subunit A/USSR/77 (H1N1) vaccine: Serological responses and clinical reactions. *J Biol Stand* 7(2):123–136.

Nicholson KG, Colegate AE, Podda A, Stephenson I, Wood J, Ypma E, Zambon MC. 2001. Safety and antigenicity of non-adjuvanted and MF59-adjuvanted influenza A/Duck/Singapore/97 (H5N3) vaccine: A randomised trial of two potential vaccines against H5N1 influenza. *Lancet* 357:1937–1943.

Obar RA, Collins CA, Hammarback JA, Shpetner HS, Vallee RB. 1990. Molecular cloning of the microtubule-associated mechanochemical enzyme dynamin reveals homology with a new family of GTP-binding proteins. *Nature* 347:256–261.

Odagiri T, Tashiro M. 1997. Segment-specific noncoding sequences of the influenza virus genome RNA are involved in the specific competition between defective interfering RNA and its progenitor RNA segment at the virion assembly step. *J Virol* 71:2138–2145.

Offringa DP, Tyson-Medlock V, Ye Z, Levandowski RA. 2000. A comprehensive systematic approach to identification of influenza A virus genotype using RT-PCR and RFLP. *J Virol Methods* 88:15–24.

Paddison PJ, Caudy AA, Bernstein E, Hannon GJ, Conklin DS. 2002. Short hairpin RNAs (shRNAs) induce sequence-specific silencing in mammalian cells. *Genes Dev* 16:948–958.

Parvin JD, Palese P, Honda A, Ishihama A, Krystal M. 1989. Promoter analysis of influenza virus RNA polymerase. *J Virol* 63:5142–5152.

Patriarca PA, Strikas RA, Gensheimer KF, Cox NJ, Fukuda K, Meltzer MI. 1999. *A Pandemic Influenza Planning Guide for State and Local Officials*. Draft 2.1. National Vaccine Program Office. Centers for Disease Control and Prevention, Atlanta, GA.

Pavlovic J, Haller O, Staeheli P. 1992. Human and mouse Mx proteins inhibit different steps of the influenza virus multiplication cycle. *J Virol* 66:2564–2569.

Perdue ML. 2003. Molecular diagnostics in an insecure world. *Avian Diseases* 47(3 Suppl):1063–1068.

Peters CJ. 2002. Many viruses are potential agents of bioterrorism. *ASM News* 68:168–173.

Potter CW. 1998. Chronicle of influenza pandemics. In: Nicholson KG, Webster RG, Hay AJ, eds. *Textbook of Influenza*. London, England: Blackwell Sciences. Pp. 3–18.

Rapp JC, Harvey AJ, Speksnijder GL, Hu W, Ivarie R. 2003. Biologically active human interferon alpha-2b produced in the egg white of transgenic hens. *Transgenic Res* 12:569–575.

Raulet DH. 1994. MHC class I-deficient mice. 1994. *Adv Immunol* 55:381–421.

Renegar KB. 1992. Influenza virus infections and immunity: A review of human and animal models. *Lab Anim Sci* 42:222–232.

Renegar KB, Small PA. 1991. Passive transfer of local immunity to influenza virus infection by 19A antibody. *J Immunol* 146:1972–1978.

Rhodes GH, Dwarki VJ, Abai AM, Felgner J, Felgner PL, Gromkowski SH, Parker SE. 1993. Injection of expression vectors containing viral genes induces cellular, humoral, and protective immunity. In: Chanock RM, Brown F, Ginsberg HS, Norrby E, eds. *Vaccines 93*. Cold Spring Harbor, NY: Cold Spring Harbor Laboratory Press. Pp. 137–141.

Rimmelzwaan GF, Baars M, van Amerongen G, van Beek R, Osterhaus AE. 2001. A single dose of an ISCOM influenza vaccine induces long-lasting protective immunity against homologous challenge infection but fails to protect Cynomolgus macaques against distant drift variants of influenza A (H3N2) viruses. *Vaccine* 20:158–163.

Robertson JS. 1979. 5' and 3' terminal nucleotide sequences of the RNA genome segments of influenza virus. *Nucleic Acids Research* 6:3745–3757.

Rodgers P, Whitby S, Dando M. 1999. Biological warfare against crops. *Sci Am* 280:70–75.

Rubinson DA, Dillon CP, Kwiatkowski AV, Sievers C, Yang L, Kopinja J, Rooney DL, Ihrig MM, McManus MT, Gertler FB, Scott ML, Van Parijs L. 2003. A lentivirus-based system to functionally silence genes in primary mammalian cells, stem cells and transgenic mice by RNA interference. *Nat Genet* 33:401–406.

Saito T, Lim W, Suzuki T, Suzuki Y, Kida H, Nishimura SI, Tashiro M. 2001. Characterization of a human H9N2 influenza virus isolated in Hong Kong. *Vaccine* 20:125–133.

Sambhara S, Kurichh A, Miranda R, Tumpey T, Rowe T, Renshaw M, Arpino R, Tamane A, Kandil A, James O, Underdown B, Klein M, Katz J, Burt D. 2001. Heterosubtypic immunity against human influenza A viruses, including recently emerged avian H5 and H9 viruses, induced by FLU-ISCOM vaccine in mice requires both cytotoxic T-lymphocyte and macrophage function. *Cell Immunol* 211:143–153.

Schnorr JJ, Schneider-Schaulies S, Simon-Jodicke A, Pavlovic J, Horisberger MA, ter Meulen V. 1993. MxA-dependent inhibition of measles virus glycoprotein synthesis in a stably transfected human monocytic cell line. *J Virol* 67:4760–4768.

Scholtissek C. 1983. Genetic relatedness of influenza viruses (RNA and protein). In: Palese P, Kingsbury DW, eds. *Genetics of Influenza Viruses*. New York, NY: Springer-Verlag. Pp. 99–126.

Scholtissek C, Burger H, Kistner O, Shortridge KF. 1985. The nucleoprotein as a possible major factor in determining host specificity of influenza H3N2 viruses. *Virology* 147:287–294.

Schulman JL, Kilbourne ED. 1965. Induction of partial specific heterotypic immunity in mice by a single infection with influenza A virus. *Bacteriol* 89:170–174.

Schwartz-Cornil I, Benureau Y, Greenberg H, Hendrickson BA, Cohen J. 2002. Heterologous protection induced by the inner capsid proteins of rotavirus requires transcytosis of mucosal immunoglobulins. *Viral* 76:8110–8117.

Scuffham PA, West PA. 2002. Economic evaluation for strategies for the control and management of influenza in Europe. *Vaccine* 20:2562–2578.

Selin LK, Nahill SR, Welsh RM. 1994. Cross-reactivities in memory cytotoxic T lymphocyte recognition of heterologous viruses. *Exp Med* 179:1933–1943.

Senne DA. 2003. Avian influenza in the Western Hemisphere including the Pacific Islands and Australia. *Avian Diseases* 47:798–805.

Seong BL, Brownlee GG. 1992. A new method for reconstituting influenza polymerase and RNA *in vitro*: A study of the promoter elements for cRNA and vRNA synthesis *in vitro* and viral rescue *in vivo*. *Virology* 186:247–260.

Sims LD, Ellis TM, Liu KK, Dyrting K, Wong H, Peiris M, Guan Y, Shortridge KF. 2003. Avian influenza in Hong Kong 1997–2002. *Avian Diseases* 47:832–838.

Slepushkin AN. 1959. The effect of a previous attack of A1 influenza on susceptibility to A2 virus during the 1957 outbreak. *Bull WHO* 20:297–301.

Slepushkin VA, Katz JM, Black RA, Gamble WC, Rota PA, Cox NJ. 1995. Protection of mice against influenza A virus challenge by vaccination with barulovirus-expressed M2 protein. *Vaccine* 13:1399–1402.

Sonoguchi T, Naito H, Hara M, Takeuchi Y, Fukumi H. 1985. Cross-subtype protection in humans during sequential overlapping and/or concurrent epidemics caused by H3N2 and H1N1 influenza viruses. *Infect Dis* 151:81–88.

Staeheli P, Horisberger MA, Haller O. 1984. Mx-dependent resistance to influenza viruses is induced by mouse interferons alpha and beta but not gamma. *Virology* 132:456–461.

Staeheli P, Haller O, Boll W, Lindenmann J, Weissmann C. 1986. Mx protein: Constitutive expression in 3T3 cells transformed with cloned Mx cDNA confers selective resistance to influenza virus. *Cell* 44:147–158.

Steinhoff MC, Fries LF, Karron RA, Clements ML, Murphy BR. 1993. Effect of heterosubtypic immunity on infection with attenuated influenza-A virus vaccines in young children. *Clin Microbiol* 31:836–838.

Strikas RA, Wallace GS, Myers MG. 2002. Influenza pandemic preparedness action plan for the United States: 2002 update. *CID* 35:590–596.

Suarez DL, Perdue ML, Cox N, Rowe T, Bender C, Huang J, Swayne DE. 1998. Comparisons of highly virulent H5N1 influenza A viruses isolated from humans and chickens from Hong Kong. *J Virol* 72:6678–6688.

Subbarao K, Klimov A, Katz J, Regnery H, Lim W, Hall H, Perdue M, Swayne D, Bender C, Huang J, Hemphill M, Rowe T, Shaw M, Xu X, Fukuda K, Cox N. 1998. Characterization of an avian influenza A (H5N1) virus isolated from a child with a fatal respiratory illness. *Science* 279:393–396.

Subbarao K, Chen H, Swayne D, Mingay L, Fodor E, Brownlee G, Xu X, Lu X, Katz J, Cox N, Matsuoka Y. 2003. Evaluation of a genetically modified reassortant H5N1 influenza A virus vaccine candidate generated by plasmid based reverse genetics. *Virology* 305:192–200.

Takada A, Kuboki N, Okazaki K, Ninomiya A, Tanaka H, Ozaki H, Itamura S, Nishimura H, Enami M, Tashiro M, Shortridge KF, Kida H. 1999. A virulent Avian influenza virus as a vaccine strain against a potential human pandemic. *Virology* 73:8303–8307.

Takada A, Matsushita S, Ninomiya A, Kawaoka Y, Kida H. 2003. Intranasal immunization with formalin-inactivated virus vaccine induces a broad spectrum of heterosubtypic immunity against influenza A virus infection in mice. *Vaccine* 21(23):3212–3218.

Talon J, Horvath CM, Polley R, Basler CF, Muster T, Palese P, Garcia-Sastre A. 2000. Activation of interferon regulatory factor 3 is inhibited by the influenza A virus NS1 protein. *J Virol* 74:7989–7996.

Taylor SF, Bender BS. 1995. Beta 2-microglobulin-deficient mice demonstrate class II MHC restricted anti-viral CD4+ but not CD8+ CTL against influenza-sensitized autologous splenocytes. *Immunol Lett* 46:67–73.

Tiley LS, Hagen M, Matthews JT, Krystal M. 1994. Sequence-specific binding of the influenza virus RNA polymerase to sequences located at the 5′ ends of the viral RNAs. *J Virol* 68:5108–5116.

Tompkins SM, Lo CY, Tumpey TM, Epstein SL. 2004. Protection against lethal influenza virus challenge by RNA interference *in vivo*. *Proc Natl Acad Sci USA* 101:8682–8686.

Topham DJ, Doherty PC. 1998. Clearance of an influenza A virus by CD4+ T-cells is inefficient in the absence of B-cells. *Virology* 72:882–885.

Topham DJ, Tripp RA, Doherty PC. 1997. CD8+ T-cells clear influenza virus by perforin or Fas dependent processes. *J Immunol* 159:5197–5200.

Treanor JJ, Wilkinson BE, Masseoud F, Hu-Primmer J, Battaglia R, O'Brien D, Wolff M, Rabinovich G, Blackwelder W, Katz JM. 2001. Safety and immunogenicity of a recombinant hemagglutinin vaccine for H5 influenza in humans. *Vaccine* 19:1732–1737.

Tumpey TM, Renshaw M, Clements JD, Katz JM. 2001. Mucosal delivery of inactivated influenza vaccine induces B-cell-dependent heterosubtypic cross-protection against lethal influenza A H5N1 virus infection. *J Virol* 75(11):5141–5150.

Turan K, Mibayashi M, Sugiyama K, Saito S, Numajiri A, Nagata K. 2004. Nuclear MxA proteins form a complex with influenza virus NP and inhibit the transcription of the engineered influenza virus genome. *Nucleic Acids Res* 32:643–652.

Ulmer JB, Donnelly JJ, Parker SE, Rhodes GH, Felgner PL, Dwarki VJ, Gromkowski SH, Deck RR, DeWitt CM, Friedman A, Hawe LA, Leander KR, Martinez D, Perry HC, Shiver JW, Montgomery DL, Liu MA. 1993. Heterologous protection against influenza by injection of DNA encoding a viral protein. *Science* 259:1745–1749.

Ulmer JB, Fu TM, Deck RR, Friedman A, Guan L, DeWitt C, Liu X, Wang S, Liu MA, Donnelly JJ, Caulfield MJ. 1998. Protective CD4+ and CD8+ T-cells against influenza virus induced by vaccination with nucleoprotein DNA. *Virology* 72:5648–5653.

van Kolfschooten F. 2003. Dutch veterinarian becomes first victim of avian influenza. *Lancet* 361:1444.

Webster RG. 2002. The importance of animal influenza for human disease. *Vaccine* 20:S16–S20.

Webster RG, Askonas BA. 1980. Cross-protection and cross-reactive cytotoxic T-cells induced by influenza virus vaccines in mice. *Eur J Immunol* 10:396–401.

Webster RG, Kawaoka Y, Taylor J, Weinberg R, Paoletti E. 1991. Efficacy of nucleoprotein and haemagglutinin antigens expressed in fowlpox virus as vaccine for influenza in chickens. *Vaccine* 9:303–308.

Webster RG, Sharp GB, Claas EC. 1995. Interspecies transmission of influenza viruses. *Am J Respir Crit Care Med* 152:S25–S30.

Wells MA, Albrecht P, Ennis FA. 1981. Recovery from a viral respiratory infection. Influenza pneumonia in normal and T deficient mice. *J Immunol* 126:1036–1041.

WHO (World Health Organization). 1999. *Influenza Pandemic Preparedness Plan. The Role of WHO and Guidelines for National or Regional Planning.* Geneva, Switzerland: WHO. [Online]. Available: http://www.who.int/csr/resources/publications/influenza/WHO_CDS_CSR_EDC_99_1/en/ [accesed December 21, 2004].

WHO. 2002. *Draft WHO Guidelines on the Use of Vaccines and Antivirals during Influenza Pandemics.* Issued 2-4 October 2002. Geneva, Switzerland: WHO. [Online]. Available: http://www.who.int/emc/diseases/flu/whoguidelines.html.

WHO. 2003. *Preparing for the Next Influenza Season in a World Altered by SARS. Disease Outbreak #l. Severe Acute Respiratory Syndrome.* Update 94 #20. 7-3-2003. [Online]. Available: http://www.who.int/csr/don/2003_07_03/en/ [accessed December 21, 2004].

Wilson TM, Logan-Henfrey L, Weller R, Kellman B. 2000. Agroterrorism, biological crimes and biological warfare targeting animal agriculture. In: Brown C, Bolin C, eds. *Emerging Diseases of Animals.* Washington, DC: ASM Press. Pp. 23–57.

Wilson TM, Gregg DA, King DJ, Noah DL, Perkins LE, Swayne DE, Inskeep W. 2001. Agroterrorism, biological crimes, and biowarfare targeting animal agriculture. The clinical, pathologic, diagnostic, and epidemiologic features of some important animal diseases. *Clin Lab Med* 21:549–591.

Wright PF, Webster RG. 2001. Orthomyxoviruses. In: Knipe DM, Howley PM, Griffin DE, eds. *Fields Virology.* 4th ed. Philadelphia, PA: Lippincott Williams & Wilkins. Pp. 1533–1579.

Xu X, Cox NJ, Bender CA, Regnery HL, Shaw MW. 1996. Genetic variation in neuraminidase genes of influenza A (H3N2) viruses. *Virology* 224:175–183.

Yetter RA, Lehrer S, Ramphal R, Small PA Jr. 1980. Outcome of influenza infection: Effect of site of initial infection and heterotypic immunity. *Infect Immun* 29:654–662.

Yewdell JW, Bennink JR, Smith GL, Moss B. 1985. Influenza A virus nucleoprotein is a major target antigen for cross-reactive anti-influenza A virus cytotoxic T-lymphocytes. *Proc Natl Acad Sci USA* 82:1785–1789.

Zambon M. 1998. Laboratory diagnosis of influenza. In: Nicholson KG, Webster RG, Hay AJ, eds. *Textbook of Influenza*. London, England: Blackwell Science. Pp. 3–18.

Zhao MQ, Arnir MK, Rice WR, Enelow RI. 2001. Type II pneumocyte-CD8+ T-cell interactions—relationship between target cell cytotoxicity and activation. *Am Respir Cell Mol Biol* 25:362–369.

Zurcher T, Pavlovic J, Staeheli P. 1992. Mouse Mx2 protein inhibits vesicular stomatitis virus but not influenza virus. *Virology* 187:796–800.

6

Beyond the Biomedical Response

OVERVIEW

An influenza pandemic will likely spawn a plethora of legal and ethical dilemmas and political and economic consequences, and its impact will depend to a large extent on the public's perception of and reaction to the crisis. This chapter presents a variety of social perspectives on the coming pandemic: economic, legal, and ethical implications of various response options; opportunities for collaboration between public and private sectors; and public communication strategies to address both interpandemic and pandemic influenza.

The chapter opens with a description of an economic model, based on the notion of preparation as an "insurance policy" against the next influenza pandemic, to calculate the investment necessary to prepare for a range of pandemic scenarios and responses. These calculations indicate the mutual exclusivity of two key goals of pandemic planning, minimizing overall mortality and minimizing economic impact, thus highlighting the need for a system by which to make such difficult choices and explain them to the public.

Focusing on the important role in mitigating pandemic influenza of both annual immunization (to build demand for flu vaccine, and therefore supply in the event of a crisis) and prompt vaccination against a pandemic strain, the chapter continues with a consideration of strategies to increase immunization uptake before and during a pandemic. In a pandemic—or even a severe annual flu season, as occurred in late 2003—public health officials face the difficult task of encouraging people with high priority to receive vaccine while persuading others to wait calmly and use nonmedical measures to reduce their exposure to infection. Limited research indicates that public officials can avoid losing their credibility in such situations by sharing the dilemmas of disease control with the public in a productive and effective way.

Current understanding about the influence and causes of panic in public crises and how to remedy its effects has been advanced through recent efforts to prepare society to deal productively with terrorism. Both the September 11, 2001, terrorist attacks and subsequent anthrax assaults in the United States demonstrated that open and informative relationships among citizens, government, and public health and safety authorities are fundamental to a population's ability to cope with unconventional health threats. In her contribution to this chapter, Monica Schoch-Spana describes a series of findings by study and research focus groups convened by the Center for Biosecurity of the University of Pittsburgh Medical Center in collaboration with Johns Hopkins University to examine governance dilemmas in bioterrorism response. These groups characterized the unique governing dilemmas posed by a major infectious outbreak and produced guidelines by which decision makers can identify opportunities to enlist public trust and cooperation in such emergencies.

Legal authority must be brought to bear on nearly every facet of pandemic preparedness, from measures designed to reduce the risk of animal-to-human transmission of disease; to surveillance and detection procedures; to medical interventions to prevent or control the spread of infection; to the imposition of voluntary or mandatory quarantine and/or isolation measures; to travel limitations, trade restrictions, and border closures. This chapter continues with an examination of the legal and ethical questions attached to major public health interventions for preventing or ameliorating pandemic influenza; it also summarizes ethical values that can inform public health practice in an emergency.

THE ECONOMIC IMPACT OF PANDEMIC INFLUENZA IN THE UNITED STATES: PRIORITIES FOR INTERVENTION

Martin I. Meltzer, Nancy J. Cox, and Keiji Fukuda[1]

Centers for Disease Control and Prevention, Atlanta, Georgia, USA

Reprinted from *Emerging Infectious Diseases*, CDC, 2003

---

[1]Address for correspondence: Martin Meltzer, National Center for Infectious Diseases, Centers for Disease Control and Prevention, Clifton Road, Mail Stop C12, Atlanta, GA 30333; fax: 404-639-3039; e-mail: qzm4@cdc.gov.

We estimated the possible effects of the next influenza pandemic in the United States and analyzed the economic impact of vaccine-based interventions. Using death rates, hospitalization data, and outpatient visits, we estimated 89,000 to 207,000 deaths; 314,000 to 734,000 hospitalizations; 18 to 42 million outpatient visits; and 20 to 47 million additional illnesses. Patients at high risk (15% of the population) would account for approximately 84% of all deaths. The estimated economic impact would be US$71.3 to $166.5 billion, excluding disruptions to commerce and society. At $21 per vaccinee, we project a net savings to society if persons in all age groups are vaccinated. At $62 per vaccinee and at gross attack rates of 25%, we project net losses if persons not at high risk for complications are vaccinated. Vaccinating 60% of the population would generate the highest economic returns but may not be possible within the time required for vaccine effectiveness, especially if two doses of vaccine are required.

Influenza pandemics have occurred for centuries, three times (1918, 1957, and 1968) in the 20th century alone. Another pandemic is highly likely, if not inevitable (Patriarca and Cox, 1997). In the 1918 influenza pandemic, more than 20 million people died (Simonsen et al., 1998). Improvements in medical care and technology since the last pandemic may reduce the impact of the next. When planning for the next pandemic, however, decision makers need to examine the following questions: Would it make economic sense to vaccinate the entire U.S. population if 15% were to become clinically ill? What if 25% were to become ill? To answer such questions, we conducted economic analyses of potential intervention scenarios.

Although many studies have examined or reviewed the economics of influenza vaccination (Campbell and Rumley, 1997; Carrat and Valleron, 1995; Jefferson and Demicheli, 1998; Kavet, 1977; Office of Technology Assessment, 1981; Patriarca et al., 1987; Riddiough et al., 1983; Schoenbaum, 1987), only one study (Schoenbaum et al., 1976), published in 1976, examined the economics of a vaccine-based intervention aimed at reducing the impact of an influenza epidemic in the United States. Our study examines the possible economic effects of the next influenza pandemic in the United States, analyzes these effects, and uses the results to estimate the costs, benefits, and policy implications of several possible vaccine-based interventions. These estimates can be used in developing national and state plans to respond to an influenza pandemic.[2] Unlike the

---

[2]A complete plan detailing a response to an influenza pandemic should include definition of a pandemic, points that will initiate various steps in the response plan, and details about deploying the intervention. While a U.S. federal influenza pandemic plan is being developed, a guide to aid state and territorial health officials in developing plans for their jurisdictions is available at http://www.cdc.gov/od/nvpo/pandemicflu.htm. Printed copies can be obtained from the author.

1976 study, ours examined the effect of varying the values of a number of key input variables. Specific objectives were to provide a range of estimates regarding the number of deaths, hospitalizations, outpatient visits, and those ill persons not seeking medical care in the next influenza pandemic; provide a cost estimate of health outcomes; estimate the potential net value of possible vaccination strategies;[3] evaluate the effect of using different criteria (e.g., death rates, economic returns due to vaccination) to set vaccination priorities; assess the economic impact of administering various doses of vaccine and of administering vaccine to different age groups and groups at risk; and calculate an insurance premium that could reasonably be spent each year for planning, preparedness, and practice.

Methods

The Model

Building a mathematical model of the spread of influenza is difficult largely because of differences in virus transmission and virulence, lack of understanding of the primary factors affecting the spread of influenza, and shortage of population-based data (Cliff and Haggett, 1993). Because of the difficulties in calculating realistic estimates of the numbers of cases in the next influenza pandemic, we used a Monte Carlo mathematical simulation model (Critchfield and Willard, 1986; Dittus et al., 1989; Dobilet et al., 1985), which uses predefined probability distributions of key input variables to calculate the number of illnesses and deaths that could result from an influenza pandemic. Some of the most important probability distributions we used describe the population-based rates of illness and death. These rates are based on illness and death rates reported in earlier influenza pandemics and epidemics. The model produces a range of estimated effects rather than a single point estimate. The model is not epidemiologic and thus does not describe the spread of the disease through a population.

Many details of the model are presented below and in Appendix I; a more detailed explanation and a complete list of all the variables used and the values assigned to the variables are available at Appendix II.

For interventions to contain and reduce the impact of an influenza pandemic, we used a societal perspective, which takes into account all benefits and all costs regardless of who receives and who pays.

---

[3]We limited our examination of possible interventions to those involving influenza vaccines. We did not consider the use of antiviral drugs for influenza prophylaxis because there may not be adequate supplies; first priority for such drugs may be for treatment; and the side effects from the drugs, particularly amantadine, make them unsuitable for long-term prophylaxis for many workers, such as drivers or heavy construction operators.

TABLE 6-1 Estimate of Age Distribution of Cases and Percentage of Population at High Risk Used to Examine the Impact of Pandemic Influenza in the United States

Age Group (yrs)	
	Percentage of All Cases[a]
0–19	40.0
20–64	53.1
65+	6.8
Totals[b]	100.0
	Percentage at High Risk[c]
0–19	6.4
20–64	14.4
65+	40.0
U.S. average[d]	15.4

[a]The actual number of cases will depend upon the assumed gross attack rate. The distribution of cases was based on lower and upper estimates of age-specific attack rates from the 1918, 1928–29, and 1957 epidemics and pandemics (Glezen, 1996).

[b]Totals do not add to exactly 100% because of rounding.

[c]Persons are categorized at high risk if they have a preexisting medical condition that makes them more susceptible to influenza-related complications. The percentages of age groups at high risk were obtained from the Working Group on Influenza Pandemic Preparedness and Emergency Response (GrIPPE, unpub. data). The Advisory Committee on Immunization Practices estimates that 27 to 31 million persons aged <65 years are at high risk for influenza-associated complications (Centers for Disease Control and Prevention, 1998).

[d]Average is an age-weighted average, using each age group's proportion of the total U.S. population.

Age Distribution and Persons at High-Risk

Since the age distribution of patients in the next pandemic is unknown, we assumed a distribution (Table 6-1) among the three age groups (0 to 19 years, 20 to 64 years, and 65 years and older).[4] Further, each age group was divided into those at high risk (persons with a preexisting medical condition making them more susceptible to complications from influenza) and those not at high risk (Table 6-1).[5] Age by itself was not considered a

---

[4]This article presents the results for one distribution of cases by age and risk group. The background paper in Appendix II, however, contains additional results obtained by using a different distribution.

[5]The Advisory Committee on Immunization Practices estimates that 27 to 31 million people ages <65 years are at high risk for influenza-associated complications (CDC, 1998). ACIP

risk factor; persons 65 years and older were assumed to have higher rates of illness and death than the rest of the population (Table 6-2).

Gross Attack Rates

In the model, we used gross attack rates (percentage of clinical influenza illness cases per population) of 15% to 35%, in steps of 5%. Infected persons who continued to work were not considered to have a clinical case of influenza, and were not included.

Illnesses and Deaths

The rates of adverse effects (outpatient visits, hospitalizations, deaths, and illnesses for which no medical care was sought), by age and risk group, were used to determine the number of persons in each category (Table 6-2) (Appendix II).

Net Returns of Vaccinating against an Influenza Pandemic

Vaccinating predefined segments of the population will be one of the major strategies for reducing the impact of pandemic influenza, and the net return, in dollars, from vaccination is an important economic measure of the costs and benefits associated with vaccination. We calculated the net return by using the following formula for each age and risk group:

$$\text{Net returns}_{\text{age, risk group}} = \text{Savings from outcomes averted in population}_{\text{age, risk group}}$$

$$- \text{cost of vaccination of population}_{\text{age, risk group}}$$

The savings from illnesses and deaths averted and the cost of vaccinations are described in Appendix I. Some input variables are described below and in Appendix II.

---

also classifies all 32 million people ≥65 years as being at elevated risk for influenza-related complications (CDC, 1998). Further, the working group on influenza pandemic preparedness and emergency response has assumed that approximately 19 million household members of persons at high risk should also be vaccinated to reduce the probability of transmission to those at high risk (GrIPPE, unpub. data, 1997).

TABLE 6-2 Variables Used to Define Distribution of Disease Outcomes of Those with Clinical Cases[a] of Influenza

Variable	Rates per 1,000 persons[b]		
	Lower	Most likely	Upper
Outpatient visits			
Not at high risk			
0–19 yrs old	165		230
20–64 yrs old	40		85
65+ yrs old	45		74
High risk			
0–19 yrs old	289		403
20–64 yrs old	70		149
65+ yrs old	79		130
Hospitalizations			
Not at high risk			
0–19 yrs old	0.2	0.5	2.9
20–64 yrs old	0.18		2.75
65+ yrs old	1.5		3.0
High risk			
0–19 yrs old	2.1	2.9	9.0
20–64 yrs old	0.83		5.14
65+ yrs old	4.0		13
Deaths			
Not at high risk			
0–19 yrs old	0.014	0.024	0.125
20–64 yrs old	0.025	0.037	0.09
65+ yrs old	0.28	0.42	0.54
High risk			
0–19 yrs old	0.126	0.22	7.65
20–64 yrs old	0.1		5.72
65+ yrs old	2.76		5.63

[a]Clinical cases are defined as cases in persons with illness sufficient to cause an economic impact. The number of persons who will be ill but will not seek medical care, are calculated as follows: Number ill$_{age}$ = (Population$_{age}$ × gross attack rate) − (deaths$_{age}$ + hospitalizations$_{age}$ + outpatients$_{age}$). The number of deaths, hospitalizations, and outpatients are calculated by using the rates presented in this table.

[b]For Monte Carlo simulations, rates are presented as lower and upper for uniform distributions, and lower, most likely, and upper for triangular distributions (Evans et al., 1993).

SOURCES: Office of Technology Assessment, 1981; Carrat and Valleron, 1995; Schoenbaum et al., 1976; Glezen, 1996; Mullooly and Barker, 1982; Barker and Mullooly, 1980; Simonsen et al., 1997; Fox et al., 1982; Glezen et al., 1987; Serfling et al., 1967; Barker and Mulooly, 1982; Glezen et al., 1982; McBean et al., 1993; Barker, 1986, and Appendix II.

Input Variables

The direct medical costs (i.e., those reimbursed by third-party payers such as health insurance companies) associated with hospitalizations, outpatient visits, and drug purchases were obtained from a proprietary database containing health insurance claims data from approximately 4 million insured persons (The MEDSTAT Group, Ann Arbor, MI) (Table 6-3). Following the methods used by McBean et al. (1993), we extracted the data for outpatient visits from the database with codes from the International Classification of Diseases, Ninth Revision (ICD-9) for pneumonia and bronchitis (ICD-9: 480–487.8), acute bronchitis (ICD-9: 466–466.1), and chronic respiratory disease (ICD-9: 490–496). Costs for inpatient care were extracted with the same codes, when recorded as the principal diagnosis and when recorded as any of the diagnoses in a patient's chart. Further, because influenza can cause patients with preexisting medical conditions to seek inpatient care, data were extracted for the inpatient costs of treating heart-related conditions (common preexisting conditions that place a person at high risk for influenza-related illness or death). Hospital costs attributed to pneumonia and bronchitis, acute bronchitis, chronic respiratory disease, and the identified heart conditions were then estimated as weighted averages (Appendix II).

The principal indirect cost was lost productivity, which was valued by using an age- and gender-weighted average wage (Table 6-3) (Haddix et al., 1996). The economic cost of a death was valued at the present net value of the average expected future lifetime earnings, weighted for gender and age (Haddix et al., 1996). All costs were standardized to 1995 US$ values.

The cost of fully vaccinating a person (i.e., administering the number of doses necessary to protect against disease) was modeled with two assumed values, approximately $21 and $62 per person fully vaccinated (Table 6-4). These costs include the cost of the vaccine, as well as its distribution and administration (health-care worker time, supplies); patient travel; time lost from work and other activities; and cost of side effects (including Guillain-Barré syndrome) (Table 6-4) (Appendix II).

Vaccine Effectiveness

The assumed levels of vaccine effectiveness used to estimate the savings gained due to a vaccine-based intervention are described in Appendix I; the equation defining savings from outcomes averted contains the rate of compliance multiplied by the assumed vaccine effectiveness. In cases requiring two doses of vaccine to satisfactorily protect against influenza-related illness and death, a person was considered compliant only after both doses.

Net Returns of Vaccination: Sensitivity Analyses

To illustrate the importance of the death rate in determining economic outcomes, we conducted further sensitivity analyses in which the death rates for persons not at high risk were one quarter or half of those used in the main analyses (Table 6-2).

Insurance Premiums

To determine how much should be spent each year to plan, prepare, and practice to ensure that mass vaccinations can take place if needed, we considered the funding of those activities as an annual insurance premium (Kaufmann et al., 1997). The premium would be used to pay for improving surveillance systems, ensuring sufficient supply of vaccine for high-priority groups (and possibly the entire U.S. population), conducting research to improve detection of new influenza subtypes, and developing emergency preparedness plans to ensure adequate medical care and maintenance of essential community services (Kaufmann et al., 1997). We calculated the premium as follows (Robinson and Barry, 1987): annual insurance premium = net returns from an intervention × the annual probability of a pandemic.

Vaccination Priorities and Distribution

During the early stages of a pandemic, the supply of influenza vaccine will likely be limited. Even if sufficient vaccine is produced to vaccinate the entire U.S. population, it will take time to administer the vaccine to all, especially if two doses are required. Because a pandemic will be caused by a new subtype of influenza, two doses of vaccine may be required. Who should receive priority for vaccination until vaccine supplies are more plentiful? To illustrate the use of the model in estimating the impact of different priorities, we created sample priority lists by using three different criteria: total deaths, risk for death, and maximizing net returns due to vaccination. In choosing the criteria for priorities, society must debate the main goal of a pandemic vaccination plan: prevent deaths, regardless of age and position in society; prevent deaths among those at greatest risk (i.e., 65 years of age); or minimize the social disruption. If the last is the goal of society, the net return due to vaccination should be used to set priorities.

The model can also be used to compare the economic consequences of plans that specify which target populations are vaccinated. To illustrate this capability, we constructed four options for prioritizing vaccine distribution. For Option A, the target population is similar to current Advisory Committee on Immunization Practices (ACIP) recommendations, with production and use of vaccine similar to current, intrapandemic recommendations (Centers for Disease Control and Prevention, 1998). We assumed 77.4

TABLE 6-3 Input Variables Used to Calculate the Economic Impact (Direct and Indirect Costs) of Health Outcomes Due to an Influenza Pandemic in the United States (in 1995 US$)

Outcome Category Item	Type of Cost	Age Group (yrs)			Sources
		0–19	20–64	65+	
Deaths					
Average age (years)		9	35	74	Assumed
PV earnings lost ($)[a]	Indirect	1,016,101	1,037,673	65,837	16, 30
Most likely ± min or max hospital costs ($)[b]	Direct	3,435 ± 2,632	7,605 ± 3,888	8,309 + 3,692	Marketscan Database; 31
Subtotal ($)[c]		1,019,536	1,045,278	74,146	
Hospitalizations					
Most likely ± min or max hospital costs ($)[b]	Direct	2,936 ± 2,099	6,016 ± 2,086	6,856 ±3,200	Marketscan Database; 31
Most likely ± min or max net pay for outpatient visits ($)[d]	Direct	74 ± 40	94 ± 70	102 ± 60	Marketscan Database; 31
Avg. copayment for outpatients visit ($)	Direct	5	4	4	Marketscan Database
Most likely ± min or max net payment for drug claims($)[e]	Direct	26 ± 9	42 ± 30	41 ± 10	Marketscan Database
Most likely ± min or max days lost[f]	Indirect	5 ± 2.7	8 ± 4.8	10 ± 5.4	Marketscan Database; 31
Value 1 day lost ($)[g]	Indirect	65	100 or 65	65	30
Subtotal ($)[c]		3,366	6,842	7,653	

325

Outpatient visits					
Avg. no. visits[h]	Direct	1.52	1.52	1.52	Marketscan Database
Most likely ± min or max net payment per visit($)[i]	Direct	49 ± 13	38 ± 12	50 ± 16	Marketscan Database
Avg. copayment for outpatient visit ($)	Direct	5	4	4	Marketscan Database
Most likely ± min or max net payment per prescription($)[j]	Direct	25 ± 18	36 ± 27	36 ± 22	Marketscan Database
Avg. prescriptions per visit	Direct	0.9	1.8	1.4	Marketscan Database
Avg. copayment per prescription ($)	Direct	3	3	3	Marketscan Database
Days lost	Indirect	3	2	5	4,5
Value 1 day lost ($)[g]	Indirect	65	100	65	30
Subtotal ($)[c]		300	330	458	
Ill, no medical care sought					
Days lost	Indirect	3	2	5	4,5
Value 1 day lost ($)[g]	Indirect	65	100	65	30
Over-the-counter drugs ($)	Direct	2	2	2	Assumed
Subtotal ($)[c]		197	202	327	

continued

TABLE 6-3 Continued

[a]Average present value (PV), using a 3% discount rate, of expected future lifetime earnings and housekeeping services, weighted by age and gender (Haddix et al., 1996) and adjusted to 1995 dollars (by multiplying by a factor of 1.07) (U.S. Bureau of the Census, 1997).

[b]Most likely, with ± defining the minimum and maximum costs for a triangular distribution (Evans et al., 1993) for Monte Carlo analysis (Critchfield and Willard, 1986; Dobilet et al., 1985; Dittus et al., 1989). The values were calculated by using cost data from Marketscan Database (The MEDSTAT Group, Ann Arbor, MI) and multiplying it by a hospital cost-to-charge ratio of 0.53. The latter ratio is a weighted average of the urban and rural (urban = 0.80, rural = 0.20) cost-to-charge ratios calculated by the Health Care Finance Administration for August 1996 (*The Federal Register*, 1996) (31 in the table).

[c]Subtotals are the totals for each category of outcome, using the most likely estimates.

[d]Most likely, with minimum and maximum values of net payments for outpatient visits up to 14 days before admission date and up to 30 days after discharge date.

[e]Net payment for drug claims associated with outpatient visits up to 14 days before admission and up to 30 days after discharge.

[f]Most likely, with ± defining the minimum and maximum days lost due to hospitalization for a triangular distribution (Evans et al., 1993) for Monte Carlo analysis (Critchfield and Willard, 1986; Dobilet et al., 1985; Dittus et al., 1989). Calculated using length of stay in hospital data from Marketscan Database (The MEDSTAT Group, Ann Arbor, MI) and adding a total of one additional day for convalescence and pre- and posthospitalization outpatient visits for 0-19 and 20-64 years of age. For 65+ years, two additional days were added to length of stay in hospital for convalescence and pre- and posthospitalization outpatient visits.

[g]For 0-19 and 65+ years age groups, a day lost to influenza was valued as equivalent to an unspecified day (Haddix et al., 1996), denoting a value for time lost by care givers and family members related to taking care of a patient in these age groups. For 20-64 years of age, 60% of days lost due to hospitalizations and related convalescence and pre- and posthospitalization outpatient visits were valued as day off work ($100/day). The remaining 40% of days lost were valued as unspecified days ($65/day). For 20-64 years of age, when patients were not hospitalized at any point during their illness (i.e., outpatient status), all days lost were assumed days off work ($100/day).

[h]The number of visits per episode of influenza is an average across all age groups. From the database, it was found that 85% of all patients had less than three outpatient visits, with an average of 1.52 visits (Appendix II).

[i]Most likely, with minimum and maximum values of net payments for outpatient visits without any specified association to hospitalizations.

[j]Most likely, with ± defining the minimum and maximum cost per prescription, with the number of prescriptions per visit.

TABLE 6-4 Cost of Vaccination[a] During an Influenza Pandemic, with Specific Costs Assigned to Side Effects of Vaccination

Item	Probability of Effect[b]	Cost of Case of Side Effect ($)[b]	Lower-Cost Scenario ($/patient)	Upper-Cost Scenario ($/patient)
Assumed cost of vaccination[a] (excluding side effects)			18	59
Side effects				
Mild[c]	0.0325	94	3.05	3.05
GBS[d]	0.000002	100,800	0.20	0.20
Anaphylaxis	0.000000157	2,490	0.01	0.01
Total cost per patient			21.26	62.26

[a]The cost of vaccination includes the cost of the vaccine, the cost of administering the vaccine, value of time spent by a person traveling to and from the place of vaccination, and patient-associated travel costs. Included in the costs of the vaccine are any costs associated with the rapid production of a larger-than-usual number of doses and the rapid delivery and correct storage of doses at vaccination sites around the country. For $18, the costs were assumed to be $10 for vaccine + administration, $4 patient time (half hour), $4 patient travel costs. For $59, the costs were assumed to be $20 for vaccine + administration (this could include the cost of two doses), $32 patient time (two trips at 2 hours per trip), and $7 patient travel costs. For comparison, a review of 10 published articles found a range of $5 to $22 per dose of vaccine, with a medium [sic] cost of $14 per dose (Jefferson and Demicheli, 1998). Additional details are provided in the background paper (see methods section). These breakdowns are illustrations only of what might be deemed reasonable estimates of time and cost. Actual costs might vary substantially and will depend on the number of doses needed to achieve a satisfactory protective response, as well as the efficiency of giving vaccinations to millions of persons.

[b]Probabilities and average cost of treating each category of side effect were derived from Office of Technology Assessment (1981).

[c]Mild side effects include sore arms due to vaccination, headaches, and other minor side effects that may require a visit to a physician or may cause the patient to miss 1 to 2 days of work.

[d]GBS = Guillain Barré syndrome.

million vaccinees. Option B targets the number of vaccinees as outlined in Option A plus approximately 20 million essential service providers (5 million health-care workers and 15 million providers of other service) (99.2 million vaccinees). Option C aims to achieve a 40% effective coverage of the entire U.S. population (106.1 million vaccinees), and Option D, 60% effective coverage of the entire U.S. population (159.2 million vaccinees).

The number of vaccine doses required to meet each option will depend on the number of doses per person needed to obtain an immune response. If two are needed, lack of compliance with a two-dose regimen will mean that the actual number of doses needed will be higher than double the target population for each option (i.e., >40% or >60% of the population will have to receive the first dose to ensure that 40% or 60% are fully vaccinated). If two doses are required, the cost per person vaccinated will increase (Table 6-4).

Findings

Illnesses and Deaths

The number of hospitalizations due to an influenza epidemic ranged from approximately 314,000 (5th percentile = 210,000; 95th percentile = 417,000) at a gross attack rate of 15% to approximately 734,000 (5th percentile = 441,000; 95th percentile = 973,000) at a gross attack rate of 35% (Figure 6-1). The mean numbers of persons requiring outpatient-based care ranged from approximately 18 million (gross attack rate of 15%) to 42 million (gross attack rate of 35%) (Figure 6-1). The mean numbers of those clinically ill not seeking medical care but still sustaining economic loss ranged from approximately 20 million (gross attack rate of 15%) to 47 million (gross attack rate of 35%) (Figure 6-1). The estimated number of deaths ranged from approximately 89,000 (5th percentile = 55,000; 95th percentile = 122,000) at a gross attack rate of 15%, which increased to approximately 207,000 deaths (5th percentile = 127,000; 95th percentile = 285,000) at a gross attack rate of 35% (Figure 6-1).

Groups at high risk (approximately 15% of the total U.S. population) (Table 6-1) would likely be disproportionately affected by an influenza pandemic. These groups accounted for approximately 85% of all deaths, with groups at high risk in the 20 to 64-year-old age group accounting for approximately 41% of total deaths (Table 6-5). Groups at high risk also accounted for 38% of all hospitalizations and 20% of all outpatient visits (Table 6-5).

Economic Impact of an Influenza Pandemic

Without large-scale immunization, the estimates of the total economic impact in the United States of an influenza pandemic ranged from $71.3 billion (5th percentile = $35.4 billion; 95th percentile = $107.0 billion) (gross attack rate of 15%) to $166.5 billion (5th percentile = $82.6 billion; 95th percentile = $249.6 billion) (gross attack rate of 35%) (Table 6-6). At any given attack rate, loss of life accounted for approximately 83% of all

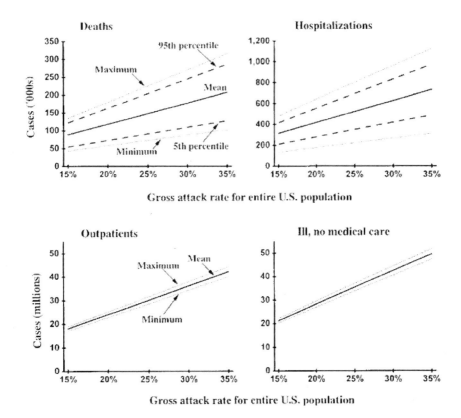

FIGURE 6-1 Impact of influenza pandemic in the United States: mean, minimum, maximum, and 5th and 95th percentiles of total death, hospitalizations, outpatients, and those ill (but not seeking medical care) for different gross attack rates. Note that for each gross attack rate, data are totals for all age groups and risk categories.

economic losses. Outpatients, persons ill but not seeking medical care, and inpatients accounted for approximately 8%, 6%, and 3%, respectively, of all economic losses (Table 6-6) (Appendix II).

Net Value of Vaccination

If it cost $21 to vaccinate a person and the effective coverage were 40%, net savings to society would result from vaccinating all age and risk groups (Figure 6-2). However, vaccinating certain age and risk groups rather than others would produce higher net returns. For example, vaccinating patients ages 20 to 64 years of age not at high risk would produce

TABLE 6-5 Impact, by Age Group, Death, Hospitalizations, and Outpatients Accounted for by Groups at High Risk During an Influenza Pandemic[a]

Category	Age Group (yrs)	Total Cases at High Risk (%)		
		Mean	5th	95th
Death	0–19	9.0	1.4	20.2
	20–64	40.9	11.1	60.9
	65 +	34.4	22.7	52.1
	Total	84.3		
Hospitalizations	0–19	4.6	2.1	7.9
	20–64	14.7	7.4	23.4
	65 +	18.3	11.0	27.6
	Total	37.6		
Outpatients	0–19	5.0	4.7	5.4
	20–64	10.4	9.8	11.0
	65 +	4.0	3.9	4.2
	Total	19.5		

[a]See Table 6-1 for distribution of groups at high and not at high risk within the U.S. population.

higher net returns than vaccinating patients ages 65 years of age and older who are at high risk (Figure 6-2). At a cost of $62 per vaccinee and gross attack rates of less than 25%, vaccinating populations at high risk would still generate positive returns (Figure 6-2). However, vaccinating populations not at high risk would result in a net loss (Figure 6-2).

Sensitivity Analyses

At a vaccination cost of $21.26 per vaccinee, reducing the death rates to half and one quarter of the initial values (Table 6-2) left positive mean net returns for all age groups not at high risk. However, at a vaccination cost of $62.26 per vaccinee, reducing death rates to half and one quarter of the initial values resulted in negative mean net returns for all age groups not at high risk. The results are much less sensitive to increases in gross attack rate than to increases in death rate. For example, assuming a cost of $62.26 per vaccinee and death rates that are half the initial rates, increasing the gross attack rate from 15% to 25% still resulted in negative net returns for all age groups, regardless of assumed level of vaccine effectiveness.

TABLE 6-6 Costs (Direct and Indirect) of Influenza Pandemic per Gross Attack Rate:[a] Deaths, Hospitalizations, Outpatients, Illnesses, and Total Costs (in 1995 US$)

	Cost per Gross Attack Rate ($ millions)				
	15%	20%	25%	30%	35%
Deaths					
Mean	59,288	79,051	98,814	118,577	138,340
5th percentile	23,800	31,733	39,666	47,599	55,532
95th percentile	94,907	126,543	158,179	189,815	221,451
Hospitalizations					
Mean	1,928	2,571	3,214	3,856	4,499
5th percentile	1,250	1,667	2,084	2,501	2,917
95th percentile	2,683	3,579	4,472	5,367	6,261
Outpatients					
Mean	5,708	7,611	9,513	11,416	13,318
5th percentile	4,871	6,495	8,119	9,742	11,366
95th percentile	6,557	8,742	10,928	13,113	15,299
Ill, no medical care sought[b]					
Mean	4,422	5,896	7,370	8,844	10,317
5th percentile	3,270	4,360	5,450	6,540	7,629
95th percentile	5,557	7,409	9,262	11,114	12,967
Grand totals					
Mean	71,346	95,128	118,910	142,692	166,474
5th percentile	35,405	47,206	59,008	70,810	82,611
95th percentile	106,988	142,650	178,313	213,975	249,638

[a]Gross attack rate = percentage of clinical influenza illness per population.

[b]Persons who become clinically ill due to influenza but do not seek medical care; illness has an economic impact (e.g., half day off work).

Implications for Policy

The amount of the insurance premium to spend on planning, preparedness, and practice for responding to the next influenza pandemic ranged from $48 million to $2,184 million per year (Table 6-7). The amount was sensitive to the probability of the pandemic, the cost of vaccinating a person, and the gross attack rate. Because higher costs of vaccination reduce net returns from an intervention, increased vaccination costs reduced the premiums. Conversely, increases in gross attack rates (all other inputs held constant) increased the potential returns from an intervention and thus the amount of premiums.

When risk for death is used as the criterion for who will be vaccinated first, persons ages 65 years and older receive top priority (Table 6-8); however, when mean net returns due to vaccination are used as the crite-

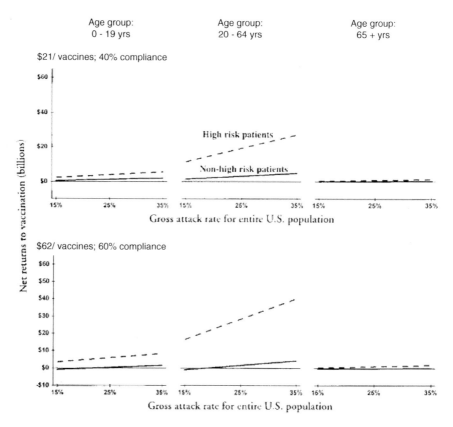

FIGURE 6-2 Mean net returns due to vaccination, by age group, for different gross attack rates and percentages of compliance. Case-age distributions are given in Table 6-1. Assumed vaccine effectiveness is the same as the high vaccine effectiveness defined in Appendix I.

rion, that group receives the lowest priority (Table 6-8). Regardless of criteria used, persons at high risk ages 0 to 19 and 20 to 64 years would always receive priority over persons not at high risk from the same age groups (Table 6-8).

While Option A would ensure positive mean net returns, Option B would result in greater mean net returns (Figure 6-3). Changing the strategy from vaccinating specific groups (Option B) to vaccinating 40% of the population decreased mean net returns (Figure 6-3). Only Option D resulted in higher mean net returns than Option B. Note, however, that the 5th and 95th percentiles for each option overlapped with those of other options. Thus, the differences in mean values between the options may not occur in practice.

TABLE 6-7 The Mean Annual Insurance Premium[a] for Planning, Preparing, and Practicing to Respond to the Next Influenza Pandemic

| Gross Attack Rate | Cost of Vaccination per Vaccinee ($) | Mean (s.d.) Insurance Premium ($ Millions) | | | | | |
| | | Low Vaccine Effectiveness[b] × 40% Compliance Probability of Pandemic | | | High Vaccine Effectiveness[b] × 60% Compliance Probability of Pandemic | | |
		1 in 30 years	1 in 60 years	1 in 100 years	1 in 30 years	1 in 60 years	1 in 100 years
15%	21	306 (122)	153 (61)	92 (37)	872 (341)	435 (170)	262 (103)
	62	162 (122)	81 (61)	48 (37)	654 (341)	326 (170)	196 (103)
25%	21	561 (204)	280 (102)	168 (61)	1,528 (569)	762 (284)	459 (171)
	62	416 (204)	207 (102)	125 (61)	1,311 (569)	653 (284)	394 (171)
35%	21	815 (286)	406 (142)	245 (86)	2,184 (796)	1,089 (397)	656 (239)
	62	670 (286)	334 (142)	201 (86)	1,967 (796)	980 (397)	591 (239)

[a]Defined here as the amount of money to be spent each year to plan, prepare, and practice to ensure that such mass vaccinations can take place if needed. See text for description of calculating premiums. The mathematically optimal allocation of such funds for each activity requires a separate set of calculations.

[b]Low and high levels of vaccine effectiveness are defined in Appendix I.

TABLE 6-8 Setting Vaccination Priorities: Which Age Group or Group at Risk Should be Vaccinated First?

Priority	Criteria for Prioritization		
	Risk for Death[a]	Total Deaths[b]	Returns Due to Vaccination
1 (top)	High risk 65+ yrs	High risk 20–64 yrs	High risk 20–64 yrs
2	Not at high risk 65+ yrs	High risk 65+ yrs	High risk 0–19 yrs
3	High risk 0–19 yrs	High risk 0–19 yrs	Not at high risk 20–64 yrs
4	High risk 20–64 yrs	Not at high risk 65+ yrs	Not at high risk 0–19 yrs
5	Not at high risk 20–64 yrs	Not at high risk 20–64 yrs	High risk 65+ yrs
6 (bottom)	Not at high risk 0–19 yrs	Not at high risk 0–19 yrs	Not at high risk 65+ yrs

[a]Priorities set by risk for death are set according to lower-limit estimates of deaths per 1,000 population for each age and risk group.

[b]The priority list using the total deaths criteria was set by examining the percentage of total deaths that each age and risk group contributed to the total deaths estimated due to a pandemic. The group with the highest percentage (i.e., contributes the largest number of deaths) is listed as having the highest priority.

Conclusions

Impact of an Influenza Pandemic

Although the next influenza pandemic in the United States may cause considerable illness and death (Figure 6-1), great uncertainty is associated with any estimate of the pandemic's potential impact. While the results can describe potential impact at gross attack rates from 15% to 35%, no existing data can predict the probability of any of those attack rates actually occurring. In addition, the groups at high risk are likely to incur a disproportionate number of deaths (Table 6-5); 50% or more of the deaths will likely occur among persons age 65 years and older (Appendix II), a distribution also found in the influenza pandemics of 1918, 1957, and 1968 (Simonsen et al., 1998).

Our results illustrate that the greatest economic cost is due to death (Table 6-6). Therefore, all other things being equal, the largest economic returns will come from the intervention(s) that prevents the largest number

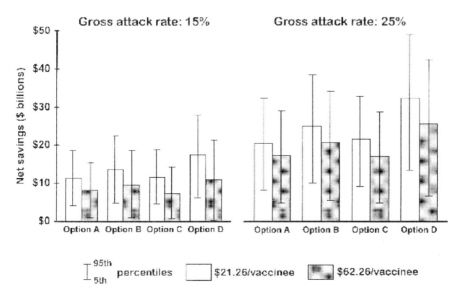

FIGURE 6-3 Four options for responding to an influenza pandemic: mean net economic returns. Notes: a) Bars show mean net returns for each option and assumed cost of vaccination. b) Option A: Similar to current Advisory Committee on Immunization Practices recommendations, with production and use similar to current, intrapandemic recommendations (CDC, 1998). Assumed approximately 77 million vaccinees. Option B: Number of vaccines as outlined in Scenario A plus 20 million essential service providers (5 million health-care workers + 15 million other service providers). Option C: Aim to achieve a 40% coverage of total U.S. population. Option D: Aim to achieve 60% coverage of total U.S. population (Appendix II).

of deaths. A limitation of the model is that, beyond the value of a lost day of work (Table 6-3), the model does not include any valuation for disruptions in commerce and society. For example, if many long-distance truck drivers were unavailable to drive for 1 or 2 weeks, there might be disruptions in the distribution of perishable items, especially food. These multiplier effects are not accounted for in this model, mainly because an estimate of an appropriate multiplier will depend on who becomes ill, how many become ill, when they become ill, and for how long they are ill.

All other factors being held constant, the net returns due to vaccination are sensitive to the combination of price and gross attack rate, with some scenarios generating negative mean returns (Figure 6-2). Further, some scenarios with a positive mean net return had a negative 5th percentile (Appendix II). The fact that negative results can be generated should serve as a warning that many interventions may not guarantee a net positive economic return.

Implications for Policy

The premium that could be spent each year for influenza pandemic response (planning, preparedness, and practice) depends most on the assumed probability of the pandemic (Table 6-7). The wide range in premiums presents a cautionary tale of the difference between possibility and probability of an influenza pandemic. What cannot be stated with any certainty are the probability of a pandemic and the number of persons who will become ill and die. Deciding the difference between possibility and probability was a key decision point in the swine flu incident of 1976–1977 (Neustadt and Fineberg, 1978).

Vaccination priorities depend on the objectives. If preventing the greatest number of deaths is the most important goal, society should ensure that those in the groups at high risk become vaccinated first, followed by those age 65 years or older who have no preexisting medical conditions making them more susceptible to complications from influenza (Table 6-8). However, if maximizing economic returns is the highest priority, persons 0 to 64 years of age, regardless of risk, should be vaccinated first (Table 6-8). Results also illustrate the need to be precise in defining the criterion used for setting priorities. For example, stating that preventing death will be the criteria used is not sufficiently precise because different priority lists can be drawn up using death rates versus total deaths (Table 6-8).

The criteria used to generate the results in Table 6-8 do not define the entire set of possible methods of setting priorities. Society may decide to use another criterion or set of criteria. Priorities for vaccination may also depend on the epidemiology of the pandemic. For example, if the strain causing the pandemic were particularly virulent among those ages 20 to 40 years, that age group may receive highest priority. Since the epidemiology of the next pandemic is unknown, any plan must allow flexibility in determining criteria for setting priorities. Table 6-8 provides a starting point for debate regarding who should be vaccinated first.

The net returns for the four scenarios modeled (Figure 6-3) further illustrate the need to clearly set criteria, goals, and objectives for a vaccine-based intervention for the next influenza pandemic. Some may state that Options C and D represent a more egalitarian means of distributing vaccine. However, egalitarianism would cost society more since the mean net returns from Options C are lower than those from Option B (Figure 6-3). Option D produces higher returns than Option B (Figure 6-3), but vaccinating 60% of the U.S. population in a short time would be difficult, especially if two doses of vaccine are required. If two doses were required, Option D would mean producing, delivering, and administering approximately 320 million doses of vaccine in a 2- to 3-month period, which has never been accomplished in the United States.

Acknowledgments

We thank Nancy Arden, Rob Breiman, Bill Jordan, Marty Meyers, Alicia Postema, Steve Schoenbaum, Larry Schonberger, Larry Sparks, and Ray Strikas for their help and encouragement.

Dr. Meltzer is senior health economist, Office of the Director, National Center for Infectious Diseases, Centers for Disease Control and Prevention. His research interests focus on assessing the economics of public health interventions such as oral raccoon rabies vaccine, Lyme disease vaccine, and hepatitis A vaccine, as well as estimating the economic burden of bioterrorism, dengue, pandemic influenza, and other infectious diseases. His research uses various methods, including Monte Carlo modeling, willingness-to-pay surveys (contingent valuation), and the use of non-monetary units of valuation, such as Disability Adjusted Life Years.

APPENDIX I

For the equation in the main text defining net returns due to vaccinations, savings from outcomes averted and the costs of vaccination are calculated as follows:

$$\text{Savings from outcomes averted}_{\text{age, risk group}} = \sum_{\text{Outcomes}} (\text{Number with outcome}_{\text{death, hospitalization, outpatient, ill, no medical care}}$$

$$\text{before intervention}_{\text{age, risk group}} \times \text{compliance}_{\text{age, risk group}}$$

$$\times \text{vaccine effectiveness}_{\text{outcomes}} \times \$\text{value of outcome}_{\text{death, hospitalization, outpatient, ill, no medical care}} \text{ prevented})$$

and;

$$\text{Cost of vaccination}_{\text{age, risk group}} = \$\text{cost/vaccinee} \times \text{population}_{\text{age, risk group}} \times \text{compliance}_{\text{age, risk group}}$$

TABLE High and Low Levels of Assumed Vaccine Effectiveness

Vaccine Effectiveness in Preventing Disease Outcomes[a,b]

Disease Outcomes	High[c]			Low[c]		
	0–19 yrs	20–64 yrs	65+ yrs	0–19 yrs	20–64 yrs	65+ yrs
Death	0.70	0.70	0.60	0.40	0.40	0.30
Hospitalization	0.55	0.55	0.50	0.55	0.55	0.50
Outpatient visits	0.40	0.40	0.40	0.40	0.40	0.40
Ill, no medical care sought	0.40	0.40	0.40	0.40	0.40	0.40

[a]Vaccine effectiveness is defined as the reduction in the number of cases in each of the age and disease categories.

[b]Within a defined age group, it was assumed that there was no difference in vaccine effectiveness between subgroups at high risk and not at high risk.

[c]The terms high and low level of effectiveness are subjective and reflect only a judgment of the levels of effectiveness in the two scenarios relative to each other.

APPENDIX II

A background paper, containing additional methodological details and results, is available electronically at the following URL: http.www.cdc.gov/ncidod/EID/vol5no5/meltzerback.htm.

INCREASING AWARENESS AND UPTAKE OF INFLUENZA IMMUNIZATION

Glen Nowak, PhD

Office of Health Communications
National Immunization Program
Centers for Disease Control and Prevention

Although much of this section focuses on the communication challenges presented by the need to increase public awareness of and uptake of seasonal influenza immunization, pandemic influenza will require similar efforts to enlist public support and cooperation. In both cases—as in most such circumstances—it is important to recognize that good communication is necessary, but not entirely sufficient, to achieving desired behavioral outcomes. Policies and incentives are also usually necessary to motivate many people to get annual flu shots (e.g., those people who believe influenza vaccination is helpful, but who are not willing to experience much inconvenience to get vaccinated).

It is crucial to note that good communication requires more than simply releasing facts, figures, and statistics to the public (Working Group on Governance Dilemmas in Bioterrorism Response, 2004). Many times, campaigns or efforts designed to achieve adoption of health promotion behaviors or recommendations rely primarily on the provision of numbers and statistics. The assumption is that people will conclude that the disease or adverse health outcome is more likely than they may have assumed. A 2004 campaign designed to increase attention and concern about deep vein thrombosis (DVT), for example, featured print ads pointing out that "DVT strikes 2 million Americans each year and that complications from this disorder cause up to 200,000 deaths per year—more than breast cancer, car crashes and AIDS combined." Although the campaign likely caused a modest increase in awareness of DVT and ways to prevent it, many (and perhaps most) people who may be affected by DVT probably remain unaware or unconvinced of this health threat. Providing numbers and statistics is helpful, but motivating people to take health-protective action requires doing more than simply listing morbidity and mortality statistics. The challenge of changing and influencing human behavior is difficult, and often far more difficult than it seems.

The 2003–2004 Flu Season:
A Recipe for Increasing Immunization Uptake

A variety of factors occurred during the 2003–2004 flu season that illustrate some of the elements and events that can significantly affect interest in, and demand for, influenza vaccine. These events occurred in a chronological fashion analogous to a "recipe" for increasing vaccine uptake. However, as the events of 2003–2004 also illustrate, many of the important ingredients in this recipe are outside the control of health officials and practitioners. For example, one factor that helped to facilitate initial media and public interest in influenza vaccination was the fact that influenza's arrival coincided with the immunization season. The convergence of influenza and the influenza vaccination season works in at least two ways to facilitate vaccination. First, it provides reporters and the media with a reason and an angle for influenza vaccination stories. Second, the presence or imminent presence of influenza not only raises the awareness, interest, and motivation levels of people, but the availability of vaccine means people can act on their concern. During that season, when people began to hear about flu, they could immediately take protective action.

A second element that helps to foster high motivation or demand for vaccine is the association of the dominant strain or initial cases of the disease with severe illness and/or outcomes. In the 2003–2004 influenza season, many of these initial cases (at least those that received significant and visible media attention) occurred among people for whom the public generally does not perceive influenza to cause serious complications. When influenza causes grave illness and death among children, healthy adults, or healthy seniors, the media are more likely to deem influenza as "news" (i.e., different and unusual enough to warrant attention). In 2003–2004, several of the initial serious influenza cases also occurred in cities and communities with large daily newspapers and major television stations, further increasing the visibility of the harm being caused by the disease. Many stories focused on individual patients or people who were deemed especially newsworthy because they did not fit the stereotypical profile of a flu casualty, such as a frail elderly person.

A third boost to immunization was provided in the 2003–2004 season when medical experts and public health authorities publicly (i.e., via press releases and the media) expressed alarm about the severity of the initial influenza cases. Many of the experts quoted in news stories predicted dire outcomes (e.g., more people than expected becoming sick with influenza) and urged influenza vaccination. Such statements, in turn, often received considerable attention and use by other media (e.g., stories on television and radio stations often cited experts who had been quoted in newspapers). It is important to note that in the 2003–2004 influenza season, the media and public health officials appeared to be working in concert. The media needed spokespeople on these issues, and public health officials needed outlets to inform the public that many people needed to receive influenza vaccination because they were susceptible to serious complications from influenza.

The 2003–2004 influenza season also illustrated the importance of "real-people" and "real-life" cases in fostering media and public interest in a vaccine-preventable disease. In November, one of the families who had a child who died from influenza held a press conference to urge other parents to get their children vaccinated. This event not only helped to boost the visibility of influenza immunization recommendations, but it also caused reporters in many parts of the country to investigate whether children in their areas were being harmed by influenza.

Although severe cases of influenza among children have occurred every year, it is relatively rare for reporters to recognize that fact or write about it. In 2003–2004, however, not only did they recognize that it could be happening in their communities, but they looked, and then wrote, about the impact influenza was having on children. The end result was increased media attention and visibility—which, in turn, fostered parent awareness and motivation. Visible, tangible, and meaningful examples of the seriousness of a vaccine-preventable disease, such as pictures of affected children and accounts of their families' grief and concern, is often highly motivating.

As a result of the confluence of all these events (i.e., flu arriving during the flu vaccination season, the initial cases causing severe illness among people not generally perceived to experience severe complications, and experts predicting a "bad" flu season), the 2003–2004 flu season was presented in the media in terms that facilitated continued media interest and that motivated public behavior. Early on, people learned or were told that it was going to be a severe flu season, a message that is more motivating than being told the flu season would be "typical" or "not so bad." This is important because while many people for whom an influenza vaccination is recommended routinely seek one, many others wait to hear or see how bad the flu season is before they take action. Heading into late November 2003, some medical and public health officials began talking about "pandemic influenza," further heightening media and public interest in both flu and flu vaccination.

For those interested in increasing the number of people who receive an annual influenza vaccination, one of the important lessons from the 2003–2004 influenza season is that several of the factors that help generate media attention to, and public demand for, flu shots are ones that cannot be affected or controlled by public health officials or medical professionals. A large amount of the media interest and consumer demand for flu vaccination is related to four factors: when influenza arrives; who is impacted in terms of illness; the severity, duration, and extent of the illness caused by the circulating strains; and people's perceptions regarding their individual (and/or family's) susceptibility to experiencing a severe case of influenza. As risk communication principles illustrate (Sandman, 1993), it is often the case that increasing the adoption of a medical recommendation (e.g., greater adoption of influenza immunization by people in at-risk groups) involves the creation of concern, anxiety, and worry. This is particularly true among people who do not routinely take the recommended action (e.g., receive an annual vaccination). There has to be some motivating level of fear before people take action, and that may play out in any number of ways. It could be a perception that many (or more) people are falling ill, a sense that the illness is especially severe, or a belief that one is vulnerable to contracting and experiencing serious illness.

Public Communication Challenges

The efforts and experiences of the past few years in trying to increase annual influenza vaccine uptake in the United States illustrates that a variety of factors must be considered as part of pandemic influenza communication planning. These factors all stem from the situation that (1) recommendations and perceptions regarding influenza vaccination are not universal, and (2) the development of effective communication plans and messages requires segmenting the audience/population based on relevant differentiating characteristics (Sandman and Lanard, 2004). People—including medical experts—have a variety of beliefs regarding the importance and value of influenza vaccination (Davis et al., 2002). This is a concern, particularly because (as will be discussed further) the so-called mass media, upon which many pandemic plans depend to disseminate information, no longer effectively reach the mass audiences (i.e., 30 percent or more of U.S. households at one time) they once did. Instead, when it comes to influenza and influenza vaccination, there are a number of distinct societal segments, each of which has different perspectives and needs that matter when it comes to developing communication messages (Sandman and Lanard, 2004). Furthermore, each segment also likely utilizes and favors different media outlets for news and information.

A key communication challenge in a pandemic will be to reduce the confusion created by mixed messages and to avoid, where possible, intentionally sending messages that provide confusing and potentially contradictory advice. Completely eliminating mixed messages from the pandemic influenza environment is likely an impossible objective. A better and more realistic objective is to utilize extensive communication and policy collaboration and partnerships to achieve highly visible, consistent recommendations and actions.

When it comes to reducing the impact and number of mixed or conflicting messages, a number of things need to be kept in mind. First, situations that involve multiple experts and organizations, differing expertise, a wide range of stakeholders (e.g., from scientists to policy makers), and a plethora of media typically lend themselves to "mixed" messages, conflicting advice, and seemingly contradictory recommendations. In many cases, a lack of scientific data or consensus help foster the presence of conflicting messages. Thus, it is important to recognize that "mixed" and "conflicting" messages are, strictly speaking, unavoidable. However, as recent examples involving avian influenza, influenza vaccine supply shortages, and Severe Acute Respiratory Syndrome (SARS) illustrate, extensive collaboration on policies and communications greatly enhances the visibility of "consensus" messages and recommendations.

Second, it's important to realize that "policies" and "behaviors" communicate—in many cases, more powerfully and effectively than words. As a result, many "mixed" or "conflicting" messages arise because patients or members of the public see or perceive a contradiction between what is being recommended and the actions of those making the recommendation. In the case of influenza vaccination, for example, one of the mixed messages that exists in the minds of many people for whom annual flu vaccination is recommended is the relatively low uptake among health care professionals (Brunell, 2004). As a result, many people assume that the vaccine must be unnecessary or ineffective, or their doctor or nurse would surely receive it.

It is also possible for messages that are designed to increase influenza immunization among people at high risk for severe illness to have unintended consequences. In the case of medical recommendations, this can happen through the use of the images and pictures used in education or public information materials. Often, posters, brochures, and television public service announcements contain pictures of people who are in, or believed to be in, the targeted population. Through focus group research, a few years ago, we learned of an "unintended" consequence related to influenza immunization education materials that targeted people 65 years old and older. In having focus group participants discuss some of the posters commonly used in the 1990s, we learned that many people in that age group did not deem these materials as relevant to them. One reason was the use of models and pictures that focused on elderly people and people in generally poor health. Healthy and active people who were 65 and older who did not seek an annual flu vaccination frequently said, "I don't need a flu shot. A flu shot is for elderly or frail people. I'm healthy and active." In their mind, most influenza vaccination materials fostered the perception that immunization was recommended for elderly people, particularly those in poor health or in nursing homes. If they didn't consider themselves to be "elderly," or if they considered themselves to be healthy and active, they tended not to believe they should get vaccinated. A more effective communication approach is to use images of healthy and active seniors and to call attention to the fact that "an annual influenza vaccination helps you stay healthy and active."

More recently the Centers for Disease Control and Prevention (CDC) recommended annual influenza vaccination for those ages 50 to 64 years and 6 to 23 months (Harper et al., 2004). In developing education materials for these groups, recent focus group research indicated that many parents and people in the newly recommended age category expect those materials to describe tangible and explicit benefits for adopting that recommendation. Their reactions could be summarized as, "There must be some reason(s) that it's now recommended that I receive an annual influenza vaccination— I'd like to know what that reason is" or "something must have changed so that I'm now in a group that is recommended for annual vaccination, what's changed?" Many parents of 6- to 23-month-olds wondered, "Why now, why the change? I didn't have an influenza vaccination when I was a child. Five years ago with my first child it wasn't necessary. What has changed that makes this necessary today?" Many of these parents believed they had no evidence from their daily experience that such a change was warranted.

Another significant pandemic (and general) influenza immunization challenge pertains to "nuanced" communications and advice. It is common, especially in circumstances that are relatively new or where broad/deep scientific and medical consensus is lacking, to develop policies, recommendations, and messages that contain caveats, clauses, and fine distinctions. In the case of policies and recommendations, this can be necessary and unavoidable. Unfortunately, when it comes to public, patient, media, and even health care practitioners, much of this "nuance" is lost and/or unrecognized. The media frequently simplify recommendations and messages, and thus fail to transmit all the nuances, while people in media and target audiences usually fail to recognize, understand, or appreciate clauses and distinctions. Furthermore, the media, health care practitioners, and the public generally prefer, and better understand, direct, simple, and clear messages. They also often fail to use or define words with the same degree of nuance as those making and putting forward the overall policies. For example, in the case of influenza vaccination, an attempt was made for a couple of years to "encourage" annual vaccination of 6- to 23- month-old children—versus "recommend" annual vaccination. Focus group research and calls from physicians and parents consistently indicated that for these groups, "encourage" and "recommend" were synonymous. Many health care professionals even asked why different words were used. More recently, focus group discussions with parents of 6- to 23-month-old children indicated that some found the reference to 23 months confusing. They asked, "Does that mean that my 2-year-old doesn't need the flu vaccination?" Clearly, we need to pay more attention to these sorts of inadvertent consequences of our well-intended and carefully crafted messages.

Three Population Segments

Our experience indicates that Americans broadly fall into three population segments with regard to influenza vaccination. One segment consists of people who routinely receive the annual influenza vaccine, including many of those whom we recommend do so. Considerable data indicate that most people 65 and older—perhaps 65 to 70 percent of those in this age group—regularly receive an annual influenza vaccination, typically relatively early in September and October.

An even larger group consists of Americans who sometimes receive an annual influenza vaccination; these also include people for whom vaccination is recommended. People in this group often monitor the flu season and make a decision each year whether there is sufficient reason to take the time and make the effort to be immunized. They appear to be swayed by factors such as information about the severity of the strain, the likelihood that they or someone they know will contract influenza, and their perceived likelihood of transmitting severe disease. Many people in this "wait and see" group ultimately will decide to get immunized, and likely do so in November or December.

Finally, there is a group of people who do not get or intend to get an influenza vaccination, and they, too, include some people for whom immunization is recommended. However, recent data suggest that most people in this group are 18 to 49 years old, so on average they have relatively low risk of flu complications. However, older people in this group often have reached their decision against immunization based on a firmly held belief or conviction—and have held their position for years (and in some cases, decades). To change their minds will require far more than telling them that 36,000 people a year die from influenza (CDC, 2004a). They probably know that influenza causes serious harm (and often have experienced influenza), but they are not convinced that the vaccine is either safe or effective; rather, many believe the vaccine will cause them to get the flu either directly or by somehow rendering their immune system more susceptible to the virus.

Targeting Pandemic Communications

In the event of a pandemic, public officials would need to tailor messages to reach the three groups (as well as other segments; see Sandman and Lanard, 2004) described above in order to respond to their individual perceptions regarding influenza immunization—and these messages would need to be conveyed through an increasingly fractured mass media. Most American households receive at least 10 television channels, and as many as 50 to 100 if they have cable or satellite service. In addition, hundreds of websites offer medical and health information. Daily newspaper readership, once a unifier of the American population, is declining, particularly among 18- to 49-year-olds. Additional factors to be considered in reaching the American public with information about pandemic influenza include:

• The increasing cultural and ethnic diversity of American society (e.g., materials and messages need to be provided in multiple languages and involve the use of multiple spokespeople).
• Variable health literacy, with crucial deficits among some populations.
• "Information overload" that divides public attention to the extent that people need to be exposed to a message 10 to 12 times (a number that has doubled over the past decade) before it receives attention, and presumably many more before people actually gain knowledge and change their behavior.

In addition, communication challenges or issues can arise when the desire/need to motivate large numbers of people to take action meets the logistical issues and challenges that arise in implementing large-scale programs (e.g., vaccinating large numbers of people). Thus, it can be relatively easy to put out messages that seemingly tell people they need to act quickly, but "not too quickly" because of an inability to accommodate demand. It is difficult to tell people that everyone needs to act, but that "we don't want everyone to act at once." Thus the message to "be afraid, but not too afraid" represents the crux of many health communication challenges. In the case of pandemic influenza, the goal is to have people understand that there are some individuals who ought to act immediately to protect their health and lives through immunization, and others who can and will need to wait until a later point (and that there are actions or steps that those who are being asked to wait can take to help reduce their risk).

To effectively develop and communicate the various messages and recommendations that will need to be used in a pandemic, a comprehensive and highly coordinated approach to communication is necessary. This will require a strong investment in research and collaborations to help determine which messages resonate, particularly among people who are not usually inclined to get an influenza vaccination. The use of less nuanced messages and advice should be investigated, coupled with the development and use of portfolios of messages and materials that recognize the cultural and racial diversity that exists in this country.

We also need to go beyond the news media in terms of developing communication plans that allow our messages greater visibility, scope, and frequency of delivery to the public (Glass and Schoch-Spana, 2002). To do so will be costly because broad coverage means getting the message across in the vast numbers of existing mass media outlets.

Finally, ensuring the effectiveness of public communication during an influenza pandemic will require a greater understanding and use of risk communication principles (Sandman, 1993). Health officials will need to learn how to share the dilemmas they face with the public in a productive and effective fashion. We are going to have to acknowledge uncertainty and gaps in scientific knowledge. When faced with the necessity of setting priorities for who will receive limited amounts of vaccine, we must be ready to provide effective coping strategies and advice to those who must wait their turn.

STRATEGIES TO REMEDY PANIC IN A PANDEMIC: LESSONS FROM BIODEFENSE

Monica Schoch-Spana, PhD

Center for Biosecurity
University of Pittsburgh Medical Center

"How will the public react to a biological attack?" is a fundamental question underpinning U.S. policy and practice in the realm of terrorism preparedness and response. Over the past 6 years, widely divergent approaches to the issue of mass responses to bioterrorism have emerged.[6] When catastrophic terrorism was a serious but postulated danger, officials frequently conceived public reactions to a biological event as part and parcel of the crisis to be contained: for example, the "worried well" who would pour into hospitals, hindering health care workers' ability to treat "real" victims. The complex realities of September 11, 2001, and the anthrax letter attacks have helped refine many authorities' understanding of the public not simply as a problem to be managed, but a constituency to be served—anxious people who need good information about the danger and what to do about it. This essay advances a third approach, encouraging authorities to place current commitments to improving public communication within a broader understanding of the governance dilemmas that bioterrorism and other health emergencies pose.

---

[6]Comments pertain to the U.S. context, though they may also have relevance elsewhere. I write from my vantage point as someone who has worked for the past 6 years with a multidisciplinary group committed to preventing the development and use of biological weapons and to advancing an adequate medical and public health response should prevention fail.

From Crowd Management to Credible Communication

Attitudes and operational approaches among U.S. decision makers and professional responders toward the public have shifted from an emphasis on containing disorder to communicating information in the bioterrorist context. Playing one-dimensional roles in hypothetical scenarios, members of the public usually surfaced as mass casualties or hysteria-driven mobs who self-evacuate affected areas or who resort to violence to gain access to scarce, potentially life-saving antibiotics and vaccines (Schoch-Spana, 2003). Prior to 2001, official response systems were often built around the notion of the public as a problem to be managed during a crisis; this bias, which remains to a certain extent today, precludes careful consideration of, and planning for, ways to solicit the cooperation of affected populations. Emphasis instead is on crowd control, not enhancing the people's ability to cope with a public health emergency.

Communication failures, however, during the serial tragedies of 2001 spurred recognition of the essential role of public outreach in managing the effects of a bioattack. Following the anthrax crisis, federal health authorities identified risk communication and health information dissemination as one of seven priority areas required to upgrade the ability of state and local health departments to respond to bioterrorism. Critical reflection on responses to the 2001 terrorist attacks also spurred the release of many helpful analyses and guidebooks for officials regarding successful communication with the media and the larger public (U.S. Department of Health and Human Services, 2002; Ethiel, 2002; CDC, 2002; Fischhoff, 2002). Practitioner and policy-maker interest in public communication remains high: Typically, two of the top five articles that are downloaded each month from the journal, *Biosecurity and Bioterrorism*, have a focus on communication (Personal communication, Jackie Fox, *Biosecurity and Bioterrorism*). U.S. and World Health Organization pandemic influenza planning similarly recognizes risk communication as a critical public health intervention (Gellin, 2004; Stöhr, 2004).

Managing Infectious Disease Threats in the Information Age

The anthrax letter scare in 2001 revealed the many communication challenges that can arise in an uncertain, evolving, large-scale health crisis that involves infectious disease.[7] Briefly reviewed here are select findings from a national, qualitative study of public communication experiences during that event (see Table 6-9) (U.S. Department of Health and Human

---

[7]For other analyses of the communication challenges presented by the anthrax attacks, see Thomas (2003); Gursky et al. (2003).

TABLE 6-9 Research Design: Public Communication During 2001
Anthrax Scare

Method	23 small, moderated, taped, and transcribed discussions held June 2002 to June 2003		
Sites	Based on proximity or distance to 2001 events; varying size and density as well as regional diversity:		
	Baltimore, MD	New York, NY	Seattle, WA
	Kansas City, MO	San Antonio, TX	Washington, DC
Subjects	Professional responders – Local political leaders, health and safety officials, doctors, nurses, journalists, and Red Cross (n = 66)	General public – Workers at risk of anthrax exposure: e.g., mail handlers, congressional and media outlet staff (n = 66) – Grassroots leaders from diverse groups and neighborhoods (n = 82)	

Services, 2002). The findings and implications drawn out in Figure 6-4 underscore that the Information Age presents both opportunities and obstacles in managing infectious disease threats. In general, communication deficits during the anthrax crisis point to the need for proactive remedies in the precrisis period.

Parallels between the anthrax scare and an influenza pandemic make the former case relevant to the larger issue of prevention and response. Like influenza, anthrax infection during fall 2001 was seen as something of an "everyman's" disease by virtue of the postal system's involvement (most people receive mail) and the inexplicable deaths of Kathy Nguyen and Ottilie Lundgren, apparent bystanders who were not members of the then-defined "at-risk" populations.[8] The September 11 attacks, too, had fostered a widespread sense of vulnerability. However, limits to generalizing from this case study exist; for example, an influenza pandemic threatens the possibility of widespread, high morbidity and mortality, a significant contrast with the U.S. anthrax experience.

*Contemporary Outbreaks Can Have Broad Impact Due to
Their Increasing "Spectacle" Quality*

In today's information-saturated environment, outbreaks affect diffuse publics without immediate epidemiological and physical involvement. Simi-

---

[8]National polling during the crisis period, for example, demonstrated that safe handling of mail was a prevalent health behavior in the United States and not one limited to crisis epicenters. See Blendon et al., 2001.

Outbreaks Have Broad Impact Due to Their Spectacle Nature	
"I was on vacation in Mexico when all of this happened, and everybody was glued to the television set watching CNN in the bar at the resort...They finally made a decision to turn off the TV...so people could enjoy their vacation." – Seniors' Advocate, Seattle, WA	Accept that outbreaks have a broad, virtual reach; approach potential "casualties" as in need of both informational and medical intervention
Responders Frequently Misdiagnose Public Demands for Health Information as 'Panic'	
"What do you mean by 'panic'? Can you give a concrete example of it?" – Facilitator "All those calls into the health department." – Responder (n.b.: paraphrase of response common across locales)	Avoid approaching high-volume demands for health information as getting in the way of 'real' public health work or 'true' epidemic containment
Expectations about Science and Government are in Conflict with Evolving Events	
"I have a natural presumption that...[if] it's the government,...everybody's going to do the most rational thing and we're going to be on top of things and everything. But I really...lost some confidence because I just got the sense that they were kind of...making it up on the fly." – Congressional Staffer, Washington, DC	Create infrastructure and protocols to move knowledge among authorities and the public more efficiently; BUT ALSO Make clear the iterative nature of understanding an organic, open-ended situation like an outbreak
Emergency Signal to the Public is Frequently Lost in All the Noise of Reporting	
"I remember feeling...like [the] media was in stream of consciousness mode and everything was without context .... Everything was just dumped on you, and you're just trying to process it. What do you do with all this information?" – Immigrant Advocate, Seattle, WA	Devise public communication plan that achieves common understanding among local residents of where and when to access and validate health information
Mainstream Media Have Limited Reach to Unfamiliar and Untrusting Publics	
"[I]n my community, I don't believe much in papers. I strongly believe in, 'Look, let's go to that place, tonight, a meeting,' and we can gather 500 without any problem." – Latino Community Organizer, New York, NY	Use grassroots leaders as key communicators to niche populations, involving them in planning prior to an emergency

FIGURE 6-4 Communication dilemmas in the Information Age: Lessons learned during 2001 anthrax scare.

larly, at the peak of the global SARS outbreak, the New York City Department of Health discovered that some residents were transposing what they were reading and seeing about Hong Kong and other hard-hit areas to conditions in New York, where the impact had been minimal (Roberts, 2003). The crisis elsewhere, that is, became the baseline for what was perceived to be happening locally. Word of, and worry about, epidemics can move readily throughout diverse populations, leading to demands on public health and safety officials and medical practitioners outside of disease epicenters.

Authorities Frequently Misdiagnose Public Demands for Health Information as "Panic"

Powder scares, anthrax exposure tests, and health information demands—by a majority of people at no or minimal risk of infection—produced excess demands on physicians, hospitals, law enforcement, and public health and safety personnel. Overburdened and confronting a lethal event, many authorities understandably interpreted such demands as "panic," that is, a problem of public irrationality or overreaction. From the vantage point of persons consciously looking for expert guidance on health matters in a novel threat situation, however, such demands are reasonable. Characterizing high-volume information requests in a crisis as panic obscures more systemic deficits within U.S. health care and public health systems, such as limited ability to ramp up activity to meet unforeseen, large-scale demand and a lower professional and institutional priority placed on health risk and crisis communication.

The Emergency "Signal" to the Public Is Frequently Lost in the "Noise" of Reporting

Officials' need and desire to convey clear and consistent messages must contend with diverse media, instantaneous reporting, and a potentially overwhelming amount of information available to the members of the public, who lack clear criteria for sorting "noise" from critical information. Research subjects reported alternating between a feast and famine of information: At certain times, they felt starved for official guidance that came out at a trickle; at other times, they felt inundated by the disparate, evolving bits of information streaming from news sources. A truly "public" broadcast system (noncommercial and noncompetitive) that provided a reliable flow of information, with regularly scheduled updates, was judged absent during the anthrax attacks and was frequently offered as the possible technological and institutional solution for the twin problems of information scarcity and overload.

Mainstream Media Have Limited Reach Among Unfamiliar and Untrusting Publics

Mass media reach the largest number of people the most quickly, and many research subjects reported that despite the overwhelming amount of information available via news reports, they still found much of what they were seeking. At the same time, grassroots civic leaders and smaller media outlets serving ethnic and immigrant communities were seen to provide a better route for reaching populations that either do not routinely use or do not trust mainstream media, or who are suspicious of official government pronouncements. In an era where information technology promises to connect everyone, "lower tech" options such as person-to-person communication networks may be the more appropriate outreach mechanism for disenfranchised populations.

Expectations About Science and Government Are in Conflict with Uncertain, Evolving Events

"*Some* government expert *somewhere* must know what to do in this kind of crisis" was an operating assumption for many research subjects when they recalled their anthrax experience. In an era where satellites can read license plate numbers, people understandably have high expectations about the ability of government officials and technical experts to "know" something. People not directly affected by the attacks posited that authorities did not provide adequate updates of emergency information either because they were acting in a deliberate, paternalistic manner and withholding information, or they were unable to convey the information efficiently out of incompetence. A third explanation—that absolute understanding of the danger and its medical aspects was lacking—was relatively absent. People directly affected by events recounted having their belief in an omniscient government undermined by firsthand experience of the tentative nature of authorities' approach to the crisis.

Communication as a Means to an End, Not an End in Itself

As 2001 demonstrated, open and informative relationships among citizens, government, and public health and safety authorities are fundamental to a population's ability to cope with unconventional health threats. Abundant communication technologies prove both benefit and burden for authorities having to contain an infectious disease threat. U.S. leaders and professional responders should be lauded for embracing effective crisis and risk communication as remedies for a potentially anxious, skeptical, and/or resistant public. Powerful cultural and technological forces—for example, computerization, media proliferation, the Internet, e-mail—make it easy, however, to think of social life merely in terms of information exchange. Authorities should be careful not to approach improved communication as the "quick social fix" for the more complex, underlying tensions that precede or emerge during bioattacks or other health crises (Sorenson, 2004).

Public communication and risk communication have become code words with which to skirt the more complex realities associated with community responses to bioterrorist and other infectious disease threats. When authorities say they want better communication with the public, what they tend to mean is public "buy-in," public compliance, and understanding—possibly even absolution—when tough choices arise for officials, such as how to distribute scarce resources in an emergency. When members of the public indicate that they want better communication from officials, what they are asking for is inclusion, consideration, and mutual respect as peer decision makers; expert guidance on which they can act; and proof that their needs have justly been considered by people in authority. As the United States gravitates toward communication as a key to bioterrorism readiness, everyone should reflect on what that communication is meant to accomplish.

Governance Dilemmas as Critical Contexts for Public Communication

The larger social and political context for public communication practice was the analytic focus of the Working Group on Governance Dilemmas in Bioterrorism Response (2004). Whether "natural" or "deliberate" in origin, a large outbreak poses unique governing dilemmas. Leaders must tend to immediate life-and-death matters such as caring for the sick, ward off socially corrosive effects like ostracism of the afflicted, and stem dramatic economic effects for victims and affected locales alike. Conflicts of interest, priority, and purpose can emerge in pursuit of these goals. The Working Group prepared a set of analytic templates for decision makers faced with these difficult situations to better prepare them to safeguard the public's trust and cooperation during a response to an infectious disease threat. The framework was intended to stave off the temptation of leaders to focus on the managerial and scientific aspects of response to the neglect of civic, social, ethical-moral, and economic dimensions that also matter to communities.

What Defines "Leadership" During an Epidemic or Biological Attack?

Five strategic goals help distinguish successful leadership during an epidemic or bioattack in twenty-first-century America. An informed and involved public, along with guidance and material support from respected leaders, can help achieve these aims:

• Limit death and suffering through proper preventive, curative, and supportive care; tend to the greater vulnerability of children, the frail elderly, and the physically compromised.
• Defend civil liberties by using the least restrictive interventions to contain an infectious agent that causes communicable disease.

• Preserve economic stability, managing the financial blow to victims as well as the near- and long-term losses of hard-hit industries, cities, and neighborhoods.

• Discourage scapegoating, hate crimes, and the stigmatization of specific people or places as "contaminated" or unhealthy.

• Bolster the ability of individuals and the larger community to rebound from unpredictable and traumatic events; provide mental health support to those who need it.

What Leadership Dilemmas May Arise in an Epidemic, and How Might They Be Averted?

Large-scale outbreaks are complex events that provoke fear and contradictory impulses. Because an epidemic's impact—illness, death, lost livelihood, disrupted commerce—is troubling to consider, leaders and the larger public may deny that a problem exists, or intervene too quickly without regard to the negative effects of their actions. Once acknowledged, an epidemic exerts immense political and social pressure for swift, decisive, visible response (Rosenberg, 1989), more so in the case of a deliberate epidemic. Apparent and sometimes genuine conflicts among strategic goals can arise. The most common dilemmas facing past leaders have been balancing disease control imperatives with those of individual liberty, economic stability, and stigma prevention (Box 6-1).

What Situations Splinter the Social Trust Necessary to Cope with Health Crises, and How Might They Be Defused?

Mutual confidence and obligation among decision makers, citizens and their leaders, and community members are the basis for achieving any and all strategic goals. Breaches of social trust, however, are a common predicament for leaders during outbreaks and are likely to arise during a bioattack (Box 6-2). Conditions that confound social trust involve preconceptions about "the government," "the public," or "the media"; the social and economic fault lines that are exacerbated by disease and dread of it; and questions about the morally defensible use of communal resources in times of crisis.

Governing successfully during large, fast-moving, lethal epidemics requires a dynamic collaboration among members of a community and the community's leaders. Officials who have realistic expectations about the societal challenges posed by large outbreaks will be better prepared to protect and actively support cooperation and trust between a community and its leaders. In the absence of an engaged public, resolution of the

BOX 6-1
Recommendations for Handling Potential Conflicts Between Strategic Response Goals

Stop disease that spreads from person to person while upholding individual freedoms

- Make response plans public before a crisis occurs; a well-informed population is more likely to cooperate with advice for reducing the spread of disease.
- Sketch out the "big picture"; make concrete the fact that personal actions can affect the safety of others—for example, remind people that staying home from work or keeping children out of school when they are ill protects others from getting sick.
- Use disease controls that respect ideals of autonomy, self-determination, and equality—public cooperation limits illness and death; public resistance does not.
- Provide goods and services that help people comply with health orders—for example, set up vaccination clinics in locations accessible to people without cars.
- Restrict civil liberties, if necessary, *only* in a transparent and equitable way.

Protect the economy while using disease controls that disrupt commerce

- Be mindful of the goal of long-term financial recovery when controlling disease; do not react based solely on the desire to avert short-term economic loss.
- Recognize public trust as precious "capital" that grows the economy—for example, if people see their health as your top priority, confidence in your efforts to safeguard the economy will follow.
- Account for the less visible and more scattered monetary impacts when making epidemic control decisions (e.g., costs of victims' health care; economic toll of stigma).

Restore social bonds when people feel at the mercy of a mysterious disease

- Express empathy for people's fears about getting sick from others; follow up with meaningful medical details that allow people to gauge personal risk accurately.
- Demonstrate compassion toward victims of disease; explain to the community at large the social costs of avoiding people out of fear, rather than out of actual danger.
- Direct law enforcement to deal appropriately with hate crimes in the event prevention fails.
- Coordinate volunteers, relief groups, and civic organizations in humanitarian response, with extra focus on assisting the most vulnerable—for example, children, the frail elderly, and disabled people of all ages.

BOX 6-2
Principles and Actions for Addressing
Social Trust Predicaments

Prevent unproductive fear, denial, or skepticism on the part of the public when delivering crisis updates

- Share what you know. Do not withhold information because you think people will panic. Creative coping is the norm; panic is the exception.
- Hold press briefings early and often to reach the public. Answering questions is not a distraction from managing the crisis; it *is* managing the crisis.
- Confirm that local health agencies and medical facilities are prepared to handle an onslaught of questions from concerned individuals, in person and by phone.
- Convey basic health facts clearly and quickly so that people have peace of mind that they are safe or so that they seek out care, if need be; similarly, brief health care and emergency workers so they have a realistic understanding about job safety.
- View rumors as a normal sign of people's need to make sense of vague or disturbing events. Refine your outreach efforts; the current ones may not be working.

Earn confidence in the use of scarce resources despite existing social and economic gaps

- Account for income disparities in response plans; anticipate the need for free or low-cost prevention and treatment.
- Make planning transparent so that the public sees that access to life-saving resources is based on medical need and not on wealth or favored status.
- Be open about eligibility criteria for goods and services, especially when tough choices arise unexpectedly—for example, which botulism attack victims will receive the limited antitoxin that exists.
- Show thorough preparations to protect vulnerable populations like children and the frail elderly, thus bolstering *everyone's* sense of security.

Maintain credibility when decisions must be made before all the facts are in

- Advise the community at the outset if crisis conditions are evolving or could be prolonged.
- Offer more detail rather than less, even when the unknowns outnumber what is known; resist the urge to reassure for the sake of reassurance alone.
- Be frank about any uncertainty regarding "facts"; describe plans to fill in knowledge gaps.
- Vary your means of reaching the public. Mix high-tech outreach (Internet, cable, network, print, radio, cell phone, automated hotlines) with contact through grassroots leaders.

immediate health crisis is rendered far more difficult, and the resilience of affected communities is diminished.

Increasing emphasis on enhanced public communication is a positive development within biodefense, and public health preparedness and response more broadly. Nonetheless, this development must be supplemented with robust discussion among leaders, and between authorities and the larger population, as to what an optimal response looks like, and from whose point of view.

Acknowledgments

The Working Group on Governance Dilemmas in Bioterrorism Response and the research focus groups—the findings of which are presented here—were convened by the Center for Biosecurity of the University of Pittsburgh Medical Center in collaboration with the Johns Hopkins University and supported under award MIPT-2003J-A-019 from the Oklahoma City Memorial Institute for the Prevention of Terrorism (MIPT) and the Office for Domestic Preparedness, Department of Homeland Security, and award 2000-10-7 from The Alfred P. Sloan Foundation. Points of view expressed in this document do not necessarily represent the official position of MIPT, the U.S. Department of Homeland Security, or the Sloan Foundation.

PUBLIC HEALTH PREPAREDNESS AND ETHICAL VALUES IN PANDEMIC INFLUENZA

Lawrence O. Gostin[9]

Georgetown University

Severe Acute Respiratory Syndrome (SARS) garnered a great deal of public attention because it was novel and its potential for spread was unknown. However, the SARS coronavirus is significantly less virulent than pandemic influenza viral infections. Influenza pandemics have occurred roughly two to three times per century, causing untold morbidity and mortality (Kolata, 1997). The Spanish influenza pandemic of 1918 caused more

[9]Lawrence O. Gostin is the John Carroll Research Professor of Law, Georgetown University; Professor of Public Health, the Johns Hopkins University; Director, Center for Law & the Public's Health (CDC Collaborating Center).

Disclaimer: Professor Gostin was a member of WHO's consultation on influenza preparedness and is working with WHO on the revision of the International Health Regulations. The views in this chapter do not necessarily reflect those of WHO. A shorter version of this chapter appears in the *Hastings Ctr Rpt* 2004;34:10–11.

than 20 million deaths in a world less than one-third the size of the current global population (Stevens et al., 2004). Modern epidemiologists now estimate that more than 50 million people died. These deaths did not occur primarily among infants and old people as suggested by conventional wisdom. Approximately half the deaths were among people in the prime of their lives. As John Barry explains in his recent book, "One cannot know with certainty, but if the upper estimate of the death toll is true as many as 8 to 10 percent of all young adults then living may have been killed by the virus. And they died with extraordinary ferocity and speed" (Barry, 2004).

The Institute of Medicine (IOM) has noted three essential prerequisites for an influenza pandemic: (1) the identification of a novel viral subtype in animal populations such as swine or poultry, (2) viral replication causing disease in humans, and (3) efficient human-to-human transmission (Institute of Medicine, 2004). The species "jump" from animals to humans could occur through a process known as "reassortment." If a person is exposed to both animal and human viral infections, the "genetic mixing" could lead to a strain that is transmissible from human to human, sometimes in ways that are highly resistant to vaccination or antiviral treatment.

Since 1997, the first two prerequisites—a novel viral strain in animals and transmission from animals to humans—have been met on four occasions. The most recent episode occurred in 2004 with H5N1 influenza found in Vietnam and Thailand (CDC, 2004b). The avian influenza outbreak resulted in the culling of large chicken populations, including farms in the United States, with severe economic and trade impacts (Dao, 2004). There is now intense interest in influenza preparedness (Webby and Webster, 2003), with major planning initiatives being undertaken by the World Health Organization (WHO, 2004a) and the IOM (2004).

The potential for pandemic spread of a "fit" influenza strain leads to intriguing ethical and legal questions about public health interventions that could severely disrupt trade, economics, travel, and personal liberty. National and global public health agencies have mooted a wide range of interventions, asking penetrating questions such as: Should intrusive powers be exercised? At what stage in the outbreak should interventions commence and with what safeguards? Planning for the next pandemic includes not simply influenza but other novel infections, both naturally occurring and intentionally disseminated (Weinstein, 2004).

This section examines the principal therapeutic and nontherapeutic public health interventions for preventing or ameliorating pandemic influenza. In each case, the hard legal and ethical questions likely to arise are explored. Thereafter, the section provides several ethical values that can help evaluate public health interventions.

Public Health Interventions to Prevent or Ameliorate Pandemic Influenza

Animal/Human Interchange

A critical early preventive strategy is to control animal populations and prevent the species jump from animals to humans (see Table 6-10). Humans are highly vulnerable to animal infections due to the close proximity of animal and human populations in farming and distribution of poultry and meat (Emanuel, 2003). Strategies to diminish the risk include separation of animal and human populations; occupational health and safety in animal work (e.g., infection control and disinfection); and control of diseased or exposed animal populations (e.g., culling).

The international community faces daunting problems in implementing these strategies. International food safety law does not emphasize animal/human interchange. The Codex Alimentarius Commission, administered by WHO and the Food and Agricultural Organization (FAO), regulates food hygiene and labeling. Codex's main concern is with the safety of the food supply and fair standards for international trade in food.[10] Occupational health and safety rules are primarily found at the national level, and country safeguards are highly variable. Countries may have a self-interest in continuing intensive farming and food distribution. These methods are cost-effective from an economic perspective, but do not necessarily result in safe practices to prevent animal-to-human transmission of disease.

Even if strong international health standards did exist, public health authorities would continue to face the problem of when to implement aggressive strategies such as culling. Premature interventions have profound economic implications affecting livelihoods and trade. However, weak or tardy interventions risk devastation to animal and human populations.

Global Surveillance

Surveillance of novel infections in humans offers early warning, providing an opportunity for a timely response (see Table 6-10). Experts recommend various surveillance activities, many of which were used in the 2003

---

[10]The Sanitary and Phytosanitary Measures Agreement is designed to promote free trade by ensuring that national measures to protect human, animal, or plant life are scientifically based and not pretexts to protect domestic markets from international competition. Taylor AL, Bettcher DW, Fluss SS, DeLand K, Yach D. International health instruments: An overview. 2002. In: Detels R, McEwen J, Beaglehole R, Tanaka H, eds. *Oxford Textbook of Public Health*. 4th ed. Oxford, England: Oxford University Press. Pp. 359–386.

TABLE 6-10 Public Health Interventions: Purposes and Values

Public Health Intervention	Purposes and Objectives	Strategies to Achieve Public Health Purpose	Ethical Issues and Recommendations
Animal/Human Interchange	Prevent "species jump" by reducing proximity of animals and humans	Separation of animals and humans; occupational health and safety; control of diseased animals	Safeguard economic interests in farming while protecting the public's health
Global Surveillance	Timely and systematic monitoring of health threats	Cover all threats of global importance; prompt country reporting; use "small-world networks"	Ensure privacy safeguards for individuals and protection of groups
Case Contact Investigations	Prevent spread of infection to contacts of infected or exposed persons	Offer counseling, vaccination, and/or treatment to infected or exposed persons	Conduct investigations with sensitivity and respect for individuals and their contacts
Vaccination and Medical Treatment	Prophylaxis, amelioration of symptoms, and/or reduced infectiousness	Offer or require vaccination or antiviral therapy to at-risk or infected persons	Balance bodily integrity with the common good; ensure fair allocation of scarce resources; make therapeutics available to developing countries

SARS outbreaks: testing and screening; health questionnaires, notices, and declarations; fever monitoring (self-monitoring, thermal scanning); and reporting and monitoring trends (Gostin et al., 2003).

Despite its importance, many countries do not conduct effective and timely surveillance. Prompt notification of an infectious disease threat can affect a country's tourism, trade, and prestige. Consequently, some governments do not respond promptly to WHO requests for information. Many countries, moreover, lack the infrastructure and resources to conduct surveillance. As a result, national surveillance activities are highly variable.

The current International Health Regulations (IHR) are weak, applying only to three diseases: cholera, plague, and yellow fever. However, WHO's draft revised IHR, if adopted, would significantly strengthen international rules for surveillance. They would apply to all health threats of interna-

TABLE 6-10 Continued

Public Health Intervention	Purposes and Objectives	Strategies to Achieve Public Health Purpose	Ethical Issues and Recommendations
Community Hygiene	Promote safer behaviors among the population	Health education on hand washing, disinfection, masks, ventilation, and avoidance of contacts	Balance health benefits with costs and cultural sensitivities; ensure equitable access
Travel and Border Controls	Prevent cross-border spread of infectious disease	Travel advisories; border restrictions; regulation of conveyances; stop-lists	Health is salient; avoid unnecessary restriction of trade; safeguard against discrimination
Decreased Social Mixing/ Increased Social Distance	Increase social distance to avoid rapid spread of infection in public settings	Close civic activities, meeting places, and transportation systems	Avoid heavy costs and diminished freedoms; deliver services to the vulnerable
Civil Confinement	Separate the infected or exposed from the healthy	Isolation; quarantine; *cordon sanitaire*	Provide due process; ensure safe and humane setting; consider compensation; gain public's trust

tional importance; mandate country notifications; gather reports from unofficial sources; and provide for real-time event management (WHO Secretariat, 2004). Global surveillance could further benefit from "small-world networks" consisting of health professionals, scientists, and nongovernmental organizations continuously monitoring disease threats (Gostin, 2004). It should be possible to supplement the surveillance provided by official sources with multiple public/private sources through the Internet and other modern communication vehicles.

Although surveillance is an essential public health strategy, even routine activities such as reporting affect privacy because government collects sensitive health information. Acute outbreaks can trigger more extreme measures such as continuous monitoring of certain populations (i.e., health care workers, immigrants, and travelers). An outbreak of a novel influenza strain will inevitably raise questions about the appropriate scope of government surveillance and its effects on privacy. Surveillance needs to take place, therefore, with privacy safeguards firmly in place.

Case Contact Investigations

Case contact investigation is a classical form of surveillance. It involves identifying infected or exposed persons and following their recent contacts. This provides an opportunity to interrupt the spread of infection (see Table 6-10). Persons exposed or infected can be offered antiviral therapy as a prophylaxis or treatment. Those who are infectious or potentially infectious can be separated from the healthy population.

Case contact investigation is ostensibly voluntary because the "index case" is under no formal obligation to reveal his or her contacts. Nevertheless, its use in sexually transmitted infections and HIV/AIDS has proved highly controversial (Bayer and Toomey, 1992). The index case may feel coerced into giving information, investigations inherently pose privacy risks, and individuals may experience stigma and discrimination. These investigations, therefore, need to be conducted with sensitivity and respect for individuals and their family, friends, or associates.

Vaccination and Medical Treatment

The dominant strategy for seasonal influenza is to use vaccinations and antiviral therapy (see Table 6-10). Recommended vaccination of high-risk populations (e.g., children and the elderly) has become standard in developed countries, and mass vaccination could be recommended in the event of a more severe outbreak. Antiviral therapy, although not as effective as vaccination, can be used for prophylaxis, alleviation of symptoms, and reduction of infectiousness (Longini et al., 2004).

Therapeutic interventions raise distinct ethical and legal concerns. Although mandating competent adults to be vaccinated or treated for their own protection is a difficult notion to espouse, the law permits a reasonable interference with bodily integrity to prevent harm to the community (Jacobson v. Massachusetts, 197 U.S. 11 [1905]).

Although officials have the legal authority to compel vaccination or treatment to protect the public, the political and ethical dimensions of doing so are complex. There is a long history of opposition to vaccinations among certain sections of the population (Spier, 2001). Anti-vaccination sentiments are not always irrational because immunizations can pose risks, as well as confer benefits. Mass vaccination to avert an influenza epidemic can go horribly wrong, as occurred with swine flu in 1976: The CDC campaign to immunize the American population cost $134 million and caused Guillain-Barré syndrome in some vaccine recipients (Neustadt and Fineberg, 1983).

When used appropriately, vaccination or treatment can confer considerable benefit to the individual and ultimately to a population. Pandemic influenza would likely result in a paucity of vaccines and antiviral medications, raising the hard problem of fair allocation of scarce resources. What ethical values should guide rationing decisions: private need (treatment of the sick); public need (prevention among vulnerable populations); maintenance of essential services (health care workers and "first responders"); or political influence (priority for those with political connections)? Justice may require that therapeutic interventions be used to benefit the most people possible, irrespective of their power or influence. This would militate toward the use of "public need" as the principal ethical value. Therapeutics, therefore, would be used primarily for prevention and targeted to those who pose the greatest risk of transmission. The ethical value of "public need" might also require use of therapeutics for emergency workers to ensure maintenance of essential services and ongoing assistance to the public. This would place private need and political influence lower on the priority scale.

The global reality is that rich countries will have much less scarcity than poor countries. The ethical question then arises as to whether developed countries would be expected to forego some of their precious stockpile of vaccines and antiviral medications for the sake of poorer countries experiencing a higher burden of morbidity and mortality from influenza. One might argue that it is in the richer country's self-interest to do so because infectious disease can and does travel across the globe. Ethical analysis would prove difficult—do developed countries have an obligation to reduce the burden of disease in developing countries? If all human life has the same worth, then it may be ethically desirable to devote therapeutic resources to poor regions experiencing higher burdens of disease. This allocation of resources is likely to have the maximum beneficial effect on morbidity and premature mortality.

Community Hygiene

One of the most valuable means of infection control is also the least intrusive. Health education to promote safer behaviors such as hand washing, disinfection, masks, ventilation, and avoidance of contacts can be highly effective (see Table 6-10). Community hygiene, although largely uncontroversial, can impose costs (e.g., purchasing and distributing equipment) and cause social unrest (e.g., exaggerated concerns about health risks). Hygiene measures are also culturally sensitive—notice the difference in mask-wearing habits in Asia as compared to North America and Europe.

Under what circumstances should public health authorities issue a national recommendation for aggressive hygiene measures given the costs and cultural expectations? Probably the most important concern would be the cost effectiveness of the hygiene measure. If a hygiene measure is clearly cost effective, then the public has the right to know how to adopt that measure in a safe way. Vulnerable members of the community may also need economic and technical assistance to ensure equitable access to essential hygiene measures. If a measure is not cost effective, then public health authorities have an obligation to inform the public about the lack of effectiveness and the risks. In some cases, such as the use of masks, the evidence for, or against, effectiveness may be unclear. In such instances, the principle of transparency may suggest that public health officials should state honestly the lack of conclusive evidence, leaving the judgment to the individual.

Travel and Border Controls

One of the first instincts in the face of infectious disease threats is to protect national borders (see Table 6-10). Consequently, international or national health agencies may issue travel advisories, establish border restrictions, or regulate conveyances such as airplanes, ships, and trains. They might similarly use "stop-lists" to prevent specified individuals or groups from traveling. The IHR afford WHO considerable authority to regulate international travel and control borders.

Travelers legitimately claim the right to know health risks, but restrictions significantly affect tourism and trade. Consequently, travel advisories can be politically charged, as were WHO advisories concerning SARS in Ontario, Canada (Krauss, 2003). A delicate balance exists between trade and health. Indeed, the draft revised IHR directs WHO to "provide security against the international spread of disease while avoiding unnecessary interference with international traffic" (WHO, 2004b).

When faced with a hard tradeoff between maximization of health or of trade, which should prevail and why? Arguably, health should take precedence over trade because of the fundamental value of human functioning and life itself. Despite the effects on tourism and trade, the public has a legitimate interest in knowing if there are health hazards in regions where they intend to travel. National and international public health agencies have an obligation to take steps that are necessary to prevent the spread of infection across borders. Thus, it would be legitimate to prevent travel of a person who poses a significant risk of transmission. What public health authorities may not do is use infectious disease control as a pretext for discrimination by targeting individuals based on their nationality, race, religion, or other status.

Decreased Social Mixing/Increased Social Distance

Most Americans take for granted the freedom to associate with others in a variety of social settings. Yet public health authorities could restrict social mixing and increase social distance to avert a serious infectious disease threat (see Table 6-10). This might involve closures of civic activities (e.g., schools, workplaces), meeting places or large gatherings (e.g., sports events, theatres, business meetings), and transportation systems (e.g., mass transit, airlines). The purpose behind restrictions on mixing is to prevent rapid spread of infection in settings where multiple people congregate.

The U.S. Constitution affords individuals the freedom to associate, but courts would likely defer to reasonable regulation of congregate settings to prevent transmission of infection (New York v. New St. Mark's Baths, 497 N.Y.S.2d 979 [1986]). As with other interventions, closures entail heavy costs in lost revenue as well as in diminished freedoms. When an infectious disease outbreak deeply affects a society's everyday activities, public health authorities will have to cogently explain the justifications for the chosen intervention and gain the public's confidence prior to implementation. Critical legal and logistical questions loom: Which authority has the power to close a venue; what criteria should be used to trigger a closure and when should the restriction be lifted; and how will services be delivered to vulnerable populations who may be at risk in an isolated residence or shelter?

Civil Confinement

The potential for a mass outbreak raises the specter of civil confinement to separate the infected or exposed from healthy individuals (see Table 6-10). This might entail isolation of infected persons, quarantine of exposed persons, or quarantine of a geographic area (*cordon sanitaire*). Civil confinements may take place in hospitals or other institutions or in a person's home. New conceptions to separate the healthy from the infectious include "sheltering in place," which public health authorities analogize to a "snow day."

Many states modernized their public health statutes in the aftermath of the terrorist attacks on September 11, 2001 (Gostin et al., 2002). Public health law reform is necessary to ensure that states and localities have the legal authority for isolation and quarantine (Gostin, 2002). In order to meet constitutional standards, state law must have clear criteria for the use of civil confinement and offer procedural due process (Greene v. Edwards, 263 S.E.2d 661 [W.Va. 1980]).

Civil confinement, of course, raises powerful civil liberties concerns. Not only is isolation or quarantine a deprivation of liberty, but enforcement can sometimes be intrusive. For example, during the SARS outbreaks, some countries used electronic bracelets, web cameras, and police. It will also be important to ensure that judicial hearings are available, particularly in a mass outbreak. Isolation or quarantine will have to take place in a humane and habitable environment. Vulnerable persons will need to be protected against reexposure to infection, offered care and treatment, and ensured the necessities of life such as safe food and water (Barbera et al., 2001). There may also be the need to consider compensation for lost work. Individuals are confined for the good of the community and have to forego their livelihood and other essential activities. Above all, public health authorities need to maintain the public's trust. To what extent would orders for civil confinement dissipate trust and reduce cooperation?

Acting Under Conditions of Uncertainty: The Key Scientific and Social Questions

Influenza pandemic preparedness requires careful consideration of the public health strategy as well as the legal and ethical implications. Several key scientific questions loom: Are specific interventions proven cost effective? What combination of measures is most cost effective? During what phase of the pandemic should interventions be implemented? When should public health measures be discontinued?

Although the foregoing interventions have been widely used, many still lack adequate evidence of cost effectiveness. Even if individual interventions are known to be cost effective, public health authorities will have to form a judgment as to the combination of measures that will be maximally effective. They will need to decide when to initiate and when to end an intervention.

The decision to intervene is a difficult one because public health authorities may be acting under conditions of scientific uncertainty. It may be unclear whether serologic tests are reliable, vaccines or treatments are safe and effective, and coercive interventions are acceptable to the population. To be effective, agencies may have to intervene at the earliest stages, before the threat level is clear. If interventions are well targeted and timed, then public health officials may prevent untold economic and human harm. However, if the interventions overreach, officials will be accused of disregarding essential economic interests and fundamental human rights.

These scientific questions are important because public health interventions do not take place in a vacuum. They raise fundamental economic, political, and legal questions that need to be considered.

Economics

As mentioned earlier, public health interventions can have dire effects on the economy. They impede individual economic freedoms to travel and pursue a business or livelihood. They also affect local, national, and regional economies through the impacts on trade, travel, tourism, and agriculture. Countries may have built-in disincentives to conduct surveillance and response in an energetic and public way.

Political

Infectious disease outbreaks can have intense sociopolitical ramifications. Diseases affect a country's prestige as well as its economy, and the electorate may hold politicians accountable. As a result, political leaders may try to deemphasize the threat or delay taking definitive action, which has occurred in numerous epidemics ranging from HIV/AIDS to SARS.

Legal and Constitutional

Infectious disease outbreaks take place in countries with vastly different legal and constitutional traditions. Public health planning may be undertaken within liberal democracies guaranteeing full protection of human rights or they may take place in less democratic, perhaps more authoritarian, societies. During the SARS outbreaks, for example, countries behaved very differently in their response to and protection of civil liberties (Sapsin et al., 2003). Infectious diseases tend to bring out the best and worst in societies. History demonstrates the potential for overreaction, stigma, and discrimination in the face of a severe epidemic (Gilman, 1999). Consequently, the legal and constitutional dimensions will be important in confronting a severe epidemic (Gostin, 2000).

Ethical Values Underpinning Public Health Preparedness: The Cross-Cutting Issues

Public health authorities have a mandate to protect the population's health. It is crucial, however, that they act ethically. Ethical values are usually too broad to determine precisely whether a particular activity is morally appropriate. Nevertheless, it should be possible to articulate several ethical values that can inform public health practice, particularly in an emergency.

Transparency

The ethical value of transparency requires officials to make decisions in an open and fully accountable manner. Government officials must be willing to make clear the basis for public health measures. They should honestly and openly inform the public about what is known and not known;

openly acknowledge when new evidence warrants reconsideration of policies; and educate the public about the goals of intervention and the steps taken to safeguard individual rights.

Protection of Vulnerable Populations

Diseases that may differentially affect segments of the population have usually imposed the additional burden of social opprobrium. Public health officials may inadvertently amplify the process as they conduct their surveillance activities. Although they may not be able to prevent stigmatization completely, officials have an obligation to take steps to mitigate the suffering that may attend their efforts by underscoring the irrationality and inequity of ethnic stereotyping. Consultation with representatives of the communities most at risk will be important for both instrumental reasons and as an expression of social solidarity. Individuals should feel a sense of participation in crucial decisions affecting their lives and communities. People place their trust in political leaders and, in return, deserve due consideration of and respect for their health and human rights.

Fair Treatment and Social Justice

Justice requires that the benefits and burdens of public health action be fairly distributed, thus precluding the unjustified encumbering of already socially vulnerable populations. Equitable public health action is based on science and assures reasoned, population-based policies. Procedural justice requires a fair and independent hearing for individuals who are subjected to burdensome public health action. Due process requirements are inherently important because fair hearings affirm the dignity of the person; due process is also instrumentally important because it ensures accurate decision making.

The Least Restrictive Alternative

International human rights law is guided by the principle of proportionality: interventions should be necessary and proportional to the risk posed (Siracusa principles, 1985). Interventions should be the least restrictive alternative necessary to prevent or ameliorate the health threat. Requiring the least restrictive/intrusive alternative represents a means to impose limits on state interventions consistent with the traditions of privacy, freedom of association, and individual liberty. The standard does not require officials to utilize less-than-optimal interventions, but rather to select the least intrusive alternative that can best achieve the identified health objective.

The Public Health Paradox

There is no way to avoid the dilemmas posed by acting without full scientific knowledge. Failure to move aggressively in the early stages of pandemic influenza can have catastrophic consequences. Actions that prove to have been unnecessary will be viewed as draconian and based on hysteria. The only safeguard is the adoption of ethical values in formulating and implementing public health decisions. Public health policy will reflect in a profound way the manner in which humane societies both implicitly and explicitly balance the common good with respect for personal rights.

REFERENCES

Barbera J, Macintyre A, Gostin L, Inglesby T, O'Toole T, DeAtley C, Tonat K, Layton M. 2001. Large-scale quarantine following biological terrorism in the United States: Scientific examination, logistic and legal limits, and possible consequences. *JAMA* 286(21):2711–2717.

Barker WH. 1986. Excess pneumonia and influenza associated hospitalization during influenza epidemics in the United States, 1970–78. *Am J Public Health* 76:761–765.

Barker WH, Mullooly JP. 1980. Impact of epidemic type A influenza in a defined adult population. *Am J Epidemiol* 112:798–813.

Barker WH, Mullooly JP. 1982. Pneumonia and influenza deaths during epidemics: Implications for prevention. *Arch Intern Med* 142:85–89.

Barry JM. 2004. *The Great Influenza: The Epic Story of the Deadliest Plague in History.* 1st ed. New York: Viking.

Bayer R, Toomey KE. 1992. HIV prevention and the two faces of partner notification. *Am J Public Health* 82:1158–1164.

Blendon RJ, Benson JM, DesRoches, CM, Herrmann MJ. 2001. *Harvard School of Public Health/Robert Wood Johnson Foundation Survey Project on Americans' Response to Biological Terrorism, Study 2: National and Three Metropolitan Areas Affected by Anthrax, November 29–December 3, 2001.* [Online]. Available: http://www.hsph.harvard.edu/press/releases/blendon/report2.pdf [accessed January 7, 2002].

Brunell PA, ed. 2004. Importance of vaccinating healthcare workers against influenza. CME monograph from *Infectious Diseases in Children.* Selected article: Piedra PA. Time has come to make vaccination mandatory. [Online]. Available: http://idinchildren.com/monograph/0402/article6.asp [accessed February 10, 2005].

Campbell DS, Rumley MA. 1997. Cost-effectiveness of the influenza vaccine in a healthy, working-age population. *J Occup Environ Med* 39:408–414.

Carrat F, Valleron A-J. 1995. Influenza mortality among the elderly in France, 1980–90: How many deaths may have been avoided through vaccination? *J Epidemiol Community Health* 49:419–425.

CDC (Centers for Disease Control and Prevention). 1998. Prevention and control of influenza: Recommendations of the Advisory Committee on Immunization Practices (ACIP). *MMWR* 47(RR-6):1–26.

CDC. 2002. *Crisis and Emergency Risk Communication.* Atlanta, GA: CDC.

CDC. 2004a. *Questions and Answers: The Disease.* [Online]. Available: http://www.cdc.gov/flu/about/qa/disease.htm.

CDC. 2004b. Outbreaks of avian influenza A (H5N1) in Asia and interim recommendations for evaluation and reporting of suspected cases—United States, 2004. *MMWR* 53(5):97–100.

Cliff AD, Haggett P. 1993. Statistical modelling of measles and influenza outbreaks. *Stat Methods Med Res* 2:43–73.
Critchfield GC, Willard KE. 1986. Probabilistic analysis of decision trees using Monte Carlo simulation. *Med Decis Making* 6:85–92.
Dao J. 2004 (February 16). Bird flu outbreak has farmers jittery. *New York Times.* Sect. A P. 12.
Davis MM, McMahon SR, Santoli JM, Schwartz B, Clark SJ. 2002. A national survey of physician practices regarding influenza vaccine. *J Gen Intern Med* 17(9):670–676.
Dittus RS, Roberts SD, Wilson JR. 1989. Quantifying uncertainty in medical decisions. *J Am Coll Cardiol* 14:23A–28A.
Dobilet P, Begg CB, Weinstein MC, Braun P, McNeil BJ. 1985. Probabilistic sensitivity analysis using Monte Carlo simulation: A practical approach. *Med Decis Making* 5:157–177.
Emanuel EJ. 2003 (May 12). Preventing the next SARS. *New York Times.* Sect. A. P. 25.
Ethiel N, ed. 2002. *Terrorism: Informing the Public.* Chicago, IL: McCormick Tribune Foundation.
Evans M, Hastings N, Peacock B. 1993. *Statistical Distributions.* 2nd ed. New York: John Wiley.
Fischhoff B. 2002. Assessing and communicating the risks of terrorism. In: Teich AH, Nelson SD, Lita SJ, eds. *Science and Technology in a Vulnerable World.* Washington, DC: American Association for the Advancement of Science. Pp. 51–64.
Fox JP, Hall CE, Cooney MK, Foy HM. 1982. Influenza virus infections in Seattle families, 1975–1979. Study design, methods and the occurrence of infections by time and age. *Am J Epidemiol* 116:212–227.
Gellin B. 2004 (June 16). *U.S. Pandemic Influenza Preparedness and Response.* Prepared for Institute of Medicine Workshop on Pandemic Influenza: Assessing Capabilities for Prevention and Response, Washington, DC: Institute of Medicine Forum on Microbial Threats.
Gilman SL. 1999. Disease and stigma. *Lancet* 354(Suppl):SIV15.
Glass TA, Schoch-Spana M. 2002. Bioterrorism and the people: How to vaccinate a city against panic. *Clin Infect Dis* 34(2):217–223.
Glezen WP. 1996. Emerging infections: Pandemic influenza. *Epidemiol Rev* 18:64–76.
Glezen WP, Payne AA, Snyder DN, Downs TD. 1982. Mortality and influenza. *J Infect Dis* 146:313–321.
Glezen WP, Decker M, Joseph SW, Mercready RG. 1987. Acute respiratory disease associated with influenza epidemics in Houston, 1981–1983. *J Infect Dis* 155:1119–1126.
Gostin LO. 2000. *Public Health Law: Power, Duty, Restraint.* Berkeley, CA, and New York, NY: University of California Press and Milbank Memorial Fund.
Gostin LO. 2002. Public health law in an age of terrorism: Rethinking individual rights and common goods. *Health Affairs* 21(6):79–93.
Gostin LO. 2004. International infectious disease law: Revision of the World Health Organization's International Health Regulations. *JAMA* 291(21):2623–2627.
Gostin LO, Sapsin JW, Teret SP, Burris S, Mair JS, Hodge JG Jr, Vernick JS. 2002. The Model State Emergency Health Powers Act: Planning and response to bioterrorism and naturally occurring infectious diseases. *JAMA* 288:622–628.
Gostin LO, Bayer R, Fairchild AL. 2003. Ethical and legal challenges posed by Severe Acute Respiratory Syndrome: Implications for the control of severe infectious disease threats. *JAMA* 290(24):3229–3237.
Gursky E, Inglesby TV, O'Toole T. 2003. Anthrax 2001: Observations on the medical and public health response. *Biosecurity and Bioterrorism* 1(2):97–110.
Haddix AC, Teutsch SM, Shaffer PA, Dunet DO. 1996. *Prevention Effectiveness.* New York: Oxford University Press.

Harper SA, Fukuda K, Uyeki TM, Cox NJ, Bridges CB; CDC Advisory Committee on Immunization Practices (ACIP). 2004 (May 28). Prevention and control of influenza: Recommendations of the Advisory Committee on Immunization Practices. MMWR Recommendations and Reports 53(RR-6):1–40.

IOM (Institute of Medicine). 2004. Learning from SARS: Preparing for the Next Disease Outbreak. 1st ed. Washington, DC: The National Academies Press.

Jefferson T, Demicheli V. 1998. Socioeconomics of influenza. In: Nicholson KG, Webster RG, Hay AJ, eds. Textbook of Influenza. London, England: Blackwell Science. Pp. 541–547.

Kaufmann AF, Meltzer MI, Schmid GP. 1997. The economic impact of a bioterrorist attack: Are prevention and postattack intervention programs justifiable? Emerg Infect Dis 3:83–94.

Kavet J. 1977. A perspective on the significance of pandemic influenza. Am J Public Health 67:1063–1070.

Kolata G. 1997 (March 21). Genetic material of virus from 1918 flu is found. New York Times. Sect. A. P. 2.

Krauss C. 2003 (April 26). The SARS epidemic: Toronto; Canada increases pressure on World Health Organization to lift travel advisory. New York Times. Sect. A. P. 8.

Longini IM Jr, Halloran ME, Nizam A, Yang Y. 2004. Containing pandemic influenza with antiviral agents. Am J Epidemiol 159(7):623–633.

McBean AM, Babish JD, Warren JL. 1993. The impact and cost of influenza in the elderly. Arch Intern Med 153:2105–2111.

Mullooly JP, Barker WH. 1982. Impact of type A influenza on children: A retrospective study. Am J Public Health 72:1008–1016.

Neustadt RE, Fineberg HV. 1978. The swine flu affair: Decision making on a slippery disease. Washington, DC: U.S. Department of Health, Education, and Welfare.

Neustadt R, Fineberg HV. 1983. The Epidemic That Never Was: Policy Making in the Swine Flu Scare. 1st ed. New York: Vintage Books.

Office of Technology Assessment, U.S. Congress. 1981. Cost Effectiveness of Influenza Vaccination. Washington, DC: Government Printing Office.

Patriarca PA, Cox NJ. 1997. Influenza pandemic preparedness plan for the United States. J Infect Dis 176(Suppl 1):S4–S7.

Patriarca PA, Arden NH, Koplan JP, Goodman RA. 1987. Prevention and control of type A influenza infections in nursing homes: Benefits and costs of four approaches using vaccination and amantadine. Ann Intern Med 107:732–740.

Riddiough MA, Sisk JE, Bell JC. 1983. Influenza vaccination: Cost-effectiveness and public policy. JAMA 249:3189–3195.

Roberts S. 2003. Communicating with the public about public health preparedness. In: DIMACS Working Group on Modeling Social Responses to Bioterrorism Involving Infectious Agents. New Brunswick, NJ: Rutgers University.

Robinson LJ, Barry PJ. 1987. The Competitive Firm's Response to Risk. New York: Macmillan.

Rosenberg CE. 1989. What is an epidemic?: AIDS in historical perspective. Daedalus 118(2):1–17.

Sandman PM. 1993. Responding to Community Outrage: Strategies for Effective Risk Communication. Fairfax, VA: American Industrial Hygiene Association.

Sandman PM, Lanard J. 2004 (October 22). Flu Vaccine Shortages: Segmenting the Audience. [Online]. Available: http://psandman.com/col/flu-1.htm.

Sapsin JW, Thompson TM, Stone L, DeLand KE. 2003. International trade, law, and public health advocacy. J Law Med Ethics 31(4):546–556.

Schoch-Spana M. 2003. Educating, informing, and mobilizing the public. In: Levy BS, Sidel VW, eds. *Terrorism and Public Health*. New York: Oxford University Press. Pp. 118–135.

Schoenbaum SC. 1987. Economic impact of influenza: The individual's perspective. *Am J Med* 82(Suppl 6A):26–30.

Schoenbaum SC, McNeil BJ, Kavet J. 1976. The swine-influenza decision. *N Eng J Med* 295:759–765.

Serfling RE, Sherman IL, Houseworth WJ. 1967. Excess pneumonia-influenza mortality by age and sex in three major influenza A2 epidemics, United States, 1957–58, 1960 and 1963. *Am J Epidemiol* 86:433–441.

Simonsen L, Clarke MJ, Williamson GD, Stroup DF, Arden NH, Schonberger LB. 1997. The impact of influenza epidemics on mortality: Introducing a severity index. *Am J Public Health* 87:1944–1950.

Simonsen L, Clarke MJ, Schonberger LB, Arden NH, Cox NJ, Fukuda K. 1998. Pandemic versus epidemic influenza mortality: A pattern of changing age distribution. *J Infect Dis* 178:53–60.

Siracusa principles on the limitation and derogation provisions in the International Covenant on Civil and Political Rights. 1985. *Hum Rights Q* 7(1):3.

Sorenson J. 2004. Commentary: Risk communication and terrorism. *Biosecurity and Bioterrorism* 2(3):229–231.

Spier RE. 2001. Perception of risk of vaccine adverse events: A historical perspective. *Vaccine* 20(Suppl 1):S78–S84.

Stevens J, Corper AL, Basler CF, Taubenberger JK, Palese P, Wilson IA. 2004. Structure of the uncleaved human H1 hemagglutinin from the extinct 1918 influenza virus. *Science* 303(5665):1866–1870.

Stöhr K. 2004 (June 16). *WHO: Priority Public Health Interventions Before and During Influenza Pandemics*. Prepared for Institute of Medicine Workshop on Pandemic Influenza: Assessing Capabilities for Prevention and Response, Washington, DC: Institute of Medicine Forum on Microbial Threats.

The Federal Register. 1996. 61(170):46301–46302.

Thomas P. 2003. *The Anthrax Attacks*. Washington, DC: The Century Foundation. [Online]. Available: http://www.homelandsec.org/WGneed/CaseStudies/full.pdf [accessed August 6, 2003].

U.S. Bureau of the Census. 1997. *Statistical Abstract of the United States: 1997*. 117th ed. Washington, DC: U.S. Bureau of the Census.

U.S. Department of Health and Human Services. 2002. *Communicating in a Crisis: Risk Communication Guidelines for Public Officials*. Washington, DC: U.S. Department of Health and Human Services.

Webby RJ, Webster RG. 2003. Are we ready for pandemic influenza? *Science* 302(5650):1519–1522.

Weinstein RA. 2004. Planning for epidemics: The lessons of SARS. *N Engl J Med* 350(23):2332–2334.

WHO (World Health Organization). 2004a. *WHO Consultation on Priority Public Health Interventions Before and During an Influenza Pandemic*. Geneva, Switzerland: WHO.

WHO. 2004b. *Intergovernmental Working Group on the Revision of the International Health Regulations*. Working paper for regional consultations. IGWG/IHR/working paper 12.2003. Geneva, Switzerland: WHO.

WHO Secretariat. 2004. *Revision of the International Health Regulations*. Publication EB113/3 Rev.1. Geneva, Switzerland: WHO.

Working Group on Governance Dilemmas in Bioterrorism Response. 2004. Leading during bioattacks and epidemics with the public's trust and help. *Biosecurity and Bioterrorism: Biodefense Strategy, Practice, and Science* 2(1):25–40.

Appendix
A

Pandemic Influenza: Assessing Capabilities for Prevention and Response

June 16–June 17, 2004
The National Academies
Lecture Room
2101 Constitution Avenue, NW (C Street Entrance)
Washington, D.C.

AGENDA

Wednesday, June 16, 2004

8:00   Continental Breakfast

8:30   **Welcome and Opening Remarks**
                 Adel Mahmoud, MD, PhD
                 Chair, Forum on Microbial Threats
                 President, Merck Vaccines

8:35   **Keynote Address: John M. Barry,** Distinguished Visiting Scholar, The Center for Bioenvironmental Research at Tulane and Xavier Universities, and author of *The Great Influenza: The Epic Story of the Deadliest Plague in History*

PLANNING AND PREPAREDNESS FOR PANDEMIC INFLUENZA

Session I: Global and National Preparedness Strategies

Moderator: Adel Mahmoud, MD, PhD, *Chair, Forum on Microbial Threats/President, Merck Vaccines*

9:05–9:35   WHO: Priority Public Health Interventions Before and During an Influenza Pandemic
Klaus Stöhr, DVM, Project Leader, Global Influenza Programme, Department of Communicable Disease Surveillance and Response, World Health Organization, Geneva

9:35–10:05   **U.S. Government Pandemic Influenza Preparedness Plan**
Bruce Gellin, MD, Director, National Vaccine Program Office, U.S. Department of Health and Human Services

10:05   *Q&A/Open Discussion*

10:30   Break

Session II: Response and Discussion of Preparedness Planning

Moderator: Stanley Lemon, MD, *Vice Chair, Forum on Microbial Threats and Dean of Medicine, The University of Texas Medical Branch at Galveston*

10:45   *Discussion Panel:* **David Fedson, MD,** Sergy Haut, France
Nancy J. Cox, PhD, Chief, Influenza Branch, CDC and Director, WHO Collaborating Centre for Surveillance, Epidemiology and Control of Influenza
Dennis Perrotta, PhD, State Epidemiologist, Texas
Peter A. Shult, PhD, Director, Communicable Disease Division and Emergency Laboratory Response, Wisconsin State Laboratory of Hygiene

11:15   *Open Discussion*

12:00   Lunch

Session III: Obstacles and Opportunities for Optimal Preparedness

Moderator: Gary Roselle, MD, *Program Director for Infectious Diseases, Department of Veterans Affairs Central Office*

1:00–1:20   Partnering with the Private Medical System
             Gordon Grundy, MD, Regional Medical Director, Aetna Inc.
1:20–1:35   *Discussion*

1:35–1:55   Vaccine Development and Production Issues
             Philip Hosbach, Vice President of New Products and
             Immunization Policy, Aventis Pasteur SA
1:55–2:10   *Discussion*

2:10–2:30   Ensuring an Adequate Stockpile of Antivirals
             Paul Brown, PhD, Global Task Force Leader for Tamiflu™
             Pandemic Planning, F. Hoffmann La-Roche, Switzerland
2:30–2:45   *Discussion*

2:45–3:05   Chasing the Elusive Virus: Preparing for the Future by
             Examining the Past
             Jeffery K. Taubenberger, MD, PhD, Chair, Department of
             Molecular Pathology, Armed Forces Institute of Pathology,
             U.S. Department of Defense
3:05–3:20   *Discussion*

3:20   Break

Session IV: Panel Discussion—Innovating Past Barriers

Moderator: Joshua Lederberg, PhD, *Nobel Laureate, Sackler Foundation Scholar, Rockefeller University*

3:30–3:45   Strategies for Control of Influenza by Targeting Broadly
             Conserved Viral Features
             Suzanne Epstein, PhD, Center for Biologics Evaluation and
             Research, Food and Drug Administration

3:45–4:10   Mathematical Modeling: Containing Pandemic Influenza
             with Vaccines and Antivirals
             Ira Longini, MD, Rollins School of Public Health, Emory
             University, Atlanta, GA
             March Lipsitch, PhD, Harvard School of Public Health,
             Boston, MA

4:10–4:25   "Insuring" for a Better Response
             Martin Meltzer, PhD, National Center for Infectious
             Diseases, U.S. Centers for Disease Control and Prevention

4:25–4:40   Coordination Between the Public and Private Sectors
             Jonathan B. Perlin, MD, PhD, MSHA, FACP, Acting Under
             Secretary for Health, Department of Veterans Affairs

4:40–5:30   *Q&A/Open Discussion*

5:30   Adjournment of the First Day

Thursday, June 17, 2004

BATTLING NATURE'S TERRORIST:
SCIENTIFIC AND PUBLIC HEALTH TOOLS

8:00   Continental Breakfast

8:30   Opening Remarks/Summary of Day 1
             Stanley Lemon, MD
             Vice Chair, Forum on Emerging Infections

Session V: Methods for the Prevention and Containment of Pandemic Influenza

Moderator: Carole Heilman, PhD, *Director, Division of Microbiology and Infectious Diseases, NIAID, NIH*

8:45–9:15   A Report from the Field: The 2003–2004 H5N1 Outbreak
             Robert Webster, PhD, Rose Marie Thomas Professor and
             Chair, Department of Infectious Diseases, St. Jude's
             Children's Research Hospital, Memphis, TN

9:15–10:15   *Discussion Panel:* Amin Soebandrio, MD, PhD, Assistant
             Deputy Minister for Research and Technology for Health
             and Medical Sciences, Indonesia
             Nguyen Tien Dzung, DVM, PhD, Head of Virology,
             National Institute for Veterinary Research, Ministry of
             Agriculture and Rural Health Development, Vietnam

Chantanee Buranathai, DVM, PhD, Chief, Emerging and
Exotic Animal Disease Section, Division of Veterinary
Epidemiology, Department of Livestock Development,
Thailand

10:15–10:40 Strategies for Preventing and Controlling Avian Influenza
and its Transmission within the Bird and Animal
Population
Dewan Sibartie, DVM, PhD, Scientific and Technical
Department, Office International des Épizooties (OIE)

10:40–11:45 Discussion Panel: Guus Koch, DVM, Central Institute for
Animal Disease Control, Wageningen University and
Research Centre, Lelystad, The Netherlands
David Swayne, DVM, PhD, Laboratory Director and
Research Leader, Southeast Poultry Research Laboratory,
U.S. Department of Agriculture
Carol Cardona, DVM, PhD, Poultry Extension
Veterinarian and Assistant Professor, Veterinary Extension,
University of California-Davis
Laurence S. Tiley, PhD, Lecturer in Molecular Virology,
Centre for Veterinary Science, University of Cambridge,
United Kingdom

11:45 Break

12:00–12:25 Enhancing Influenza Surveillance: From the Global to the
Local Perspective
Nancy J. Cox, PhD, Chief, Influenza Branch, Centers for
Disease Control and Prevention and Director, WHO
Collaborating Centre for Surveillance, Epidemiology and
Control of Influenza
12:25–1:00 Discussion

1:00 Lunch

Session VI: Panel Discussion—Priorities for Improving Preparedness

Moderator: Frederick Sparling, MD, Professor of Medicine,
Microbiology, and Immunology, University of North Carolina

2:00–2:20   Pandemic Influenza and Mortality: Past Evidence and
             Projections for the Future
             Lone Simonsen, PhD, Office of Global Affairs, National
             Institute of Allergy and Infectious Diseases, National
             Institutes of Health
2:20–2:40   Increasing Awareness and Uptake of Influenza
             Immunization
             Glen Nowak, PhD, Office of Health Communications,
             National Immunization Program, CDC
2:40–3:00   Public Communication Strategies to Remedy Panic in a
             Pandemic
             Monica Schoch-Spana, PhD, Center for Biosecurity,
             University of Pittsburgh Medical Center
3:00–3:20   Preparing the Legal System for Pandemic Influenza
             Larry Gostin, JD, Center on Law and the Public's Health,
             Georgetown University

3:20   *Open Discussion*

5:00   Closing Remarks/Adjourn

DISCUSSANTS-AT-LARGE

David Bell, MD, Senior Medical Officer, Office of the Director, National
Center for Infectious Diseases, Centers for Disease Control and
Prevention

Timothy Booth, MD, Director, Viral Diseases Division, National Microbiology Laboratory, Health Canada, Canadian Science Centre for
Human and Animal Health, Winnipeg, Ontario

Kathy Coelingh, PhD, Senior Director of Scientific and Regulatory
Affairs, MedImmune Vaccines, Mountain View, CA

Jack Croddy, Senior Advisor, Office of Diplomacy, U.S. Department of
State

William M. Egan, PhD, Acting Director, Office of Vaccines, Center for
Biologics Evaluation and Research, U.S. Food and Drug Administration

Geoffrey Evans, MD, Medical Officer, Vaccine Injury Compensation
Program, Health Resources and Services Administration, U.S. Department of Health and Human Services

Harold Foster, Deputy Director, Office of International Health Affairs,
U.S. Department of State

Adolfo Garcia–Sastre, PhD, Associate Professor, Department of Microbiology, Mount Sinai School of Medicine, New York

Kathleen F. Gensheimer, MD, MPH, State Epidemiologist and Director, Medical Epidemiology Section, Maine Bureau of Health, Department of Human Services

Robert A. Heckert, DVM, PhD, National Program Leader, Animal Health, Agricultural Research Service, U.S. Department of Agriculture

Charles Hoke, MD, Walter Reed Army Institute of Research, U.S. Army Medical Research and Materiel Command

Yanzhong Huang, PhD, Assistant Professor and Director, Center for Global Health Studies, John C. Whitehead School of Diplomacy and International Relations, Seton Hall University

Dominick Iacuzio, F. Hoffman La-Roche

George Kemble, PhD, Senior Director of Research, MedImmune Vaccines, Mountain View, CA

Richard F. Kingham, JD, Partner, Covington and Burling, Washington, DC, and London

David J. Lipman, MD, Director, National Center for Biotechnology Information, National Library of Medicine, National Institutes of Health

Nina Marano, DVM, MPH, Dipl. ACVPM, Associate Director for Veterinary Medicine and Public Health National Center for Infectious Diseases, Centers for Disease Control and Prevention

James T. Matthews, PhD, Director, External Research and Development, Aventis Pasteur Group, Swiftwater, PA

Michael McGuire, F. Hoffman La-Roche

Mark Miller, MD, Division of International Epidemiology and Population Studies, Fogarty International Center, National Institutes of Health

Arnold Monto, MD, Professor of Epidemiology, Director of the University of Michigan Bioterrorism Preparedness Initiative, School of Public Health, University of Michigan, Ann Arbor

Stuart Nightingale, MD, Senior Advisor, Office of the Assistant Secretary for Public Health Emergency Preparedness, U.S. Department of Health and Human Services

Tara O'Toole, MD, MPH, Center for Biosecurity, University of Pittsburgh Medical Center

Michael Perdue, PhD, Research Leader, Environmental Microbial Safety Laboratory, Animal & Natural Resources Institute, Agricultural Research Service, U.S. Department of Agriculture

Sara Radcliffe, MPH, Director, Science Policy and Bioethics, Biotechnology Industry Organization

Stewart Simonson, Assistant Secretary for Public Health Emergency Preparedness, Office of Public Health Emergency Preparedness, U.S. Department of Health and Human Services

Eve Slater, MD, former Assistant Secretary for Health, U.S. Department of Health and Human Services

Rick Smith, MD, Office of Special Programs, Healthcare Emergency Preparedness, Health Resources and Services Administration, U.S. Department of Health and Human Services

Kanta Subbarao, MD, Senior Investigator, Respiratory Viruses Section, National Institute for Allergy and Infectious Diseases, National Institutes of Health

Susan C. Trock, DVM, MPH, DACVPM (Epi), New York State Department of Agriculture and Markets

Clara Witt, VMD, MPH, Global Emerging Infections Surveillance System, U.S. Department of Defense

Appendix
B

Selected Bibliography

LEARNING FROM THE PAST: PANDEMICS AND OTHER THREATS TO PUBLIC HEALTH

Henzler DJ, Kradel DC, Davison S, Ziegler AF, Singletary D, DeBok P, Castro AE, Lu H, Eckroade R, Swayne D, Lagoda W, Schmucker B, Nesselrodt A. 2003. Epidemiology, production losses, and control measures associated with an outbreak of avian influenza subtype H7N2 in Pennsylvania (1996–98). *Avian Diseases* 47(Suppl 3):1022–1036.

Kobasa D, Takada A, Shinya K, Hatta M, Halfmann P, Theriault S, Suzuki H, Nishimura H, Mitamura K, Sugaya N, Usui T, Murata T, Maeda Y, Watanabe S, Suresh M, Suzuki T, Suzuki Y, Feldmann H, Kawaoka Y. 2004. Enhanced virulence of influenza A viruses with the haemagglutinin of the 1918 pandemic virus. *Nature* 431(7009):703–707.

Neuraminidase Inhibitor Susceptibility Network. 2004. NISN statement on antiviral resistance in influenza viruses. *Weekly Epidemiological Record* 79(33):306–308.

Simonsen L, Fukuda K, Schonberger LB, Cox NJ. 2000. The impact of influenza epidemics on hospitalizations. *Journal of Infectious Diseases* 181(3):831–837.

Snacken R, Kendal AP, Haaheim LR, Wood JM. 1999. The next influenza pandemic: Lessons from Hong Kong, 1997. *Emerging Infectious Diseases* 5(2):195–203.

Stevens J, Corper AL, Basler CF, Taubenberger JK, Palese P, Wilson IA. 2004. Structure of the uncleaved human H1 hemagglutinin from the extinct 1918 influenza virus. *Science* 303(5665):1866–1870.

Tumpey TM, Garcia-Sastre A, Mikulasova A, Taubenberger JK, Swayne DE, Palese P, Basler CF. 2002. Existing antivirals are effective against influenza viruses with genes from the 1918 pandemic virus. *Proceedings of the National Academy of Sciences USA* 99(21):13849–13854.

Tumpey TM, Garcia-Sastre A, Taubenberger JK, Palese P, Swayne DE, Basler CF. 2004. Pathogenicity and immunogenicity of influenza viruses with genes from the 1918 pandemic virus. *Proceedings of the National Academy of Sciences USA* 101(9):3166–3171.

Webby RJ, Webster RG. 2003. Are we ready for pandemic influenza? *Science* 302(5650):1519–1522.

GLOBAL PREVENTION OF AND PREPARATION
FOR PANDEMIC INFLUENZA

Health Canada. 2004. Table of contents, preface, and introduction. In: *Canadian Pandemic Influenza Plan*. Pp. i–vii, 3–14. [Online]. Available: http://www.hc-sc.gc.ca/pphb-dgspsp/cpip-pclcpi/ [accessed June 8, 2004].

Health, Welfare and Food Bureau, The Government of Hong Kong SAR. 2004. *Prevention of Avian Influenza: Consultation on Long-term Direction to Minimize the Risk of Human Infection*. [Online]. Available: http://www.hwfb.gov.hk/download/consult/040402_feh/e_avian_flu.pdf [accessed May 2004].

WHO (World Health Organization). 2004. *National Influenza Pandemic Plans*. [Online]. Available: http://www.who.int/csr/disease/influenza/nationalpandemic/en/print.html [accessed June 7, 2004].

WHO. 2004. *WHO Consultation on Priority Public Health Interventions Before and During an Influenza Pandemic*. Geneva, Switzerland: WHO Department of Communicable Disease Surveillance and Response.

WHO. 2004. *WHO Guidelines on the Use of Vaccines and Antivirals During Influenza Pandemics*. WHO/CDS/CSR/RMD/2004.8. Geneva, Switzerland: WHO. [Online]. Available: http://www.who.int/csr/resources/publications/influenza/WHO_CDS_CSR_RMD_2004_8/en [accessed December 16, 2004].

PREPARING THE UNITED STATES FOR PANDEMIC INFLUENZA

Amendment to the Public Health Service Act to ensure an adequate supply of vaccines. S. 371, 108th Congress, 1st Session (2003).

Earls MJ, Hearne SA. 2004. *Facing the Flu: From the Bird Flu to a Possible Pandemic, Why Isn't America Ready?* Issue Report by Trust for America's Health. [Online]. Available: http://healthyamericans.org/reports/files/AvianFlu.pdf [accessed December 20, 2004].

Harper SA, Fukuda K, Uyeki TM, Cox NJ, Bridges CB; Centers for Disease Control and Prevention Advisory Committee on Immunization Practices. 2004, May 28. Prevention and control of influenza: Recommendations of the Advisory Committee on Immunization Practices. *MMWR Recommendations and Reports* 53(RR-6):1–40.

Improved Vaccine Affordability and Availability Act. S. 754, 108th Congress, 1st Session (2003).

Slater EE. 2004. Industry and government perspective in influenza control. *Texas Heart Institute Journal* 31(1):42–44.

The Flu Protection Act of 2004. S. 2038, 108th Congress, 2d Session (2004).

STATE AND LOCAL PREPARATION MEASURES

Gensheimer KF, Meltzer MI, Postema AS, Strikas RA. 2003. Influenza pandemic preparedness. *Emerging Infectious Diseases* 9(12):1645–1648.

Glaser CA, Gilliam S, Thompson WW, Dassey DE, Waterman SH, Saruwatari M, Shapiro S, Fukuda K. 2002. Medical care capacity for influenza outbreaks, Los Angeles. *Emerging Infectious Diseases* 8(6):569–574.

Misegades L. 2002. *Nature's Terrorist Attack: Pandemic Influenza*. Preparedness planning for state health officials. Washington, DC: Association of State and Territorial Health Officials.

State of California Hospital Bioterrorism Preparedness Program: 2003 Implementation Plan. 2003. Emergency Medical Services Authority, Department of Health Services, State of California. Pp. 1–6, 35–36.

Texas Department of Health. 2004, January 15. *Texas Department of Health Pandemic Influenza Plan [Draft].* [Online]. Available: http://www.cste.org/specialprojects/ Influenza%20Pandemic%20State%20Plans/TxPanFluPlan1.15.2004.pdf [accessed December 20, 2004].

STRATEGIES TO PREVENT AND CONTROL TRANSMISSION AMONG BIRDS AND OTHER ANIMALS

Bulaga LL, Garber L, Senne DA, Myers TJ, Good R, Wainwright S, Trock S, Suarez DL. 2003. Epidemiologic and surveillance studies on avian influenza in live-bird markets in New York and New Jersey, 2001. *Avian Diseases* 47(Suppl 3):996–1001.

Buranathai C. 2004 (June 16–17). *Information Sheet 1: Summary of Avian Influenza Outbreak in Thailand, 2004.* Prepared for Institute of Medicine (IOM) Forum on Microbial Threats workshop: Pandemic Influenza: Assessing Capabilities for Prevention and Response, Washington, DC.

Buranathai C. 2004 (June 16–17). *Information Sheet 2: Avian Influenza Outbreak in Thailand: Virological Aspects.* Prepared for IOM Forum on Microbial Threats workshop: Pandemic Influenza: Assessing Capabilities for Prevention and Response, Washington, DC.

Buranathai C. 2004 (June 16–17). *Information Sheet 3: Avian Influenza Outbreak in Thailand: Detection of H5N1 from Cats and Tigers.* Prepared for IOM Forum on Microbial Threats workshop: Pandemic Influenza: Assessing Capabilities for Prevention and Response, Washington, DC.

Buranathai C. 2004 (June 16–17). *Information Sheet 4: Avian Influenza Outbreak in Thailand: Movement Control.* Prepared for IOM Forum on Microbial Threats workshop: Pandemic Influenza: Assessing Capabilities for Prevention and Response, Washington, DC.

Buranathai C. 2004 (June 16–17). *Information Sheet 5: Avian Influenza Outbreak in Thailand: Current Policies.* Prepared for IOM Forum on Microbial Threats workshop: Pandemic Influenza: Assessing Capabilities for Prevention and Response, Washington, DC.

Cardona C. 2002. Recommendations to prevent the spread and/or introduction of avian influenza virus. *Fact Sheets & Information: Poultry.* UC Davis School of Veterinary Medicine Cooperative Extension. [Online]. Available: http://www.vetmed.ucdavis.edu/ vetext/INF-PO_AI-Recommendations.pdf [accessed June 8, 2004].

Cardona C. Undated. Avian influenza: AI recommendations. *Fact Sheets & Information: Poultry.* UC Davis School of Veterinary Medicine Cooperative Extension. [Online]. Available: http://www.vetmed.ucdavis.edu/vetext/INF-PO_AI.html [accessed May 20, 2004].

Centers for Disease Control and Prevention (CDC). 2004, February 13. Outbreaks of avian influenza A (H5N1) in Asia and interim recommendations for evaluation and reporting of suspected cases—United States, 2004. *MMWR* 53(5):97–100.

Ehlers M, Moller M, Marangon S, Ferre N. 2003. The use of Geographic Information System (GIS) in the frame of the contingency plan implemented during the 1999–2001 avian influenza (AI) epidemic in Italy. *Avian Diseases* 47(Suppl 3):1010–1014.

Fouchier RA, Osterhaus AD, Brown IH. 2003. Animal influenza virus surveillance. *Vaccine* 21(16):1754–1757.

Guan Y, Poon LL, Cheung CY, Ellis TM, Lim W, Lipatov AS, Chan KH, Sturm-Ramirez KM, Cheung CL, Leung YH, Yuen KY, Webster RG, Peiris JS. 2004. H5N1 influenza: A protean pandemic threat. *Proceedings of the National Academy of Sciences USA* 101(21):8156–8161.

Halvorston D, Capua I, Cardona C, Frame D, Karunakaran D, Marangon S, Ortali G, Roepke D, Woo-ming B. 2003, March. *The Economics of Avian Influenza Control.* Presented at the Western Poultry Disease Conference.

Koopmans M, Wilbrink B, Conyn M, Natrop G, van der Nat H, Vennema H, Meijer A, van Steenbergen J, Fouchier R, Osterhaus A, Bosman A. 2004. Transmission of H7N7 avian influenza A virus to human beings during a large outbreak in commercial poultry farms in the Netherlands. *Lancet* 363(9409):587–593.

Liu M, Guan Y, Peiris M, He S, Webby RJ, Perez D, Webster RG. 2003. The quest of influenza A viruses for new hosts. *Avian Diseases* 47(3 Suppl):849–856.

Myers TJ, Rhorer MD, Clifford J. 2003. USDA options for regulatory changes to enhance the prevention and control of avian influenza. *Avian Diseases* 47(Suppl 3):982–987.

Neumann G, Hatta M, Kawaoka Y. 2003. Reverse genetics for the control of avian influenza. *Avian Diseases* 47(Suppl 3):882–887.

Pearson JE. 2003. International standards for the control of avian influenza. *Avian Diseases* 47:972–975.

Pharo HJ. 2003. The impact of new epidemiological information on a risk analysis for the introduction of avian influenza viruses in imported poultry meat. *Avian Diseases* 47(Suppl 3):988–995.

Scientific Committee on Animal Health and Welfare, Health & Consumer Protection Directorate-General, European Commission. 2000. *The Definition of Avian Influenza: The Use of Vaccination Against Avian Influenza.*

Sims LD, Ellis TM, Liu KK, Dyrting K, Wong H, Peiris M, Guan Y, Shortridge KF. 2003. Avian influenza in Hong Kong, 1997–2002. *Avian Diseases* 47(Suppl 3):832–838.

Sims LD, Guan Y, Ellis TM, Liu KK, Dyrting K, Wong H, Kung NY, Shortridge KF, Peiris M. 2003. An update on avian influenza in Hong Kong, 2002. *Avian Diseases* 47(Suppl 3):1083–1086.

Spackman E, Senne DA, Bulaga LL, Myers TJ, Perdue ML, Garber LP, Lohman K, Daum LT, Suarez DL. 2003. Development of real-time RT-PCR for the detection of avian influenza virus. *Avian Diseases* 47(Suppl 3):1079–1082.

Stöhr K. 2003. The WHO global influenza program and its animal influenza network. *Avian Diseases* 47:934–938.

Symposium Organizing Committee. 2003. Recommendations of the Fifth International Symposium on Avian Influenza. *Avian Diseases* 47(Suppl 3):1260–1261.

Tran TH, Nguyen TL, Nguyen TD, Luong TS, Pham PM, Nguyen VC, Pham TS, Vo CD, Le TQ, Ngo TT, Dao BK, Le PP, Nguyen TT, Hoang TL, Cao VT, Le TG, Nguyen DT, Le HN, Nguyen KT, Le HS, Le VT, Christiane D, Tran TT, Menno de J, Schultsz C, Cheng P, Lim W, Horby P, Farrar J; World Health Organization International Avian Influenza Investigative Tea. 2004. World Health Organization International Avian Influenza Investigative Team. Avian influenza A (H5N1) in 10 patients in Vietnam. *New England Journal of Medicine* 350(12):1179–1188.

van der Goot JA, Koch G, de Jong MC, van Boven M. 2003. Transmission dynamics of low- and high-pathogenicity A/Chicken/Pennsylvania/83 avian influenza viruses. *Avian Diseases* 47(Suppl 3):939–941.

Webster R. 2004. Wet markets—a continuing source of Severe Acute Respiratory Syndrome and influenza? *Lancet* 363:234–236.

World Health Organization. 2004, March 2. *Avian Influenza A(H5N1)—Update 31: Situation (Poultry) in Asia: Need for a Long-Term Response, Comparison with Previous Outbreaks.* [Online]. Available: http://www.who.int/csr/don/2004_03_02/en/print.html [accessed June 7, 2004].

BIOMEDICAL APPROACHES TO PREVENTING OR CONTROLLING A PANDEMIC

Antivirals

Bowles SK, Lee W, Simor AE, Vearncombe M, Loeb M, Tamblyn S, Fearon M, Li Y, McGeer A; Oseltamivir Compassionate Use Program Group. 2002. Use of oseltamivir during influenza outbreaks in Ontario nursing homes, 1999–2000. *Journal of the American Geriatric Society* 50(4):608–616.

Cooper NJ, Sutton AJ, Abrams KR, Wailoo A, Turner D, Nicholson KG. 2003. Effectiveness of neuraminidase inhibitors in treatment and prevention of influenza A and B: Systematic review and meta-analyses of randomised controlled trials. *British Medical Journal* 326(7401):1235.

Ferguson NM, Mallett S, Jackson H, Roberts N, Ward P. 2003. A population-dynamic model for evaluating the potential spread of drug-resistant influenza virus infections during community-based use of antivirals. *Journal of Antimicrobial Chemotherapy* 51(4):977–990.

Hayden FG. 2001. Perspectives on antiviral use during pandemic influenza. *Philosophical Transactions of the Royal Society of London, Series B, Biological Sciences* 356(1416):1877–1884.

Kaiser L, Wat C, Mills T, Mahoney P, Ward P, Hayden F. 2003. Impact of oseltamivir treatment on influenza-related lower respiratory tract complications and hospitalizations. *Archives of Internal Medicine* 163(14):1667–1672.

Kati WM, Montgomery D, Carrick R, Gubareva L, Maring C, McDaniel K, Steffy K, Molla A, Hayden F, Kempf D, Kohlbrenner W. 2002. In vitro characterization of A-315675, a highly potent inhibitor of A and B strain influenza virus neuraminidases and influenza virus replication. *Antimicrobial Agents and Chemotherapy* 46(4):1014–1021.

Longini IM Jr, Halloran ME, Nizam A, Yang Y. 2004. Containing pandemic influenza with antiviral agents. *American Journal of Epidemiology* 159(7):623–633.

Monto AS. 2003. The role of antivirals in the control of influenza. *Vaccine* 21(16):1796–1800.

Oxford J, Balasingam S, Lambkin R. 2004. A new millennium conundrum: How to use a powerful class of influenza anti-neuraminidase drugs (NAIs) in the community. *Journal of Antimicrobial Chemotherapy* 53(2):133–136.

Peltola VT, McCullers JA. 2004. Respiratory viruses predisposing to bacterial infections: Role of neuraminidase. *Pediatric Infectious Disease Journal* 23(Suppl 1):S87–S97.

Zambon M, Hayden FG; Global Neuraminidase Inhibitor Susceptibility Network. 2001. Position statement: Global Neuraminidase Inhibitor Susceptibility Network. *Antiviral Research* 49(3):147–156.

Vaccines

Adis Data Information BV. 2003. Influenza virus vaccine live intranasal—MedImmune vaccines: CAIV-T, influenza vaccine live intranasal. *Drugs R&D* 4(5):312–319.

Chen Z. 2004. Influenza DNA vaccine: An update. *Chinese Medical Journal* 117(1):125–132. [Online]. Available: http://www.cmj.org/information/full.asp?pmid=20041125 [accessed June 8, 2004].

Epstein SL, Tumpey TM, Misplon JA, Lo CY, Cooper LA, Subbarao K, Renshaw M, Sambhara S, Katz JM. 2002. DNA vaccine expressing conserved influenza virus proteins protective against H5N1 challenge infection in mice. *Emerging Infectious Diseases* 8(8):796–801.

Fedson DS. 2004. Vaccination for pandemic influenza: A six point agenda for interpandemic years. *Pediatric Infectious Disease Journal* 23(Suppl 1):S74–S77.

Ferguson NM, Galvani AP, Bush RM. 2003. Ecological and immunological determinants of influenza evolution. *Nature* 422(6930):428–433.

Glezen WP. 2004. Control of influenza. *Texas Heart Institute Journal* 31(1):39–41.

Hoch D. 2004, May. Influenza pandemic preparedness: The European vaccine manufacturers' perspective. *ESWI Bulletin.* [Online]. Available: http://www.eswi.org/ [accessed June 8, 2004].

Jin H, Zhou H, Lu B, Kemble G. 2004. Imparting temperature sensitivity and attenuation in ferrets to A/Puerto Rico/8/34 influenza virus by transferring the genetic signature for temperature sensitivity from cold-adapted A/Ann Arbor/6/60. *Journal of Virology* 78(2):995–998.

Kemble G, Greenberg H. 2003. Novel generations of influenza vaccines. *Vaccine* 21(16):1789–1795.

Lambert LC, Kim S. 2004, May. Pandemic preparedness: Developing a clinical trial research plan. *ESWI Bulletin.* [Online]. Available: http://www.eswi.org/ [accessed June 8, 2004].

McElhaney JE, Aoki FY. 2004, May. FluMist™: History and future. *ESWI Bulletin.* [Online]. Available: http://www.eswi.org/ [accessed June 8, 2004].

Palese P, García-Sastre A. 2002. Influenza vaccines: Present and future. *Journal of Clinical Investigation* 110(1):9–13.

Webby RJ, Perez DR, Coleman JS, Guan Y, Knight JH, Govorkova EA, McClain-Moss LR, Peiris JS, Rehg JE, Tuomanen EI, Webster RG. 2004. Responsiveness to a pandemic alert: Use of reverse genetics for rapid development of influenza vaccines. *Lancet* 363(9415):1099–1103.

LEGAL ISSUES IN THE PREVENTION AND CONTROL OF A PANDEMIC

Barbera J, Macintyre A, Gostin L, Inglesby T, O'Toole T, DeAtley C, Tonat K, Layton M. 2001. Large-scale quarantine following biological terrorism in the United States: Scientific examination, logistic and legal limits, and possible consequences. *Journal of the American Medical Association* 286(21):2711–2717.

Epstein RA. 2003, Summer. Let the shoemaker stick to his last: A defense of the "old" public health. *Perspectives in Biology and Medicine* 46(Suppl 3):S138–S159.

Fedson, DS. 2004 (June 16–17). *Reverse Genetics, Intellectual Property and Influenza Vaccination.* Prepared for IOM Forum on Microbial Threats workshop: Pandemic Influenza: Assessing Capabilities for Prevention and Response, Washington, DC.

Gostin LO. 2004. International infectious disease law: Revision of the World Health Organization's International Health Regulations. *Journal of the American Medical Association* 291(21):2623–2627.

Gostin LO, Bayer R, Fairchild AL. 2003. Ethical and legal challenges posed by Severe Acute Respiratory Syndrome: Implications for the control of severe infectious disease threats. *Journal of the American Medical Association* 290(24):3229–3237.

Gostin LO, Bloche MG. 2003. The politics of public health: A response to Epstein. *Perspectives in Biology and Medicine* 46(Suppl 3):S160–S175.

Mair JS, Mair M. 2003. Vaccine liability in the era of bioterrorism. *Biosecurity and Bioterrorism: Biodefense Strategy, Practice, and Science* 1(3):169–184.

IMPROVING PREPAREDNESS: SURVEILLANCE, PREDICTION, AND COMMUNICATION

Brunell PA, ed. 2004, February. Importance of Vaccinating Healthcare Workers Against Influenza. CME monograph from *Infectious Diseases in Children*. Selected articles: Eickhoff TC, Keys to compliance; Piedra PA, Time has come to make vaccination mandatory; The literature's message; Glezen WP, Influenza past and present. [Online]. Available: http://idinchildren.com/monograph/0402/cmei.pdf [accessed June 8, 2004].

Cain KP, Blitz SG. 2004. Integration of clinical practice, publicity, and policy: A shot in the arm for influenza control. *American Journal of Managed Care* 10(1):11–12.

Davis MM, McMahon SR, Santoli JM, Schwartz B, Clark SJ. 2002. A national survey of physician practices regarding influenza vaccine. *Journal of General Internal Medicine* 17(9):670–676.

Fraser C, Riley S, Anderson RM, Ferguson NM. 2004. Factors that make an infectious disease outbreak controllable. *Proceedings of the National Academy of Sciences USA* 101(16):6146–6151.

Gensheimer KF, Fukuda K, Brammer L, Cox N, Patriarca PA, Strikes RA. 2002. Preparing for pandemic influenza: The need for enhanced surveillance. *Vaccine* 20(Suppl 2): S63–S65.

Glass TA, Schoch-Spana M. 2002. Bioterrorism and the people: How to vaccinate a city against panic. *Clinical Infectious Diseases* 34(2):217–223.

Mooney JD, Holmes E, Christie P. 2002. Real-time modelling of influenza outbreaks: A linear regression analysis. *Eurosurveillance Monthly* 7(12):184–187. [Online]. Available: http://www.eurosurveillance.org/em/v07n12/0712-225.asp [accessed June 8, 2004).

Participants of the WHO Consultation on Global Priorities in Influenza, 2002 May 6–7. 2003. *The Global Agenda on Influenza Surveillance and Control*. [Online]. Available: http://www.who.int/csr/disease/influenza/csrinfluenzaglobalagenda/en/print.html [accessed June 7, 2004].

Pavlin J. *Epidemiologic Surveillance in Developing Countries*. Global Emerging Infections System, U.S. Department of Defense.

Perdue ML. 2003. Molecular diagnostics in an insecure world. *Avian Diseases* 47(Suppl 3):1063–1068.

Schoch-Spana M. 2000. Implications of pandemic influenza for bioterrorism response. *Clinical Infectious Diseases* 31(6):1409–1413.

Schopflocher DP, Russell ML, Svenson LW, Thu-Ha N, Mazurenko I. 2004. Pandemic influenza planning: Using the U.S. Centers for Disease Control and Prevention FluAid software for small area estimation in the Canadian context. *Annals of Epidemiology* 14:73–76.

Shult PA, Kirk C. 2003. Laboratory-based surveillance for influenza: Role of the Wisconsin State Laboratory of Hygiene. *Wisconsin Medical Journal* 102(6):26–30.

Simonsen L, Clarke MJ, Schonberger LB, Arden NH, Cox NJ, Fukuda K. 1998. Pandemic versus epidemic influenza mortality: A pattern of changing age distribution. *Journal of Infectious Diseases* 178(1):53–60.

Working Group on Governance Dilemmas in Bioterrorism Response. 2004. Leading during bioattacks and epidemics with the public's trust and help. *Biosecurity and Bioterrorism: Biodefense Strategy, Practice, and Science* 2(1):25–40.

World Health Organization. 2004. *WHO Global Influenza Surveillance Network*. [Online]. Available: http://www.who.int/csr/disease/influenza/surveillance/en/print.html [accessed June 7, 2004].

Appendix
C

The Critical Path to
New Medical Products*

On March 16, the Food and Drug Administration (FDA) released a report addressing the recent slowdown in innovative medical therapies submitted to the FDA for approval, "*Innovation/Stagnation: Challenge and Opportunity on the Critical Path to New Medical Products.*" That report describes the urgent need to modernize the medical product development process—the Critical Path—to make product development more predictable and less costly.

According to Acting FDA Commissioner Lester M. Crawford, "A new focus on updating the tools currently used to assess the safety and efficacy of new medical products will very likely bring tremendous public health benefits." Because of its unique vantage point, the FDA can work with outside experts in companies, patient groups, and the academic community to coordinate, develop, and/or disseminate solutions to Critical Path problems, to improve the efficiency of product development industry-wide. Through this initiative, the FDA will take the lead in the development of a national Critical Path Opportunities List, to bring concrete focus to these tasks.

We will develop this list through extensive consultation with private and public stakeholders. To this end, we are establishing an open public docket to obtain input on the most pressing scientific and/or technical hurdles causing major delays and other problems in the drug, device, and/or biologic development process, as well as proposed approaches to their

---

*From http://www.fda.gov/oc/initiatives/criticalpath/

solution. In addition, FDA will make internal changes to intensify its ability to surface and address crucial issues and to support high-priority critical path research efforts.

Challenge and Opportunity on the Critical Path to New Medical Products (March 2004)
- Full Report (PDF) Available: http://www.fda.gov/oc/initiatives/criticalpath/whitepaper.html
- White Paper Executive Summary Available: http://www.fda.gov/oc/initiatives/criticalpath/whitepaper.html#execsummary
- Critical Path News Release Available: http://www.fda.gov/bbs/topics/news/2004/NEW01035.html

Appendix
D

Forum Members, Speakers, and Staff Biographies

FORUM MEMBERS

ADEL A.F. MAHMOUD, M.D., Ph.D. *(Chair)*, is President of Merck Vaccines at Merck & Co., Inc. He formerly served Case Western Reserve University and University Hospitals of Cleveland as Chairman of Medicine and Physician-in-Chief from 1987 to 1998. Prior to that, Dr. Mahmoud held several positions, spanning 25 years, at the same institutions. Dr. Mahmoud and his colleagues conducted pioneering investigations on the biology and function of eosinophils. He prepared the first specific anti-eosinophil serum, which was used to define the role of these cells in host resistance to helminthic infections. Dr. Mahmoud also established clinical and laboratory investigations in several developing countries, including Kenya, Egypt, and The Philippines, to examine the determinants of infection and disease in schistosomiasis and other infectious agents. This work led to the development of innovative strategies to control those infections, which have been adopted by the World Health Organization (WHO) as selective population chemotherapy. In recent years, Dr. Mahmoud turned his attention to developing a comprehensive set of responses to the problems associated with emerging infections in the developing world. He was elected to membership of the American Society for Clinical Investigation in 1978, the Association of American Physicians in 1980, and the Institute of Medicine of the National Academy of Sciences in 1987. He received the Bailey K. Ashford Award of the American Society of Tropical Medicine and Hygiene in 1983, and the Squibb Award of the Infectious Diseases Society of America in 1984. Dr. Mahmoud currently serves as Chair of the Forum on Emerging Infections and is a member of the Board on Global Health, both of the Institute of Medicine. He also chairs the U.S. Delegation to the U.S.-Japan Cooperative Medical Science Program.

STANLEY M. LEMON, M.D. *(Vice-Chair)*, is Dean of the School of Medicine at the University of Texas Medical Branch at Galveston. He received his undergraduate degree in biochemical sciences from Princeton University summa cum laude, and his M.D. with honors from the University of Rochester. He completed postgraduate training in internal medicine and infectious diseases at the University of North Carolina at Chapel Hill, and is board-certified in both. From 1977 to 1983, he served with the U.S. Army Medical Research and Development Command, directing the Hepatitis Laboratory at the Walter Reed Army Institute of Research. He joined the faculty of the University of North Carolina School of Medicine in 1983, serving first as Chief of the Division of Infectious Diseases, and then Vice Chair for Research of the Department of Medicine. In 1997, Dr. Lemon moved to the University of Texas Medical Branch as Professor and Chair of the Department of Microbiology & Immunology. He was subsequently appointed Dean *pro tem* of the School of Medicine in 1999, and permanent Dean of Medicine in 2000. Dr. Lemon's research interests relate to the molecular virology and pathogenesis of the positive-stranded RNA viruses responsible for hepatitis C and hepatitis A. He is particularly interested in the molecular mechanisms controlling replication of these RNA genomes and related mechanisms of disease pathogenesis. He has published over 180 papers, and numerous textbook chapters related to hepatitis and other viral infections, and has a longstanding interest in vaccine development. He has served previously as Chair of the Anti-Infective Drugs Advisory Committee and the Vaccines and Related Biologics Advisory Committee of the U.S. Food and Drug Administration, and is past Chair of the Steering Committee on Hepatitis and Poliomyelitis of WHO's Programme on Vaccine Development. He presently serves as Chairman of the U.S. Hepatitis Panel of the U.S.-Japan Cooperative Medical Science Program, and recently chaired an Institute of Medicine study committee related to vaccines for the protection of the military against naturally occurring infectious disease threats.

DAVID ACHESON, M.D., is Chief Medical Officer at the Center for Food Safety and Applied Nutrition, U.S. Food and Drug Administration (FDA). He received his medical degree at the University of London. After completing internships in general surgery and medicine, he continued his postdoctoral training in Manchester, England, as a Wellcome Trust Research Fellow. He subsequently was a Wellcome Trust Training Fellow in Infectious Diseases at the New England Medical Center and at the Wellcome Research Unit in Vellore, India. Dr. Acheson was Associate Professor of

THE THREAT OF PANDEMIC INFLUENZA

Medicine, Division of Geographic Medicine and Infectious Diseases, New England Medical Center, until 2001. He then joined the faculties of the Department of Epidemiology and Preventive Medicine and Department of Microbiology and Immunology at the University of Maryland Medical School. Currently at the FDA, his research concentration is on foodborne pathogens and encompasses a mixture of molecular pathogenesis, cell biology, and epidemiology. Specifically, his research focuses on Shiga toxin-producing *E. coli* and understanding toxin interaction with intestinal epithelial cells using tissue culture models. His laboratory has also undertaken a study to examine Shiga toxin-producing *E. coli* in food animals in relation to virulence factors and antimicrobial resistance patterns. More recently, Dr. Acheson initiated a project to understand the molecular pathogenesis of *Campylobacter jejuni*. Other studies have undertaken surveillance of diarrheal disease in the community to determine causes, outcomes, and risk factors of unexplained diarrhea. Dr. Acheson has authored/co-authored over 72 journal articles, and 42 book chapters and reviews, and is coauthor of the book *Safe Eating* (Dell Health, 1998). He is reviewer of more than 10 journals and is on the editorial board of *Infection and Immunity* and *Clinical Infectious Diseases*. Dr. Acheson is a Fellow of the Royal College of Physicians, a Fellow of the Infectious Disease Society of America, and holds several patents.

RUTH L. BERKELMAN, M.D., is the Rollins Professor and Director, Center for Public Health Preparedness and Research at the Rollins School of Public Health at Emory University. She came to Emory University in 2000 following 20 years with the Centers for Disease Control and Prevention (CDC), where she had served as an Assistant Surgeon General both in the position as Senior Adviser to the Director, CDC, and as Deputy Director, National Center for Infectious Diseases. In the mid-1990s, she led CDC's efforts to address the threat of emerging infectious diseases. Her career began as an Epidemic Intelligence Service (EIS) Officer, and her expertise is primarily in infectious diseases and disease surveillance. Dr. Berkelman is board certified in pediatrics and internal medicine, and is a graduate of Harvard Medical School. She is active in the Infectious Diseases Society of America and the American Epidemiologic Society, and she currently serves on the Policy and Scientific Affairs Board of the American Society of Microbiology. She also consults with the Nuclear Threat Initiative on reduction of the threat of biologic weapons.

ENRIQUETA C. BOND, Ph.D., is President of the Burroughs Wellcome Fund. Dr. Bond received her undergraduate degree from Wellesley College, her M.A. from the University of Virginia, and her Ph.D. in molecular biology and biochemical genetics from Georgetown University. She is a member of the Institute of Medicine, the American Association for the Advancement of Science, the American Society for Microbiology, and the American Public Health Association. Dr. Bond serves on the Council of the Institute of Medicine as its Vice-Chair; she chairs the Board of Scientific Counselors for the National Center for Infectious Diseases at the Centers for Disease Control and Prevention, and she chairs the Institute of Medicine's Clinical Research Roundtable. She serves on the Board and Executive Committee of the Research Triangle Park Foundation, and on the Board of the Medicines for Malaria Venture. Prior to being named President of the Burroughs Wellcome Fund in 1994, Dr. Bond served on the staff of the Institute of Medicine since 1979, becoming the Institute's Executive Officer in 1989.

STEVEN J. BRICKNER, Ph.D., is Research Advisor, Antibacterials Chemistry, at Pfizer Global Research and Development. He received his Ph.D. in organic chemistry from Cornell University and was a NIH Postdoctoral Research Fellow at the University of Wisconsin-Madison. Dr. Brickner is a medicinal chemist with nearly 20 years of research experience in the pharmaceutical industry, all focused on the discovery and development of novel antibacterial agents. He is an inventor/co-inventor on 21 U.S. patents, and has published numerous scientific papers, primarily within the area of the oxazolidinones. Prior to joining Pfizer in 1996, he led a team at Pharmacia and Upjohn that discovered and developed linezolid, the first member of a new class of antibiotics to be approved in the last 35 years.

NANCY CARTER-FOSTER, M.S.T.M., is Senior Advisor for Health Affairs for the U.S. Department of State, Assistant Secretary for Science and Health, and the Secretary's Representative on HIV/AIDS. She is responsible for identifying emerging health issues and making policy recommendations for U.S. government foreign policy concerns regarding international health, and coordinates the Department's interactions with the nongovernmental community. She is a member of the National Academy of Sciences Institute of Medicine's Forum on Infectious Diseases, and a member of the Infectious Diseases Society of America (IDSA), and the American Association of the Advancement of Science (AAAS). She has helped bring focus to global health issues in U.S. foreign policy and brought a national security focus to global health. In prior positions as Director for Congressional and Legislative Affairs for the Economic and Business Affairs Bureau of the U.S. Department of State, and Foreign Policy Advisory to the Majority WHIP U.S. House of Representatives, Trade Specialist Advisor to the House of Representatives Ways and Means Trade Subcommittee, and consultant to the World Bank, Asia Technical Environment Division, Ms. Carter-Foster has worked on a wide variety of health, trade, and environmental issues amass-

THE THREAT OF PANDEMIC INFLUENZA

ing in-depth knowledge and experience in policy development and program implementation.

GAIL H. CASSELL, Ph.D., is Vice President, Scientific Affairs, Distinguished Lilly Research Scholar for Infectious Diseases, Eli Lilly & Company. Previously, she was the Charles H. McCauley Professor and (since 1987) Chair, Department of Microbiology, University of Alabama Schools of Medicine and Dentistry at Birmingham, a department which, under her leadership, has ranked first in research funding from the National Institutes of Health since 1989. She is a member of the Director's Advisory Committee of the Centers for Disease Control and Prevention. Dr. Cassell is past President of the American Society for Microbiology (ASM) and is serving her third 3-year term as Chairman of the Public and Scientific Affairs Board of ASM. She is a former member of the National Institutes of Health Director's Advisory Committee and a former member of the Advisory Council of the National Institute of Allergy and Infectious Diseases. She has also served as an advisor on infectious diseases and indirect costs of research to the White House Office on Science and Technology and was previously Chair of the Board of Scientific Counselors of the National Center for Infectious Diseases, Centers for Disease Control and Prevention. Dr. Cassell served 8 years on the Bacteriology-Mycology-II Study Section and served as its Chair for 3 years. She serves on the editorial boards of several prestigious scientific journals and has authored over 275 articles and book chapters. She has been intimately involved in the establishment of science policy and legislation related to biomedical research and public health. Dr. Cassell has received several national and international awards and an honorary degree for her research on infectious diseases.

JESSE L. GOODMAN, M.D., M.P.H., was Professor of Medicine and Chief of Infectious Diseases at the University of Minnesota, and is now serving as Deputy Director for the FDA Center for Biologics Evaluation and Research, where he is active in a broad range of scientific, public health, and policy issues. After joining the FDA commissioner's office, he has worked closely with several centers and helped coordinate FDA's response to the antimicrobial resistance problem. He was Co-Chair of a recently formed federal interagency task force which developed the national Public Health Action Plan on antimicrobial resistance. He graduated from Harvard College and attended the Albert Einstein College of Medicine followed by internal medicine, hematology, oncology, and infectious diseases training at the University of Pennsylvania and University of California, Los Angeles, where he was also Chief Medical Resident. He received his M.P.H. from the University of Minnesota. He has been active in community public health activities, including creating an environmental health partnership in St. Paul,

Minnesota. In recent years, his laboratory's research has focused on the molecular pathogenesis of tickborne diseases. His laboratory isolated the etiological intracellular agent of the emerging tickborne infection, human granulocytic ehrlichiosis, and identified its leukocyte receptor. He has also been an active clinician and teacher and has directed or participated in major multicenter clinical studies. He is a Fellow of the Infectious Diseases Society of America and, among several honors, has been elected to the American Society for Clinical Investigation.

EDUARDO GOTUZZO, M.D., is Principal Professor and Director at the Instituto de Medicina Tropical "Alexander von Humbolt," Universidad Peruana Cayetan Heredia (UPCH), in Lima, Peru. He is also Chief of the Department of Infectious and Tropical Diseases at the Cayetano Heredia Hospital and Adjunct Professor of Medicine at the University of Alabama–Birmingham School of Medicine. Dr. Gotuzzo has proven to be an active member in numerous international societies such as President of the Latin America Society of Tropical Disease (2000–2003), member of the Scientific Program of Infectious Diseases Society of America (2000–2003), member of the International Organizing Committee of the International Congress of Infectious Diseases (1994–Present), President Elect of the International Society for Infectious Diseases (1996–1998), and President of the Peruvian Society of Internal Medicine (1991–1992). He has published over 230 articles and chapters as well as six manuals and one book. Recent honors and awards include being named an Honorary member of American Society of Tropical Medicine and Hygiene (since 2002), Associated Member of National Academy of Medicine (since 2002), Honorary Member of Society of Internal Medicine (since 2000), Distinguished Visitor, Faculty of Medical Sciences, University of Cordoba, Argentina (since 1999), and the Golden Medal for "Outstanding Contribution in the field of Infectious Diseases," awarded by the Trnava University, Slovakia (1998), among many others.

CHRISTINE M. GRANT, J.D., M.B.A., is New Jersey's immediate past Commissioner of Health and Senior Services. Chris Grant, is a nationally recognized expert in healthcare and pharmaceutical financing and public health crises. She has had careers in government business and philanthropy and degrees in business, law, and science. As a cabinet member with Governor Whitman, she was New Jersey's Chief Health Official and had responsibility for a 2,000-person, $2 billion agency between 1999 and 2001. She is currently the Vice President of Policy and Government Relations for Aventis Pasteur, the world's largest vaccine company. Her previous work at the company included the creation of a center of activity known as Public Business. She is now working on a number of domestic and global issues including the creation of collaborative systems to manage a global or pandemic influenza outbreak.

MARGARET A. HAMBURG, M.D., is Vice President for Biological Programs at Nuclear Threat Initiative (NTI), a charitable organization working to reduce the global threat from nuclear, biological, and chemical weapons. Dr. Hamburg is in charge of the biological program area. Before taking on her current position, Dr. Hamburg was the Assistant Secretary for Planning and Evaluation, U.S. Department of Health and Human Services, serving as a principal policy advisor to the Secretary of Health and Human Services with responsibilities including policy formulation and analysis, the development and review of regulations and/or legislation, budget analysis, strategic planning, and the conduct and coordination of policy research and program evaluation. Prior to this, she served for almost 6 years as the Commissioner of Health for the City of New York. As chief health officer in the nation's largest city, Dr. Hamburg's many accomplishments included the design and implementation of an internationally recognized tuberculosis control program that produced dramatic declines in tuberculosis cases; the development of initiatives that raised childhood immunization rates to record levels; and the creation of the first public health bioterrorism preparedness program in the nation. She completed her internship and residency in Internal Medicine at the New York Hospital/Cornell University Medical Center and is certified by the American Board of Internal Medicine. Dr. Hamburg is a graduate of Harvard College and Harvard Medical School. She currently serves on the Harvard University Board of Overseers. She has been elected to membership in the Institute of Medicine, the New York Academy of Medicine, and the Council on Foreign Relations, and is a Fellow of the American Association for the Advancement of Science and the American College of Physicians.

CAROLE A. HEILMAN, Ph.D., is Director of the Division of Microbiology and Infectious Diseases (DMID) of the National Institute of Allergy and Infectious Diseases (NIAID). Dr. Heilman received her B.S. in biology from Boston University in 1972, and earned her M.S. and Ph.D. in microbiology from Rutgers University in 1976 and 1979, respectively. Dr. Heilman began her career at the National Institutes of Health as a Postdoctoral Research Associate with the National Cancer Institute where she carried out research on the regulation of gene expression during cancer development. In 1986, she came to NIAID as the influenza and viral respiratory diseases program officer in DMID and, in 1988, she was appointed chief of the respiratory diseases branch where she coordinated the development of acellular pertussis vaccines. She joined the Division of AIDS as Deputy Director in 1997 and was responsible for developing the Innovation Grant

Program for Approaches in HIV Vaccine Research. She is the recipient of several notable awards for outstanding achievement. Throughout her extramural career, Dr. Heilman has contributed articles on vaccine design and development to many scientific journals and has served as a consultant to the World Bank and WHO in this area. She is also a member of several professional societies, including the Infectious Diseases Society of America, the American Society for Microbiology, and the American Society of Virology.

DAVID L. HEYMANN, M.D., is currently the Executive Director of the World Health Organization (WHO) Communicable Diseases Cluster. From October 1995 to July 1998 he was Director of the WHO Programme on Emerging and Other Communicable Diseases Surveillance and Control. Prior to becoming director of this program, he was the chief of research activities in the Global Programme on AIDS. From 1976 to 1989, prior to joining WHO, Dr. Heymann spent 13 years working as a medical epidemiologist in sub-Saharan Africa (Cameroon, Ivory Coast, the former Zaire, and Malawi) on assignment from the CDC in CDC-supported activities aimed at strengthening capacity in surveillance of infectious diseases and their control, with special emphasis on the childhood immunizable diseases, African hemorrhagic fevers, pox viruses, and malaria. While based in Africa, Dr. Heymann participated in the investigation of the first outbreak of Ebola in Yambuku (former Zaire) in 1976, then again investigated the second outbreak of Ebola in 1977 in Tandala, and in 1995 directed the international response to the Ebola outbreak in Kikwit. Prior to 1976, Dr. Heymann spent 2 years in India as a medical officer in the WHO Smallpox Eradication Programme. Dr. Heymann holds a B.A. from the Pennsylvania State University, an M.D. from Wake Forest University, and a diploma in Tropical Medicine and Hygiene from the London School of Hygiene and Tropical Medicine, and completed practical epidemiology training in the EIS training program of the CDC. He has published 131 scientific articles on infectious diseases in peer-reviewed medical and scientific journals.

JAMES M. HUGHES, M.D., received his B.A. in 1966 and M.D. in 1971 from Stanford University. He completed a residency in internal medicine at the University of Washington and a fellowship in infectious diseases at the University of Virginia. He is board-certified in internal medicine, infectious diseases, and preventive medicine. He first joined CDC as an Epidemic Intelligence Service officer in 1973. During his CDC career, he has worked primarily in the areas of foodborne disease and infection control in health care settings. He became Director of the National Center for Infectious Diseases in 1992. The center is currently working to address domestic and global challenges posed by emerging infectious diseases and the threat of bioterrorism. He is a member of the Institute of Medicine and a fellow of the American College of Physicians, the Infectious Diseases Society of America, and the American Association for the Advancement of Science. He is an Assistant Surgeon General in the Public Health Service.

GERALD T. KEUSCH, M.D., is Provost and Dean for Global Health at Boston University (BU) and BU School of Public Health. He is a graduate of Columbia College (1958) and Harvard Medical School (1963). After completing a residency in internal medicine, fellowship training in infectious diseases, and two years as an NIH Research Associate at the SEATO Medical Research Laboratory in Bangkok, Thailand, Dr. Keusch joined the faculty of Mt. Sinai School of Medicine in 1970, where he established a laboratory to study the pathogenesis of bacillary dysentery and the biology and biochemistry of Shiga toxin. In 1979, he moved to Tufts Medical School and New England Medical Center in Boston, to found the Division of Geographic Medicine, which focused on the molecular and cellular biology of tropical infectious disease. In 1986, he integrated the clinical infectious diseases program into the Division of Geographic Medicine and Infectious Diseases, continuing as Division Chief until 1998. He has worked in the laboratory and in the field in Latin America, Africa, and Asia on basic and clinical infectious diseases and HIV/AIDS research. From 1998 to 2003 he was Associate Director for International Research and Director of the Fogarty International Center at the NIH. Dr. Keusch is a member of the American Society for Clinical Investigation, the Association of American Physicians, the American Society for Microbiology, and the Infectious Diseases Society of America (IDSA). He is the recipient of the Squibb (1981), Finland (1997), and Bristol (2002) Awards of the IDSA. In 2002 he was elected to the Institute of Medicine of the National Academies.

LONNIE KING, D.V.M., is Dean of the College of Veterinary Medicine, Michigan State University. Dr. King's previous positions include both Associate Administrator and Administrator of the USDA Animal and Plant Health Inspection Service (APHIS) and Deputy Administrator for USDA/APHIS/Veterinary Services. Before his government career, Dr. King was in private practice. He also has experience as a field veterinary medical officer, station epidemiologist, and staff assignments involving Emergency Programs and Animal Health Information. Dr. King has also directed the American Veterinary Medical Association's Office of Governmental Relations, and is certified in the American College of Veterinary Preventive Medicine. He has served as President of the Association of American Veterinary Medicine Colleges, and currently serves as Co-Chair of the National Commission on Veterinary Economic Issues, Lead Dean at Michigan State University for food safety with responsibility for the National Food Safety and Toxicology Center, the Institute for Environmental Toxicology, and the Center for Emerging Infectious Diseases. He is also co-developer and course leader for science, politics, and animal health policy. Dr. King received his B.S. and D.V.M. degrees from Ohio State University, and his M.S. degree in epidemiology from the University of Minnesota. He has also completed the Senior Executive Program at Harvard University, and received an M.P.A. from American University. Dr. King previously served on the Committee for Opportunities in Agriculture, the Steering Committee for a Workshop on the Control and Prevention of Animal Diseases, and the Committee to Ensure Safe Food from Production to Consumption.

JOSHUA LEDERBERG, Ph.D., is Professor emeritus of Molecular Genetics and Informatics and Sackler Foundation Scholar at The Rockefeller University, New York, New York. His lifelong research, for which he received the Nobel Prize in 1958, has been in genetic structure and function in microorganisms. He has a keen interest in international health and was Co-Chair of a previous Institute of Medicine Committee on Emerging Microbial Threats to Health (1990–1992) and currently is Co-Chair of the Committee on Emerging Microbial Threats to Health in the 21st Century. He has been a member of the National Academy of Sciences since 1957 and is a charter member of the Institute of Medicine.

JOSEPH MALONE, M.D., the director of the Department of Defense Global Emerging Infection System (DoD-GEIS), completed the CDC's EIS program in June 2003. He graduated from Boston University School of Medicine in 1980, and trained in internal medicine and infectious diseases at Naval Hospitals in San Diego, and Bethesda, MD, leading to board certification. He was a staff physician at the Naval Hospitals in San Diego, CA, and Bethesda, MD. He deployed to Guantanamo Bay, Cuba, in support of Operation Safe Harbor and was attached to Surgical Team 1 during Operation Desert Shield. He later directed the Infectious Disease Division and HIV unit at the Naval Medical Center at Portsmouth, VA, from 1996–1996. In 1999 he worked for the Disease Surveillance Program (in affiliation with DoD-GEIS) at the U.S. Naval Medical Research Unit No. 3 in Cairo, Egypt. While at CDC's EIS program he was deployed to New York City to assist in the emergency public health response after the September 11, 2001, attacks, assisted in the public health response to documented anthrax contamination in Kansas City, and was the acting state epidemiologist for the State of Missouri from February–June 2003. Captain Malone has several military awards, including the HHS/USPHS Crisis Response Service Award. He is an Associate Professor at the Uniformed Services University of Health Sciences and holds the Certificate of Knowledge in Travelers' Health and Tropical Medicine from the American Society of Tropical Medicine and Hygiene. He has over 20 publications.

LYNN MARKS, M.D., is board-certified in internal medicine and infectious diseases. He was on faculty at the University of South Alabama College of Medicine in the Infectious Diseases Department focusing on patient care, teaching, and research. His academic research interest was on the molecular genetics of bacterial pathogenicity. He subsequently joined SmithKline Beecham's (now GlaxoSmithKline) anti-infectives clinical group and later progressed to global head of the Consumer Healthcare division Medical and Regulatory group. He then returned to pharmaceutical research and development as global head of the Infectious Diseases Therapeutic Area Strategy Team for GlaxoSmithKline.

STEPHEN S. MORSE, Ph.D., is Director of the Center for Public Health Preparedness at the Mailman School of Public Health of Columbia University, and a faculty member in the Epidemiology Department. Dr. Morse recently returned to Columbia from 4 years in government service as Program Manager at the Defense Advanced Research Projects Agency (DARPA), where he co-directed the Pathogen Countermeasures program and subsequently directed the Advanced Diagnostics program. Before coming to Columbia, he was Assistant Professor (Virology) at The Rockefeller University in New York, where he remains an adjunct faculty member. Dr. Morse is the editor of two books, *Emerging Viruses* (Oxford University Press, 1993; paperback, 1996) (selected by *American Scientist* for its list of "100 Top Science Books of the 20th Century"), and *The Evolutionary Biology of Viruses* (Raven Press, 1994). He currently serves as a Section Editor of the CDC journal *Emerging Infectious Diseases* and was formerly an Editor-in-Chief of the Pasteur Institute's journal *Research in Virology*. Dr. Morse was Chair and principal organizer of the 1989 NIAID/NIH Conference on Emerging Viruses (for which he originated the term and concept of emerging viruses/infections); served as a member of the Institute of Medicine-National Academy of Sciences' Committee on Emerging Microbial Threats to Health (and chaired its Task Force on Viruses), and was a contributor to its report, *Emerging Infections* (1992); was a member of the IOM's Committee on Xenograft Transplantation; currently serves on the Steering Committee of the IOM's Forum on Emerging Infections, and has served as an adviser to WHO, PAHO (Pan-American Health Organization), FDA, the Defense Threat Reduction Agency (DTRA), and other agencies. He is a Fellow of the New York Academy of Sciences and a past Chair of its Microbiology Section. He was the founding Chair of ProMED (the nonprofit international Program to Monitor Emerging Diseases) and was one of the originators of ProMED-mail, an international network inaugurated by ProMED in 1994 for outbreak reporting and disease monitoring using the Internet. Dr. Morse received his Ph.D. from the University of Wisconsin-Madison.

MICHAEL T. OSTERHOLM, Ph.D., M.P.H., is Director of the Center for Infectious Disease Research and Policy at the University of Minnesota where he is also Professor at the School of Public Health. Previously, Dr. Osterholm was the state epidemiologist and Chief of the Acute Disease Epidemiology Section for the Minnesota Department of Health. He has received numerous research awards from the NIAID and CDC. He served as principal investigator for the CDC-sponsored Emerging Infections program in Minnesota. He has published more than 240 articles and abstracts on various emerging infectious disease problems and is the author of the best selling book, *Living Terrors: What America Needs to Know to Survive the Coming Bioterrorist Catastrophe*. He is past President of the Council of State and Territorial Epidemiologists. He currently serves on the National Academy of Sciences, IOM Forum on Emerging Infections. He has also served on the IOM Committee on Food Safety, Production to Consumption and the IOM Committee on the Department of Defense Persian Gulf Syndrome Comprehensive Clinical Evaluation Program, and as a reviewer for the IOM report on chemical and biological terrorism.

GEORGE POSTE, Ph.D., D.V.M., is Director of the Arizona Biodesign Institute and Dell E. Webb Distinguished Professor of Biology at Arizona State University. From 1992 to 1999 he was Chief Science and Technology Officer and President, Research and Development of SmithKline Beecham (SB). During his tenure at SB he was associated with the successful registration of 29 drug, vaccine, and diagnostic products. He is Chairman of diaDexus and Structural GenomiX in California and Orchid Biosciences in Princeton. He serves on the Board of Directors of AdvancePCS and Monsanto. He is an advisor on biotechnology to several venture capital funds and investment banks. In May 2003 he was appointed as Director of the Arizona Biodesign Institute at Arizona State University. This is a major new initiative combining research groups in biotechnology, nanotechnology, materials science, advanced computing, and neuromorphic engineering. He is a Fellow of Pembroke College Cambridge and Distinguished Fellow at the Hoover Institution and Stanford University. He is a member of the Defense Science Board of the U.S. Department of Defense and in this capacity he Chairs the Task Force on Bioterrorism. He is also a member of the National Academy of Sciences Working Group on Defense Against Bioweapons. Dr. Poste is a Board Certified Pathologist, a Fellow of the Royal Society, and a Fellow of the Academy of Medical Sciences. He was awarded the rank of Commander of the British Empire by Queen Elizabeth II in 1999 for services to medicine and for the advancement of biotechnology. He has published over 350 scientific papers, co-edited 15 books on cancer, biotechnology, and infectious diseases and serves on the editorial boards of multiple technical journals. He is invited routinely to be the keynote speaker at a wide variety of academic, corporate, investment, and government meetings to discuss the impact of biotechnology and genetics on health care and the challenges posed by bioterrorism. Dr. Poste is married with three children. His personal interests are in military history, photography, automobile racing, and exploring the wilderness zones of the American West.

GARY A. ROSELLE, M.D., received his M.D. from Ohio State University School of Medicine in 1973. He served his residency at Northwestern University School of Medicine and his Infectious Diseases fellowship at the University of Cincinnati School of Medicine. Dr. Roselle is the Program Director for Infectious Diseases for the VA Central Office in Washington, D.C., as well as the Chief of the Medical Service at the Cincinnati VA Medical Center. He is a Professor of Medicine in the Department of Internal Medicine, Division of Infectious Diseases at the University of Cincinnati College of Medicine. Dr. Roselle serves on several national advisory committees. In addition, he is currently heading the Emerging Pathogens Initiative for the Department of Veterans Affairs. Dr. Roselle has received commendations from the Cincinnati Medical Center Director, the Under Secretary for Health for the Department of Veterans Affairs, and the Secretary of Veterans Affairs for his work in the infectious diseases program for the Department of Veterans Affairs. He has been an invited speaker at several national and international meetings, and has published over 80 papers and several book chapters.

JANET SHOEMAKER is director of the American Society for Microbiology's Public Affairs Office, a position she has held since 1989. She is responsible for managing the legislative and regulatory affairs of this 42,000-member organization, the largest single biological science society in the world. She has served as principal investigator for a project funded by the National Science Foundation (NSF) to collect and disseminate data on the job market for recent doctorates in microbiology and has played a key role in American Society for Microbiology (ASM) projects, including the production of the ASM *Employment Outlook in the Microbiological Sciences* and *The Impact of Managed Care and Health System Change on Clinical Microbiology*. Previously, she held positions as Assistant Director of Public Affairs for ASM, as ASM coordinator of the U.S./U.S.S.R. Exchange Program in Microbiology, a program sponsored and coordinated by the National Science Foundation and the U.S. Department of State, and as a freelance editor and writer. She received her baccalaureate, cum laude, from the University of Massachusetts, and is a graduate of the George Washington University programs in public policy and in editing and publications. She has served as Commissioner to the Commission on Professionals in Science and Technology, and as the ASM representative to the ad hoc Group for Medical Research Funding, and is a member of Women in Government Relations, the American Society of Association Executives, and the American Association for the Advancement of Science. She has co-authored published articles on research funding, biotechnology, biological weapons control, and public policy issues related to microbiology.

P. FREDERICK SPARLING, M.D., is J. Herbert Bate Professor emeritus of Medicine, Microbiology and Immunology at the University of North Carolina (UNC) at Chapel Hill, and is Director of the North Carolina Sexually Transmitted Infections Research Center. Previously, he served as Chair of the Department of Medicine and Chair of the Department of Microbiology and Immunology at UNC. He was President of the Infectious Disease Society of America in 1996–1997. He was also a member of the Institute of Medicine's Committee on Microbial Threats to Health (1991–1992). Dr. Sparling's laboratory research is in the molecular biology of bacterial outer membrane proteins involved in pathogenesis, with a major emphasis on gonococci and meningococci. His current studies focus on the biochemistry and genetics of iron-scavenging mechanisms used by gonococci and meningococci and the structure and function of the gonococcal porin proteins. He is pursuing the goal of a vaccine for gonorrhea.

SPEAKERS

DAVID M. BELL, M.D., is Senior Medical Officer, Office of the Director, National Center for Infectious Diseases, CDC, Atlanta. He served as consultant to WHO in 2003 as the CDC-WHO liaison for SARS and in 2004 to assist in containment of avian influenza, as the WHO "focal point" for developing recommendations to reduce community and international transmission (e.g., quarantines, closing schools, screening at borders). From 1997–2003 Dr. Bell coordinated CDC's programs to combat antimicrobial resistance and was Co-Chair of the U.S. Federal Task Force that produced and implemented a U.S. government action plan to combat this prob¹ ..⸱. He assisted in developing the WHO Global Strategic Plan for C⸱ ..nment of Antimicrobial Resistance, in part by serving as Chair of ⸱ ⸱. HO consultation that developed global principles for antibiotic u⸱ ⸱n food animals. From 1987–1997 Dr. Bell directed CDC's programs ⸱o prevent HIV transmission in health care settings. Previously he directed the Diagnostic Virology Laboratory at the University of Tennessee and practiced general pediatrics. Dr. Bell is a member of the FDA Anti-Infective Drugs Advisory Committee and the Infectious Diseases Society of America's Committee on National and Global Public Health. He is co-author of over 90 scientific publications, Associate Editor of the *Emerging Infectious Diseases Journal*, and Clinical Assistant Professor of Pediatric Infectious Diseases at Emory University. Dr. Bell graduated from Princeton University and Harvard Medical School. His medical training included residency at Boston Children's Hospital, the Epidemic Intelligence Service Program at CDC, and fellowship in pediatric infectious diseases at the University of Rochester.

CAROL J. CARDONA, D.V.M., Ph.D., is an Assistant Professor and an Assistant Specialist in Cooperative Extension at the University of California, Davis. She received her B.S. in biology from Hanover College in 1984 and her D.V.M. degree from Purdue University in 1990. In 1992, Dr. Cardona completed a residency in avian diseases and became a diplomate of the American College of Poultry Veterinarians. Dr. Cardona earned her Ph.D. degree from Michigan State University in 1997. After postdoctoral study at Cornell University, Dr. Cardona began her career at the University of California, Davis in a position split between research and extension education. Soon after she joined the faculty at the University of California, Davis, the California poultry industry was hit with an outbreak of H6N2 avian influenza. Dr. Cardona helped the poultry industry develop a widely implemented surveillance and control program. She has studied the use of vaccine in commercial poultry populations, the response of commercial strains of chickens to H6N2 avian influenza virus in commercial settings, and the epidemiology of avian influenza in commercial poultry populations. Dr. Cardona is a member of the American Association of Avian Pathologists, the American Society for Microbiology, and the World Veterinary Poultry Association.

NGUYEN TIEN DZUNG, D.V.M., Ph.D., is Head of the Virology Department of the National Institute for Veterinary Researchs (NIVR) in Hanoi, Vietnam. He received his D.V.M. from the Havana University (Cuba) in 1973. After graduation he worked in the NIVR on diagnostic technique and vaccine development for Classical Swine Fever. He enjoyed a fellowship in France where he earned the Diplome of General Microbiology from the Paris Pasteur Institute (option Virology) and then the Diplome of Doctorat in Biotechnology and Analysis of Natural Substances from the Tours University in France in 1986. Back in Vietnam he was nominated Head of the Virology Department of the NIVR in 1988 and responsible for conducting research on the major viral diseases of animals in Vietnam. Many of his studies dealt with viral diagnosis techniques, vaccine development, and epidemiological surveillance. Dr. Nguyen was the principal scientific adviser for fighting against avian influenza outbreak in Vietnam during 2003–2004.

BRUCE G. GELLIN, M.D., M.P.H., is Director of the National Vaccine Program Office (NVPO). He is one of our nation's top experts on vaccines and infectious diseases. Before joining NVPO, Dr. Gellin was the Director of the National Network for Immunization Information, an organization he founded to be a resource for up-to-date, authoritative information about vaccines and immunizations. Dr. Gellin has had broad experience in public health aspects of infectious diseases and has held positions at the NIAID (NIH), the CDC, the Rockefeller Foundation, and Johns Hopkins University School of Public Health. In addition, he has been a regular consultant to the World Health Organization. He is board certified in internal medicine and infectious diseases and is currently on the faculty at Columbia University School of Public Health, George Washington University School of Medicine, and Vanderbilt University Schools of Medicine and Nursing. Dr. Gellin is a graduate of the University of North Carolina (Morehead Scholar), Cornell University Medical College, and the Columbia University School of Public Health, and is an infectious disease expert with training in epidemiology. He has written extensively about public health aspects of infectious diseases in medical and non-medical texts and the peer-reviewed medical literature. He is an editor of the *Clinical Infectious Diseases Journal*'s special section on vaccines and has been a reviewer for over a dozen medical journals. He also served as a medical advisor to *Encyclopedia Britannica*.

LAWRENCE O. GOSTIN, J.D., LL.D. (Hon.), is the John Carroll Research Professor at Georgetown University Law Center; Professor of Public Health at the Johns Hopkins University; and Director of the Center for Law & the Public's Health at the Johns Hopkins and Georgetown Universities (CDC Collaborating Center "Promoting Public Health Through Law") (http://www.publichealthlaw.net). He is a Research Fellow at the Centre for Socio-Legal Studies, Oxford University. Professor Gostin is an elected lifetime Member of the IOM and serves on the IOM Board on Health Promotion and Disease Prevention. Professor Gostin also consults for the WHO and UNAIDS. Professor Gostin has lead major law reform initiatives for the U.S. government including the Model Emergency Health Powers Act (MEHPA) to combat bioterrorism and other emerging health threats. Professor Gostin received the Rosemary Delbridge Memorial Award from the National Consumer Council (United Kingdom) for the person "who has most influenced Parliament and government to act for the welfare of society." He also received the Key to Tohoko University (Japan) for distinguished contributions to human rights in mental health. Professor Gostin's latest books are: *The AIDS Pandemic: Complacency, Injustice, and Unfulfilled Expectations* (University of North Carolina Press, 2004); *The Human Rights of Persons with Intellectual Disabilities: Different But Equal* (Oxford

University Press, 2003); *Public Health Law and Ethics: A Reader* (University of California Press and Milbank Memorial Fund, 2002); *Public Health Law: Power, Duty, Restraint* (University of California Press and Milbank Memorial Fund, 2000).

GORDON W. GRUNDY, M.D., M.B.A., is Regional Medical Director for Aetna Inc. in the northeast. Dr. Grundy has primary health plan responsibility for medical management activities in New England, New York, and northern New Jersey. He also oversees regional quality management activities including NCQA accreditation. Prior to joining Aetna in 1999, Dr. Grundy served as medical director for Yale Preferred Health and HealthChoice of Connecticut for 3 years. He graduated from the University of Colorado in 1966 and received his medical degree from the University of Rochester (NY) School of Medicine in 1970. After serving as a staff associate with the National Cancer Institute, he completed residency training in pediatrics at the Yale-New Haven Hospital in 1975. During his 21-year career as a pediatrician, Dr. Grundy also earned an M.B.A. in health care management from the University of New Haven in 1992. Dr. Grundy currently sits on the Board of Directors of the Alliance for the Prudent Use of Antibiotics (APUA), an international organization dedicated to improving antimicrobial effectiveness and containing drug resistance. He is a Fellow of the American Academy of Pediatrics and holds memberships in the American Medical Association, the Connecticut State Medical Society and the American College of Physician Executives.

MARK LIPSITCH, D. PHIL., is Associate Professor of Epidemiology and Immunology & Infectious Diseases at the Harvard School of Public Health. He studied philosophy at Yale University and received his D.Phil. in zoology from Oxford in 1995. He did postdoctoral work with Bruce Levin at Emory University and at the CDC from 1995–1999. His research in the population biology of infectious diseases has focused on antimicrobial resistance in community- and hospital-acquired pathogens, and on the population dynamics of *Streptococcus pneumoniae*. Recent work has involved development of methods for detecting and predicting malaria epidemics, as well as analyses of the 1918 influenza pandemic and the 2003 SARS epidemic. He also maintains a laboratory research program, focusing on the population biology of *S. pneumoniae* and on the role of host immunity in determining interactions among strains of this organism. At Harvard he teaches courses in the Epidemiology Department on mathematical modeling of disease transmission and on methods for infectious disease epidemiology. He has recently received outstanding young investigator awards from the Ellison Medical Foundation, the American Society for Microbiology, and the Pharmaceutical Research and Manufacturers' Association

Foundation. He is an Associate Editor of the *American Journal of Epidemiology* and *Emerging Themes in Epidemiology*.

IRA M. LONGINI, JR., Ph.D., is Professor of Biostatistics, Rollins School of Public Health, Emory University. He received a Ph.D. in Biometry at the University of Minnesota in 1977. Dr. Longini began his career with the International Center for Medical Research and Training and the Universidad del Valle in Cali, Colombia, where he works on tropical infectious disease problems. He has been at Emory since 1984. His research interests are in the area of stochastic processes applied to epidemiological problems. He has specialized in the mathematical and statistical theory of epidemics—a process that involves constructing and analyzing mathematical models of disease transmission and disease progression and the analysis of infectious disease data based on these models. He has worked extensively in the design, analysis, and interpretation of vaccine trials. This research has been carried out jointly with faculty members and collaborators at other universities, the CDC, the Los Alamos National Laboratory, and NIH. Dr. Longini has worked extensively on the analysis of epidemics of influenza, HIV, cholera, dengue fever, rhinovirus, rotavirus, and measles. Dr. Longini is also working with the NIH and the CDC on mathematical and statistical models for the control of a possible bioterrorist attack with an infectious agent such as smallpox, and other natural infectious disease threats such as pandemic influenza and SARS. Dr. Longini is author or co-author of 100 scientific papers, and he has won a number of awards for excellence in research, including the Howard M. Temin Award in Epidemiology for Scientific Excellence in the Fight Against HIV/AIDS. He is a Fellow of the American Statistical Association.

ARNOLD S. MONTO, M.D., is Professor of Epidemiology at the University of Michigan in Ann Arbor and is Director of the University of Michigan Bioterrorism Preparedness Initiative. The major focus of his work has been the epidemiology, prevention, and treatment of acute infections. Respiratory infections, in particular influenza, have been a major interest, with special reference to the evaluation of vaccines and the assessment of the value of antivirals such as amantadine, rimantadine, and the neuraminidase inhibitors. Dr. Monto was closely involved in the U.S. HCFA-sponsored studies, which made influenza vaccine a covered benefit for older individuals. He has also studied other approaches to influenza vaccine use, particularly to control transmission of virus in the community and in nursing homes. He is currently involved in assessing the efficacy of the neuraminidase inhibitors in prophylaxis and therapy of influenza and internationally in evaluating the relative efficacy of hepatitis A vaccine in post-exposure prophylaxis. Dr. Monto has served for periods of time in the Acute Respiratory Infection program at WHO, Geneva, and as Scholar in Residence at IOM/NRC. He has also been a member of the National Advisory Allergy and Infectious Diseases Council. He is now President of the American Epidemiological Society.

DENNIS M. PERROTTA, Ph.D., CIC., is the Texas State Epidemiologist, and Scientific Director of the Center for Public Health Preparedness and Response, Texas Department of Health. He is doctorally trained in epidemiology, board certified in infection control, and has worked in public health, for more than 22 years spanning a wide range of subject areas including bioterrorism, asthma, influenza control, environmental health and infectious disease epidemiology. He has served as President of the Council of State and Territorial Epidemiologists and as President of the Armed Forces Epidemiological Board. He served on the 1997–1999 IOM Committee to Improve Civilian Medical Response to Chemical and Biological Terrorism and is facilitating state health department efforts regarding bioterrorism preparedness. He is Adjunct Associate Professor at the University of Texas School of Nursing and the three schools of public health in Texas. He is the principal investigator on three major bioterrorism and emerging infections grants.

LONE SIMONSEN, Ph.D., is a senior epidemiologist at NIAID at NIH in Bethesda, Md. She received her Ph.D. in population biology from University of Massachusetts in 1991 in the area of mathematical modeling in infectious diseases. Dr. Simonsen then joined the EIS program at the CDC where she worked as an epidemiologist in the Influenza Branch during 1992–1996. Subsequently she worked as an epidemiologist for WHO and UNAIDS in Geneva during 1997–2000 on technical issues relating to global surveillance and burden of TB, drug resistance, and HIV/AIDS. After returning to the United States, Dr. Simonsen joined NIAID in May 2000 to conduct research in infectious disease epidemiology. She has contributed broadly to developing the field of quantitative epidemiology of infectious diseases, in particular mathematical modeling tools needed to study seasonal variations in disease outcomes to better estimate burden of disease for influenza, rotavirus, and malaria. She has recently undertaken several studies to better quantify the benefits of elderly influenza vaccination efforts as well as the risk of intussusception following rotavirus immunization of infants. Her primary focus of research since 1992 has been studies on the impact of pandemic and epidemic influenza; she has published numerous scientific papers in this area.

DAVID E. SWAYNE, D.V.M., Ph.D., is Director of the Southeast Poultry Research Laboratory (SEPRL), Agricultural Research Service, U.S. Department of Agriculture (USDA). SEPRL is USDA's national laboratory that conducts research on exotic and emerging poultry diseases, including avian influenza. He received his B.S. in domestic animal biology from University of Arkansas (1980), Ph.D. in veterinary medicine and M.S. in veterinary pathology from the University of Missouri (1984), and Ph.D. in veterinary pathology from the University of Georgia (1987). Dr. Swayne began his career as an Assistant and Associate Professor in Veterinary Pathobiology at The Ohio State University (1987–1994), where he studied pathogenicity and pathogenesis of low pathogenic avian influenza viruses in poultry, especially the avian influenza viruses from wild birds. In 1994, he joined SEPRL in his current position. His research has focused on understanding the pathobiology of influenza virus infections in poultry and other birds, development of vaccines and vaccination control programs, and prediction of the emergence of high from low pathogenicity avian influenza viruses. Dr. Swayne is a member of the American Veterinary Medical Association, American Association of Avian Pathologists, World Veterinary Poultry Association, and U.S. Animal Health Association. He is a diplomate of the American College of Veterinary Pathologists and American College of Poultry Veterinarians. He serves as an avian influenza expert and consultant for the World Organization of Animal Health (Office International des Épizooties [OIE]).

JEFFREY K. TAUBENBERGER, M.D., Ph.D., serves as Chief of the Department of Molecular Pathology at the Armed Forces Institute of Pathology in Washington, D.C., a position he has held since 1994. He received his M.D. in 1986 and Ph.D. in 1987 from the Medical College of Virginia, and did a residency in pathology at the National Cancer Institute. His clinical activities involve diagnostic molecular genetics. He holds dual board certifications in anatomic pathology and in molecular genetic pathology from the American Board of Pathology and the American Board of Medical Genetics. His clinical interests are chiefly in the development and implementation of molecular diagnostic assays for neoplasia and infectious diseases. His research interests include (1) influenza virus biology and surveillance, including characterization of the 1918 influenza virus that killed 40 million people; (2) biology of other RNA viruses including SARS and marine mammal morbilliviruses; and (3) gene expression during early lymphocyte differentiation. He is the recipient of numerous awards and is a frequent speaker at national and international meetings, including multiple keynote addresses. He has published over 80 papers in such journals as *Science* and the *Proceedings of the National Academy of Sciences*, and has written twelve book chapters. His work has been funded by grants from the National Institutes of Health, the Veterans Administration, the Environmental Protection Agency, and the American Registry of Pathology. He is currently the principal investigator on two NIH grants to characterize the 1918 influenza virus. His 1918 influenza work has generated national and international publicity since 1997.

FORUM STAFF

STACEY L. KNOBLER is Director of the Forum on Microbial Threats at IOM and a senior program officer for the Board on Global Health (BGH). She has served as the director of the BGH study, *Neurological, Psychiatric, and Developmental Disorders in Developing Countries* and as a research associate for the Board's earlier studies on *The Assessment of Future Scientific Needs for Live Variola (Smallpox) Virus and Cardiovascular Disease in Developing Countries*. Previously, Ms. Knobler has held positions as a Research Associate at the Brookings Institution, Foreign Policy Studies Program, and as an Arms Control and Democratization Consultant for the Organization for Security and Cooperation in Europe in Vienna and Bosnia-Herzegovina. She has also worked as a research and negotiations analyst in Israel and Palestine. Ms. Knobler received her baccalaureate, summa cum laude, in political science and molecular genetics from the University of Rochester, and her M.P.A from Harvard University. She has conducted research and published on issues that include biological and nuclear weapons control, foreign aid, health in developing countries, poverty and public assistance, and the Arab-Israeli peace process.

ELIZABETH KITCHENS, Ph.D., is a Research Associate for IOM's Forum on Microbial Threats. Prior to joining the Forum, Elizabeth was a Christine Mirzayan Science and Technology Policy Graduate Fellow at The National Academies. In December 2003, she was awarded a Ph.D. in molecular and cellular biology from the University of California, Berkeley, where she studied the developmental process of T-cells. She received a B.S. from the University of California, San Diego, in biochemistry and cell biology. Elizabeth recently joined the staff at IOM in September 2004.

KATHERINE A. OBERHOLTZER is Research Assistant for IOM's Board on Global Health. She recently played a key role in the development and production of the BGH study, *Microbial Threats to Health: Emergence, Detection, and Response*. Katherine received her B.S. in integrated science and technology with a concentration in biotechnology from James Madison University in 2000. She is currently pursuing her Professional Editing Certificate at the George Washington University. Katherine has worked as the Meeting Coordinator for the Maryland AIDS Education and Training Center of the Institute of Human Virology at the University of Maryland, Baltimore. Katherine joined the staff at IOM in December 2000.

LAURA SIVITZ, M.S.J., joined the staff of IOM in 2002 as the research associate in an 18-month study on prion diseases. She played a leadership role in the development, production, and dissemination of the report *Advancing Prion Science: Guidance for the National Prion Research Program.* In November 2003, she joined the staff of the Forum on Microbial Threats in the Board on Global Health at IOM. Previously, Ms. Sivitz had served as a technology reporter for *Washington Techway* magazine; as the science-writer intern for *Science News*; as the Washington correspondent for the *York Daily Record* of Pennsylvania; and as a science, legal, and business reporter for the Medill News Service of Chicago. She won a National Science Foundation fellowship in 1994 to conduct research at the University of Pennsylvania on piezoelectric ceramics for use in mammography systems. Ms. Sivitz received her B.A. in physics from Bryn Mawr College in 1996 and her M.S. in journalism from Northwestern University in 2001.